Thyroid Disease: Updates from Diagnosis to Treatment

Thyroid Disease: Updates from Diagnosis to Treatment

Guest Editors

Luca Giovanella
Petra Petranović Ovčariček

Basel • Beijing • Wuhan • Barcelona • Belgrade • Novi Sad • Cluj • Manchester

Guest Editors
Luca Giovanella
Nuclear Medicine and
Thyroid Diseases
University Hospital of Zurich
Zurich
Switzerland

Petra Petranović Ovčariček
Department of Oncology and
Nuclear Medicine
University Hospital Center
Sestre Milosrdnice
Zagreb
Croatia

Editorial Office
MDPI AG
Grosspeteranlage 5
4052 Basel, Switzerland

This is a reprint of the Special Issue, published open access by the journal *Journal of Clinical Medicine* (ISSN 2077-0383), freely accessible at: https://www.mdpi.com/journal/jcm/special_issues/1716S77H3Z.

For citation purposes, cite each article independently as indicated on the article page online and as indicated below:

Lastname, A.A.; Lastname, B.B. Article Title. *Journal Name* **Year**, *Volume Number*, Page Range.

ISBN 978-3-7258-5865-1 (Hbk)
ISBN 978-3-7258-5866-8 (PDF)
https://doi.org/10.3390/books978-3-7258-5866-8

Contents

About the Editors

Luca Giovanella

Luca Giovanella is a renowned specialist in endocrinology and nuclear medicine, directing both the nuclear medicine department and thyroid-parathyroid clinical unit at Clinica Moncucco in Lugano, Switzerland. He holds a professorship in nuclear medicine at the University of Zurich, Switzerland. Since 2021, he has chaired the EANM Thyroid Committee. His extensive research portfolio includes over 500 peer-reviewed publications focusing primarily on thyroid disorders, and he has contributed to the development of multiple clinical guidelines for thyroid and parathyroid diseases.

Petra Petranović Ovčariček

Petra Petranović Ovčariček is an experienced nuclear medicine specialist practicing at the University Hospital Center Sestre Milosrdnice in Zagreb, Croatia, where she also holds the position of Assistant Professor at the University of Zagreb School of Medicine. Her clinical expertise centers on thyroid and parathyroid disorders. She actively participated as a member of the EANM Thyroid Committee from 2019 to 2024 and has served as their Guidelines representative since 2021.

Journal of
Clinical Medicine

MDPI

Editorial

Clinical Advances in Thyroid Disease Assessment and Management

Petra Petranović Ovčariček [1,2,*] and Luca Giovanella [3,4]

1 Department of Oncology and Nuclear Medicine, University Hospital Center Sestre Milosrdnice, 10000 Zagreb, Croatia
2 School of Medicine, University of Zagreb, 10000 Zagreb, Croatia
3 Gruppo Ospedaliero Moncucco, Department of Nuclear Medicine, 6900 Lugano, Switzerland; luca.giovanella.md@gmail.com
4 Department of Nuclear Medicine, University Hospital Zurich, University of Zurich, 8091 Zurich, Switzerland
* Correspondence: p.petranovic@gmail.com; Tel.: +385-1-3787654

Thyroid disorders affect millions worldwide, with differentiated thyroid cancer (DTC) representing the most common endocrine malignancy. Detection rates have risen substantially, largely due to the widespread use of ultrasonography (US), creating new diagnostic and therapeutic challenges in DTC management. Current clinical practice relies heavily on sonographic features of thyroid nodules and structured reporting systems such as American College of Radiology Thyroid Imaging, Reporting and Data System (ACR TI-RADS). However, the variability in outcomes among similar imaging categories underscores the need for improved assessment methods. Likewise, the quantification of treatment response and long-term outcomes, previously a barrier to individualized therapy, is being addressed through the integration of molecular and demographic predictors into clinical algorithms.

1. Improving Nodule Risk Assessment

Currently used risk stratification models rely predominantly on imaging characteristics, often overlooking patient-specific factors. Integrating demographic and clinical variables such as age, gender, and size of the nodule into classification systems may improve predictive precision. Recent research has shown measurable improvements in thyroid nodule risk stratification when patient-specific factors are integrated into imaging-based classification systems [1]. Age has emerged as a strong independent predictor of malignancy, with odds ratios decreasing consistently with advancing age across all ACR TI-RADS categories. In a cohort of 1128 nodules, malignancy rates varied markedly by age group, with younger patients exhibiting a higher risk even within lower ACR TI-RADS. Nodule size remains a critical determinant, with larger nodules carrying higher malignancy rates independent of sonographic score. These findings support adjusted thresholds for recommending fine needle aspiration, particularly for sonographically "indeterminate" nodules, based on patient age and gender.

2. Thyroid Cancer Epidemiological Changes

An analysis of 94,892 patients from the Surveillance, Epidemiology, and End Results (SEER) database (2001–2020) revealed significant epidemiological changes [2]. The proportion of patients aged $\geq$ 60 years increased by 4.2%, that of males increased by 2.1%, and papillary thyroid carcinoma (PTC) cases increased by 5.3% in the 2011–2020 cohort compared with 2001–2010. Regional disease presentation rose by 3.7%, reflecting potential changes in both detection practices and disease biology. Although survival improved by 8% in the later cohort, this difference is not statistically significant. Key prognostic factors included stage, age, gender, and histopathological subtype. Patients with the follicular variant of PTC demonstrated the most favourable outcome (HR: 0.78), while those

 https://doi.org/10.3390/jcm14217510

with anaplastic tumors and thyroid sarcomas showed the poorest prognosis (HR: 9.61), as expected.

3. Radioiodine Therapy: Modulating Clinical Indications

Radioiodine therapy remains a cornerstone in thyroid disease management. In benign conditions, its therapeutic scope is still expanding. The authors of a recent study involving patients with large toxic multinodular goiter treated with 20 mCi (740 MBq) of ^{131}I reported a mean thyroid volume reduction of 36% at six months, accompanied by a 12.8% increase in tracheal diameter [3]. These findings support the use of ^{131}I as an effective alternative to surgery, even in managing large goiters.

In DTC, a risk-adapted approach to ^{131}I therapy has become standard practice. Treatment intent, whether ablative, adjuvant, or therapeutic, is now guided by individualized risk assessment. Post-therapy ^{131}I scintigraphy provides essential staging information, underscoring the theranostic role of ^{131}I [4]. Personalized therapy selection approaches consider both stimulation methods and administered activity, optimized according to patient-specific parameters.

4. Advances in Biomarker Development and Validation

Analytical challenges in thyroid biomarker measurement have limited the wide clinical adoption of promising markers. New-generation calcitonin (CT) immunoassays have addressed long-standing issues related to pre-analytical degradation and inter-assay variability [5–7]. Procalcitonin has emerged as a robust alternative or complementary marker to CT, particularly valuable when CT levels are indeterminate [8].

Evaluation of biomarker kinetics provides additional insights: CT and carcinoembryonic antigen (CEA) doubling times shorter than six months indicate poor prognosis, whereas values exceeding two years are associated with favourable outcomes. Novel biomarkers, such as pro-gastrin-releasing peptide (ProGRP) and CA19-9, are under investigation for monitoring advanced disease and assessing therapeutic response [9].

5. Autoimmune Thyroid Disease and Pregnancy

Recent clinical studies have clarified optimal timing for conception after ^{131}I therapy in women with Graves' disease. TRAb levels may remain elevated for up to two years post-treatment, with the risk of hyperthyroidism declining over time: 8.8% when conception occurs within 6–12 months, 5.5% at 12–18 months, and 3.6% for 18–24 months [10].

Third-trimester TRAb levels above 10 U/L are the principal risk factor for neonatal hyperthyroidism. Regarding anti-thyroid drugs, propylthiouracil increases fetal malformation risk by approximately 1.1–1.6% above baseline, while thiamazole increases risk by 2–3% depending on dose. These findings inform preconception counseling and individualize management during pregnancy [11].

6. Redifferentiation Therapy in Radioiodine-Refractory DTC

Pharmacological redifferentiation therapies are redefining the management of radioiodine-refractory DTC. These strategies primarily target the MAPK signaling pathway to restore sodium iodide symporter expression, thereby re-establishing radioiodine avidity [12]. Clinical trials involving the use of MEK and BRAF inhibitors have demonstrated renewed radioiodine uptake in previously refractory tumors, offering a potential shift from palliative to disease-modifying treatment [13–21].

7. Management of Rare Thyroid Disorders

Resistance to thyroid hormone (RTH) remains a rare but clinically significant condition, often complicating perioperative care. Mutations in thyroid hormone receptor genes (THRα or THRβ) result in elevated thyroid hormone levels with non-suppressed TSH and a mixed clinical phenotype with features of either hypothyroidism or hyperthyroidism. A recent case report described successful perioperative management in a pediatric patient with complex congenital heart disease and RTH [22]. Thiamazole administration selectively mitigated thyroid hormone effects on α-receptors, enabling safe cardiac surgery. This case exemplifies the importance of individualized strategies for managing rare endocrine disorders with complex comorbidities.

8. Knowledge Gaps and Future Research Directions

The authors of future studies should integrate molecular and genomic profiling into clinical decision-making algorithms. Validation of genetic and epigenetic predictors in large, diverse cohorts will improve risk stratification and identify novel therapeutic targets.

Artificial intelligence and machine learning offer substantial promise for enhancing diagnostic accuracy. Multimodal data integration, including imaging, molecular, and clinical features, could strengthen risk assessment and treatment selection. In addition, prospective validation of AI tools is an important research priority.

Long-term, population-based follow-up studies are essential to confirm the clinical utility of new diagnostic and therapeutic strategies. Establishing biobanks and standardized outcome registries will facilitate this progress. Finally, cost-effectiveness analyses are needed to guide the adoption of novel technologies.

9. Conclusions

Recent advances in thyroid medicine have led to measurable improvements in diagnosis, risk assessment, and treatment outcomes. The integration of patient-specific parameters with imaging-based classifications enhances thyroid nodule characterization. Biomarker development continues to refine both diagnostic precision and disease monitoring.

Epidemiological data reveal evolving disease patterns, while innovation in radioiodine and redifferentiation therapy expands therapeutic possibilities. Despite this progress, however, challenges persist in standardizing protocols, validating biomarkers, and achieving a true personalization of treatment.

The studies presented in this Special Issue provide evidence-based insights into the evolving domains. Continued collaborations among researchers, clinicians, and healthcare systems will be essential to translate these advances into routine clinical practice and to achieve the ultimate goal: improved patient outcomes through precision-based thyroid care.

Author Contributions: Conceptualization, P.P.O. and L.G.; methodology, P.P.O. and L.G.; investigation, P.P.O. and L.G.; data curation, P.P.O. and L.G.; writing—original draft preparation, P.P.O. and L.G.; writing—review and editing, P.P.O. and L.G. All authors have read and agreed to the published version of the manuscript.

Funding: This research received no external funding.

Institutional Review Board Statement: Not applicable.

Informed Consent Statement: Not applicable.

Data Availability Statement: Not applicable.

Conflicts of Interest: The authors declare no conflicts of interest.

References

1. Angelopoulos, N.; Androulakis, I.; Askitis, D.P.; Valvis, N.; Paparodis, R.D.; Petkova, V.; Boniakos, A.; Zianni, D.; Rizoulis, A.; Bantouna, D.; et al. Integrating Clinical Parameters into Thyroid Nodule Malignancy Risk: A Retrospective Evaluation Based on ACR TI-RADS. *J. Clin. Med.* **2025**, *14*, 5352. [CrossRef]
2. Doğan, Ö.; Ahmed, M.A.; Ekinci, Ö.B.; Yıldız, A.; Dogan, I. Evaluation of Changes in Clinicopathological Features and Prognosis in Patients with Thyroid Cancer. *J. Clin. Med.* **2025**, *14*, 1482. [CrossRef]
3. Yazici Demir, K.; Kaya, Z.; Dayanan, R.; Mercantepe, T.; Mercantepe, F. Does Radioactive Iodine Treatment Affect Thyroid Size and Tracheal Diameter? *J. Clin. Med.* **2025**, *14*, 115. [CrossRef] [PubMed]
4. Campennì, A.; Siracusa, M.; Ruggeri, R.M. Oldie but Goldie: The Fundamental Role of Radioiodine in the Management of Thyroid Cancer. *J. Clin. Med.* **2024**, *13*, 6400. [CrossRef] [PubMed]
5. Mater, A.; Boelen, A.; Heijboer, A.C.; Hillebrand, J.J. Insights into the Stability of Serum Calcitonin and a Comparison of Three Serum Calcitonin Immunoassays. *Clin. Chim. Acta* **2026**, *579*, 120603. [CrossRef]
6. Mater, A.; Boelen, A.; Heijboer, A.C.; Hillebrand, J.J. Thyroglobulin and Calcitonin Measurements: Pitfalls and Future Perspectives. *J. Endocrinol.* **2024**, *264*, e240156. [CrossRef] [PubMed]
7. Moretti, G.; Troiani, E.; Sarlo, F.; Baroni, S.; Urbani, A. Analytical Performance Evaluation of a New Calcitonin Assay. *J. Appl. Lab. Med.* **2022**, *7*, 568–574. [CrossRef]
8. Codrich, M.; Biasotto, A.; D'Aurizio, F. Circulating Biomarkers of Thyroid Cancer: An Appraisal. *J. Clin. Med.* **2025**, *14*, 1582. [CrossRef]
9. Giovanella, L.; D'Aurizio, F.; Petranović Ovčariček, P. Circulating Biomarkers in Medullary Thyroid Carcinoma: Bridging Laboratory Complexities and Clinical Application Through Algorithm Design. *J. Clin. Med.* **2025**, *14*, 5645. [CrossRef]
10. Dietlein, M.; Schmidt, M.; Drzezga, A.; Kobe, C. Radioiodine Therapy of Graves' Disease in Women with Childbearing Potential and the Pre-Conceptional Counseling About Antithyroid Drugs. *J. Clin. Med.* **2025**, *14*, 1667. [CrossRef]
11. Bogović Crnčić, T.; Ćurko-Cofek, B.; Batičić, L.; Girotto, N.; Tomaš, M.I.; Kršek, A.; Krištofić, I.; Štimac, T.; Perić, I.; Sotošek, V.; et al. Autoimmune Thyroid Disease and Pregnancy: The Interaction Between Genetics, Epigenetics and Environmental Factors. *J. Clin. Med.* **2024**, *14*, 190. [CrossRef]
12. Petranović Ovčariček, P.; Tuncel, M.; Aghaee, A.; Campennì, A.; Giovanella, L. Redifferentiation Therapies in Thyroid Oncology: Molecular and Clinical Aspects. *J. Clin. Med.* **2024**, *13*, 7021. [CrossRef]
13. Buffet, C.; Wassermann, J.; Hecht, F.; Leenhardt, L.; Dupuy, C.; Groussin, L.; Lussey-Lepoutre, C. Redifferentiation of Radioiodine-Refractory Thyroid Cancers. *Endocr. Relat. Cancer* **2020**, *27*, R113–R132. [CrossRef] [PubMed]
14. Dunn, L.A.; Sherman, E.J.; Baxi, S.S.; Tchekmedyian, V.; Grewal, R.K.; Larson, S.M.; Pentlow, K.S.; Haque, S.; Tuttle, R.M.; Sabra, M.M.; et al. Vemurafenib Redifferentiation of BRAF Mutant, Rai-Refractory Thyroid Cancers. *J. Clin. Endocrinol. Metab.* **2019**, *104*, 1417–1428. [CrossRef] [PubMed]
15. Rothenberg, S.M.; Daniels, G.H.; Wirth, L.J. Redifferentiation of Iodine-Refractory BRAF V600E-Mutant Metastatic Papillary Thyroid Cancer with Dabrafenib-Response. *Clin. Cancer Res.* **2015**, *21*, 5640–5641. [CrossRef]
16. Iravani, A.; Solomon, B.; Pattison, D.A.; Jackson, P.; Ravi Kumar, A.; Kong, G.; Hofman, M.S.; Akhurst, T.; Hicks, R.J. Mitogen-Activated Protein Kinase Pathway Inhibition for Redifferentiation of Radioiodine Refractory Differentiated Thyroid Cancer: An Evolving Protocol. *Thyroid* **2019**, *29*, 1634–1645. [CrossRef]
17. Burman, B.; Tuttle, R.M.; Grewal, R.K.; Sherman, E.J.; Baxi, S.S.; Boucai, L.; Sabra, M.; Fish, S.; Pentlow, K.S.; Haque, S.; et al. Phase 2 of Trametinib plus Radioiodine in RAS-Mutant and Wild-Type, Radioiodine-Refractory Thyroid Cancer (ETCTN9446). *J. Clin. Oncol.* **2022**, *40*, 6089. [CrossRef]
18. Leboulleux, S.; Benisvy, D.; Taieb, D.; Attard, M.; Bournaud, C.; Terroir-Cassou-Mounat, M.; Lacroix, L.; Anizan, N.; Schiazza, A.; Garcia, M.E.; et al. MERAIODE: A Phase II Redifferentiation Trial with Trametinib and 131I in Metastatic Radioactive Iodine Refractory RAS Mutated Differentiated Thyroid Cancer. *Thyroid* **2023**, *33*, 1124–1129. [CrossRef]
19. Weber, M.; Kersting, D.; Riemann, B.; Brandenburg, T.; Führer-Sakel, D.; Grünwald, F.; Kreissl, M.C.; Dralle, H.; Weber, F.; Schmid, K.W.; et al. Enhancing Radioiodine Incorporation into Radioiodine-Refractory Thyroid Cancer with MAPK Inhibition (ERRITI): A Single-Center Prospective Two-Arm Study. *Clin. Cancer Res.* **2022**, *28*, 4194–4202. [CrossRef]
20. Leboulleux, S.; Do Cao, C.; Zerdoud, S.; Attard, M.; Bournaud, C.; Lacroix, L.; Benisvy, D.; Taïeb, D.; Bardet, S.; Terroir-Cassou-Mounat, M.; et al. A Phase II Redifferentiation Trial with Dabrafenib-Trametinib and 131I in Metastatic Radioactive Iodine Refractory BRAF p.V600E-Mutated Differentiated Thyroid Cancer. *Clin. Cancer Res.* **2023**, *29*, 2401–2409. [CrossRef]

21. Ho, A.L.; Dedecjus, M.; Wirth, L.J.; Tuttle, R.M.; Inabnet, W.B.; Tennvall, J.; Vaisman, F.; Bastholt, L.; Gianoukakis, A.G.; Rodien, P.; et al. Selumetinib Plus Adjuvant Radioactive Iodine in Patients with High-Risk Differentiated Thyroid Cancer: A Phase III, Randomized, Placebo-Controlled Trial (ASTRA). *J. Clin. Oncol.* **2022**, *40*, 1870–1878. [CrossRef] [PubMed]
22. Fedorczak, A.; Kruk, B.; Mazurek-Kula, A.; Kępczyński, Ł.; Stawerska, R. Resistance to Thyroid Hormone in a Boy with a Severe, Complex, Congenital Heart Defect (CHD) Requiring Multiple Cardiac Surgeries—Whether and How to Prepare Child for the Surgery. *J. Clin. Med.* **2025**, *14*, 1209. [CrossRef]

Journal of
Clinical Medicine

MDPI

Article

Oldie but Goldie: The Fundamental Role of Radioiodine in the Management of Thyroid Cancer

Alfredo Campennì [1,*], Massimiliano Siracusa [1] and Rosaria Maddalena Ruggeri [2]

[1] Unit of Nuclear Medicine, Department of Biomedical and Dental Sciences and Morpho-Functional Imaging, University of Messina, 98125 Messina, Italy; m.siracusadr@alice.it
[2] Endocrinology Unit, Department of Human Pathology of Adulthood and Childhood DETEV, University of Messina, 98125 Messina, Italy; rmruggeri@unime.it
* Correspondence: acampenni@unime.it; Tel.: +39-090-2217367

Abstract: Background/Objectives: The management of differentiated thyroid cancer (DTC) patients has undergone a major paradigm shift in past years, especially regarding the role of a careful postoperative disease assessment both in deciding for or against the use of iodine-131 therapy (i.e., patients' selection) and in selecting the correct goal of the treatment: ablative, adjuvant or therapeutic. Furthermore, diagnostic and risk-oriented uses of iodine isotopes (i.e., $^{123/124/131}I$) should always be considered during both postoperative assessment and follow-up of DTC patients to improve early staging and response assessment to initial treatments, respectively. The present review summarizes current (and real-life-related) evidence and the emerging perspectives on the therapeutic, diagnostic, and theragnostic use of radioiodine isotopes. **Methods**: A review of the pertinent literature was performed in PubMed, Web of Science, and Scopus without language restrictions or time limits and using one or more fitting search criteria and terms. **Results**: According to the literature evidence and real-life clinical practice, a risk-oriented postoperative iodine-131 therapy remains pivotal for most DTC patients and improves early disease staging through post-therapy functional imaging (i.e., theragnostic aim). Accordingly, the goal of iodine-131 therapy, the optimal strategy (empiric vs. dosimetric approach), the appropriate stimulation method [i.e., levothyroxine (L-T4) withdrawal vs. recombinant human thyrotropin (rhTSH) administration] and, finally, the suggested radioiodine activity to deliver for iodine-131 therapy (RIT) should be personalized, especially in metastatic DTC patients. **Conclusions**: The evidence related to the diagnostic and theragnostic use of iodine isotopes leads to a significant improvement in the postoperative risk stratification and staging of DTC patients in addition to a more accurate assessment of the response to initial treatments. In conclusion, radioiodine is really an *oldie but goldie* radiotracer. It has both a current fundamental role and a future perspective for the more careful management of DTC patients.

Keywords: iodine-131; iodine-123; iodine-124; radioiodine therapy; theragnostic; diagnostic functional imaging; differentiated thyroid cancer

1. Introduction

The first therapeutic application of iodine-131 was successfully administered for the first time more than 80 years ago by Doctor Saul Hertz to treat a young female patient affected by hyperthyroidism due to Graves' disease (GD). Since then, millions of patients worldwide have been receiving iodine-131 therapy (RIT) for the definitive treatment of autoimmune (i.e., GD) or non-autoimmune hyperthyroidism [i.e., toxic (multi)-nodular goiter (TMNG/TNG, respectively)], such as through post-surgical therapy of DTC. Iodine-131 decays by β-electrons and emits an electromagnetic photon (i.e., gamma-ray). Based on these physical characteristics, iodine-131 can be considered the first theragnostic agent in nuclear medicine: its gamma-ray emission is used to observe and quantify iodine distribution and kinetics within the target (e.g., thyroid gland or remnant). In contrast, its β-particle emission (β-radiation) produces a therapeutic effect. The physical characteristics of this oldie but goldie radiotracer are useful for the correct clinical, diagnostic, and therapeutic management of DTC patients.

Differentiated thyroid cancer, a follicular cell-originating tumor, is the most frequent thyroid malignancy, and its incidence has been increasing in recent decades with an overall increased annual incidence of about 3% [1–3].

The most common DTC histotype is represented by papillary thyroid carcinoma (PTC), accounting for more than 80% of all thyroid malignancies with a significant prevalence of both small tumors and female patients [1,4–9].

In DTC patients, the standard of care involves risk-oriented thyroid surgery, postoperative iodine-131 therapy (p-RIT), and both individualized long-term follow-up and levothyroxine therapy tailored according to the patients' risk of relapse [1,10–15]. The goal of postoperative RIT should always be marked as follows: thyroid remnant ablation, adjuvant therapy, and treatment of known metastases.

According to Avram et al. [16], (p-RIT) can be planned by two different empirical approaches: (i) the "functional imaging-guided approach" (i.e., theragnostic approach), based on information obtained with a postoperative diagnostic radioiodine (^{123}I, ^{131}I, ^{124}I) scan, or (ii) the "risk-adapted approach", based on the local standard of care and the evaluation of clinical–pathological factors other than imaging evidence. Additionally, the dosimetric approach could also be taken into account, at least for patients in whom RIT is performed for ablative or therapeutic purposes.

In addition, RIT represents the primary treatment modality in advanced DTC patients affected by loco-regional and/or distant iodine-avid metastases detected at post-therapy radioiodine scan or during follow-up [10,12,17]. In such patients, radioiodine activity is sometimes preferably chosen by a dosimetric approach using the so-called lesion-based (primarily targeting *efficacy*) or blood-based (primarily targeting *safety*) methods [16,18].

Finally, a risk-adapted use of diagnostic whole-body scintigraphy (Dx-WBS) with radioiodine isotopes (^{131}I or ^{123}I) (i.e., functional imaging) should always be considered in selected DTC patients both for better assessing the response to initial treatments (i.e., thyroid surgery and RIT) and during late follow-up, as already reported [19–23].

The present review aims to discuss current (and real-life-related) evidence and emerging perspectives on the therapeutic, diagnostic, and theragnostic use of radioiodine isotopes.

2. Methods

Starting from the review query, we carried out a literature search of Embase, PubMed/MEDLINE, and Scopus with the purpose of extracting any significant published studies based on the diagnostic, therapeutic, and theragnostic role of radioiodine isotopes. No restrictions regarding either the year of the papers' release or their language were applied. We used one or more fitting search criteria and terms. The combination terms used for this research are listed below: (A) "Radioiodine therapy" OR "Diagnostic radioiodine" AND (B) "Radioiodine isotopes" or "Radioiodine" AND (C) "differentiated thyroid cancer" OR "thyroid cancer" OR "Radioiodine functional imaging" OR "follow-up" OR "theragnostic".

3. Diagnostic Functional Imaging

The use of diagnostic iodine-131 whole-body scintigraphy (Dx-WBS) has been limited in recent years since some authors argue that it is less sensitive than pT-WBS in detecting metastases other than producing the so-called "stunning effect" of iodine-avid tissue [23–25].

However, this criticism should no longer be taken into account for at least two main reasons: (i) technological improvement in nuclear medicine instrumentation [i.e., SPECT/CT imaging (hybrid imaging)], image acquisition and reconstruction protocols, with the resulting possibility to administer lower ($\leq$74 MBq) iodine-131 activity, thus reducing the risk of a stunning effect and increasing the diagnostic performance, especially in terms of sensitivity and specificity, and (ii) the wider availability of iodine isotopes other than iodine-131 (i.e., $^{123/124}$I), which are able to produce higher-quality imaging, avoiding the stunning effect, and with the consequent further improvement of the diagnostic performance [23,25].

Accordingly, diagnostic functional imaging using different iodine isotopes (e.g., $^{131}/^{123}/^{124}$I) can be used during the postoperative assessment of DTC patients to improve their risk stratification and early staging. Thus, the decision-making process can be enhanced in deciding for or against RIT and in choosing its correct purpose (e.g., "functional imaging-guided approach"; see the specific paragraph).

Currently, iodine-131 or iodine-123 Dx-WBS is more frequently used in the follow-up of DTC patients as part of the diagnostic procedures (e.g., laboratory test and nUS) to evaluate the response to initial therapies (e.g., thyroid surgery and RIT) or in DTC patients with recurrent disease [12].

According to the 2015 ATA guidelines, the use of iodine-131 or iodine-123 Dx-WBS at the time of the first follow-up (i.e., response assessment) should be reserved for patients with (1) positive TgAb; (2) poorly informative pT-WBS (e.g., due to the presence of large thyroid remnant); or (3) high-risk DTC [10]. Some authors have also reported on the usefulness of Dx-WBS in patients with metastases at pT-WBS and/or primary malignancy in the isthmus [12,26]. In particular, the isthmus topography of malignant thyroid nodules is an independent risk factor for having both metastatic disease at initial diagnosis and persistent disease at the time of the first follow-up (i.e., response assessment), as already described [26–32]. Accordingly, in such patients, a more aggressive follow-up, including diagnostic functional imaging, should always be considered [8,26].

Recently, the shared guidelines between the American and European Association of Nuclear Medicine (SNMMI and EANM, respectively) [16] considered important the use of Dx-WBS to (1) establish a new baseline after RIT [33]; (2) determine interval response to RIT; and (3) assess the patient's thyroid cancer status. Along with laboratory tests (i.e., basal and stimulated-Tg testing) and cross-sectional anatomic imaging, the results of follow-up DxWBS contribute to the dynamic risk restratification of DTC patients.

To date, Dx-WBS (regardless of the iodine isotopes used) should always be integrated by hybrid imaging (i.e., $^{123/131}$I-Dx-WBS-SPECT/CT) to significantly improve the diagnostic performance of the functional imaging, especially in detecting micro-metastases involving the lymph nodes of the central compartment (i.e., VI Robbins' level) in patients with negative nUS but a less than excellent response to initial therapies [i.e., bio-chemical indeterminate or biochemical incomplete response (BIndR or BIR, respectively)] [12,34]. In such patients, $^{123/131}$I-Dx-WBS-SPECT/CT is able to change the response assessment from BIndR/BIR (better prognosis) to structural incomplete response (SIR, worse prognosis), thus significantly modifying their further clinical, diagnostic, and therapeutic management, as recently described [35].

Recently, a basal Tg value $\geq$ 0.39 ng/mL has been suggested for selecting patients to address ^{123}I-Dx-WBS-SPECT/CT to further increase the diagnostic performance of functional imaging and reduce the number of cases that cannot be used [35].

To date, the use of rhTSH (i.e., exogenous stimulation on L-T4 therapy) is supported as the preferred strategy to perform $^{123}/^{131}$I-Dx-WBS-SPECT/CT, which can reduce patients' discomfort while maintaining the diagnostic accuracy of functional imaging [8,21,22,36].

4. Postoperative Iodine-131 Therapy (p-RIT)

The goal of RIT can only be established once the postoperative disease status has been assessed by integrating the histopathological report and the so-called "local factors" (i.e., clinical, laboratory, and imaging parameters, which can be different from patient to patient). Accordingly, the first administration of ^{131}I therapeutic activity (i.e., p-RIT) can be used for the following reasons: (1) to destroy normal thyroid tissue remnants in DTC patients classified as low-risk for having persistent/recurrent disease according to the histopathological report (i.e., ablative aim); (2) to irradiate suspected but unproved (e.g., by imaging studies) loco-regional and/or distant metastatic disease in low-to-intermediate or intermediate risk DTC patients (adjuvant aim); or (3) to treat loco-regional and/or distant metastatic disease already noted by imaging studies (therapeutic aim) [16,37].

Noteworthily, p-RIT is used in low-risk DTC patients to simplify their long-term follow-up, which is always necessary in such patients, by using serum thyroglobulin (Tg) monitoring [associated with thyroglobulin antibody (TgAb) measurement] and neck-ultrasound (nUS) (if needed) [38].

However, in such patients, p-RIT can also be used for an early functional (re)staging based on theragnostic information obtained by ^{131}I post-therapy whole-body scintigraphy (pT-WBS), ideally associated with SPECT/CT (Figure 1). Indeed, unexpected loco-regional (i.e., micro-lymph node metastases) and/or distant metastases (more rarely) can be noted in low-risk DTC with undetectable or low Tg levels (in the absence of TgAb) and negative nUS [7,12,39–47] (Figure 2). However, false positive radioiodine uptake can be sometimes noted at pT-WBS due to inflammatory or benign disease, as well as some malignant lesions, as already described [48,49]. Noteworthily, the use of hybrid imaging (i.e., SPECT/CT), as a complement to planar imaging, significantly improves the "diagnostic" performance of pT-WBS, reducing the number of either false positive (i.e., radioiodine pitfalls) or false negative results [20,21,36,50].

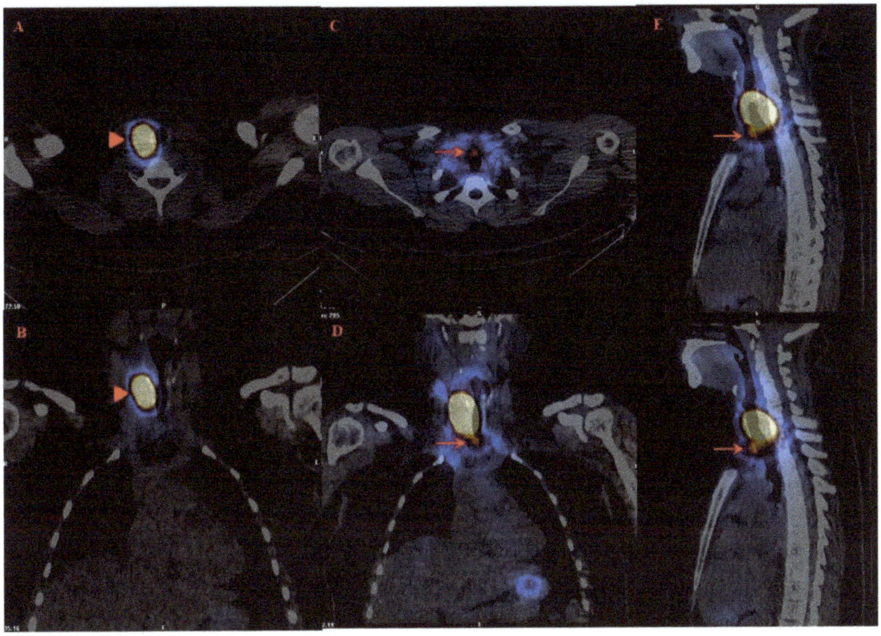

Figure 1. A twenty-six-year-old woman affected by multifocal papillary thyroid carcinoma (12 mm in maximum size), follicular variant, located in the lower part of the left lobe (pT1b(m), Nx, Mx). Postoperative neck-ultrasonography (nUS) performed within three months after thyroid surgery did not show any thyroid remnant and/or suspicious or pathological loco-regional lymph node. The patient underwent rhTSH-aided (standard protocol) iodine-131 therapy (RIT) with ablative purpose (2.2 GBq). At RIT, the peaks of TSH 65 µIU/mL, TgAb 13.6 IU/mL, and basal and stimulated Tg values (day 1, 3, and 5) were <0.04, 3.2, and 10.3 ng/mL, respectively. (**A**,**B**) pT-WBS (anterior and posterior views) and static images (anterior and posterior views) of the neck–thoracic region were obtained two days after RIT. An intense radioiodine uptake consistent with thyroid remnant parenchyma was noted in the right thyroid bed ((**A**,**B**) arrowheads). In addition, a small-sized radioiodine avid lymph node metastasis (red arrows) located in the pre-tracheal region (i.e., VI Robbins' level) was noted (**C**–**E**).

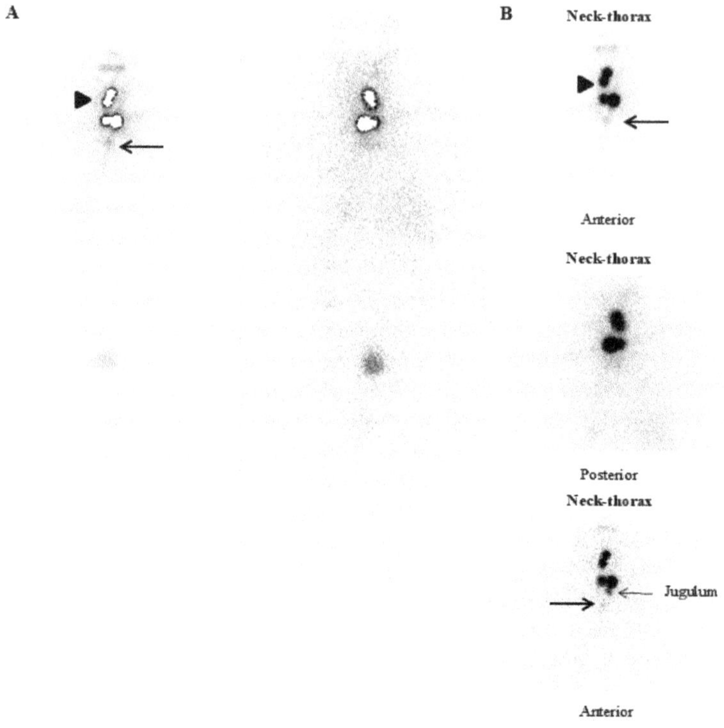

Figure 2. A fifty-two-year-old man affected by papillary thyroid carcinoma (24 mm in maximum size), classical variant, located in the left lobe (pT2, Nx, Mx). Postoperative neck-ultrasonography (nUS) performed within three months after thyroid surgery did not show any thyroid remnant and/or suspicious or pathological loco-regional lymph node. The patient underwent rhTSH-aided (standard protocol) iodine-131 therapy (RIT) with ablative purpose (2.2 GBq). (**A**,**B**): pT-WBS (anterior and posterior views) and static images (anterior and posterior views) of the neck–thoracic region were obtained two days after RIT. Three areas of intense radioiodine uptake (arrowheads) consistent with thyroid remnants were noted in the thyroid bed. In addition, a slight but focal radioiodine uptake consistent with lymph node metastasis was observed immediately below both the thyroid remnant and jugulum region (black arrows). At RIT, the peaks of TSH 111 µIU/mL, TgAb < 10 IU/mL, and basal and stimulated Tg values (days 1, 3, and 5) were always <0.15 ng/mL.

Although some different points of view exist between endocrinologists and nuclear medicine physicians on the use of p-RIT in lower-risk DTC patients, a strict cooperation within a multidisciplinary team is mandatory for better defined local standards of care. All in all, p-RIT therapy should be considered under the following conditions:

1. Tumor diameter greater than 20 mm: The risk of locoregional and/or distant metastatic disease at diagnosis/initial treatment increases with tumor size, becoming significant for lesions > 2 cm [8,51–55]. The ATA guidelines also report that, in these patients, the risk of structural disease persistence/recurrence (and therefore a more severe prognosis) increases significantly, rising from 1 to 2% in unifocal microcarcinomas to 5% for tumors measuring between 2 and 4 cm [10].
2. Tumor diameter between 10 and 20 mm, multifocal/bilateral: The risk of structural disease persistence/recurrence is not negligible, affecting up to 6% of patients with multifocal and/or bilateral tumors [10,56].

3. Isthmic location: The isthmic location has emerged as an additional and independent risk factor for both the presence of locoregional or distant metastases at diagnosis/initial treatment and disease persistence one year after initial treatments [26,57].
4. Presence of thyroid residue and/or locoregional metastases on postoperative ultrasound and/or functional imaging: Thyroid residue visible on morphological and/or functional imaging (indicating a suboptimal surgery) increases the risk of disease persistence/recurrence, which grows as its size increases, and also limits the diagnostic value of thyroglobulin (Tg) during follow-up. Additionally, the identification of locoregional lymph node metastases on ultrasound imaging indicates radioiodine therapy (with a therapeutic intent) [37].
5. Measurable postoperative basal and/or stimulated thyroglobulin; positive anti-thyroglobulin antibodies: RIT should also be considered for patients with basal and/or stimulated Tg (endogenous or exogenous stimulation using recombinant TSH, rhTSH) above the local institutional cut-off and, in any case, above 2 and 5 ng/mL, respectively [10,16,58,59]. Moreover, RIT should always be considered in patients with positive anti-thyroglobulin antibodies (AbTg). In fact, the positivity of AbTg makes the follow-up of patients more difficult and less reliable, limiting both the diagnostic accuracy and the clinical significance of Tg measurements [10,16,58,59]. The AbTg value is also important since the commonly reported reference cut-offs refer to the adult population with an intact thyroid. Therefore, the use of the Limit of Quantification (LoQ) or the Limit of Detection (LoD) has been proposed to exclude the presence of potentially interfering AbTg [60,61].
6. Presence of locoregional and/or distant metastases on postoperative functional whole-body imaging and "hybrid" imaging ($^{131\text{-}123}$I-Dx-imaging): Postoperative diagnostic functional imaging (^{123}/^{131}I-Dx-imaging) provides information that changes the histopathological risk class in 15% of DTC patients. The use of ^{123}/^{131}I-Dx-imaging, by revealing the presence of locoregional and/or distant metastases, could modify the clinical management of a significant number of patients, indicating the need for ^{131}I therapy with therapeutic intent [16].

In addition to the parameters considered above, the decision for or against the use of RIT for low-to-intermediate risk DTC patients should also take into account local factors that differ among patients according to their demographic, clinical, economic, and social characteristics and provenience. Thus, based on technical–methodological availability, expertise for follow-up, and patient preferences, RIT should always be taken into account when the following cases occur:

a. Less than optimal pre- and postoperative neck-US evaluation;
b. Less than optimal thyroid surgery (i.e., low-volume thyroid surgeon);
c. Poorly informative histological report (i.e., not a standardized report);
d. Positive anti-thyroglobulin antibody;
e. Limited access to referral centers;
f. Patient's will to maximize the therapeutic process to reduce anxiety related to disease recurrence, considering that the goal of cancer treatment is not only to prolong survival but also to maintain and improve the quality of life.

Finally, ^{131}I therapy represents the main treatment option in DTC patients with iodine-avid metastases, and up to 50% of such patients obtain a complete remission or stabilization for a long-term period after RIT, thus having a favorable impact on both overall survival and disease-free survival [62–65]. The remaining patients are declared to be radioactive iodine refractory (RAI-R) and, as a consequence, RIT is no longer justified [66]. The absence of the sodium iodide symporter (NIS) in the membrane of thyroid cells leads to RAI-R. This is due to gene mutation or rearrangement. Accordingly, the aberrant activation of signal pathways results in the abnormal expression of thyroid-specific genes, leading to RAI-R [67]. In such patients, to date, there are few available and alternative therapies that can be used for the treatment of local (e.g., surgical approach, external beam radiation therapy, interventional radiological procedures) or systemic (e.g., tyrosine kinase inhibitors—TKIs) metastatic disease [12]. The choice of the alternative therapy depends on the loco-regional spread of the tumor as well as the number, size, and location of metastatic disease [12]. Finally, it is important to consider the emerging role of the second-line TKIs (i.e., BRAF and MEK inhibitors) as agents able to restore or enhance radioiodine uptake in RAI-R patients, offering the possibility of a de novo use of RIT [12].

4.1. Postoperative Iodine-131 Therapy (p-RIT) Planning (Empiric Approach)

Two empirical approaches can be used to perform p-RIT.

The *"functional imaging-guided approach"* is based on results obtained by postoperative $^{131/123}$I diagnostic scintigraphy (pDx-WBS) (i.e., theragnostic approach). This approach can significantly improve the postoperative risk stratification and staging of DTC patients by evaluating the topography and extension of iodine-avid thyroid tissue regardless of their initial risk class assigned, according to the 2015 American Thyroid Association [10,16]. In particular, *a functional imaging-guided approach* can be instrumental in the decision-making process of low(er)-risk DTC patients in whom a selective use of RIT is indicated [17,68]. Indeed, a negative pDx-WBS (i.e., no radioiodine uptake or thyroid remnant only) in patients with undetectable Tg value and negative TgAb can lead to either avoiding RIT or reducing radioiodine activity using low instead of moderate approaches. Conversely, a positive pDx-WBS (i.e., unexpected loco-regional and/or distant metastatic disease) corresponds to RIT changing the aim from ablative to therapeutic, thus using higher radioiodine activities that could be personalized by a dosimetric approach [16,69]. In such patients, ^{124}I-PET/CT can be considered an alternative functional imaging method to $^{131/123}$I pDx-WBS due to its favorable characteristics and higher sensitivity in detecting metastases, even if it is more expensive and less readily available [70,71]. In summary, the *"functional imaging-guided approach"* for planning p-RIT is the paradigm of thyroid cancer theragnostics [16,68].

The *"risk-adapted approach"* is based on the accurate evaluation of clinical–pathological factors and institutional protocols [16]. In particular, in patients affected by low- to intermediate-risk DTC, both the decision for or against the use of RIT and the chosen purpose (i.e., ablative or adjuvant) depend on the histological report (accurately evaluated since, to date, a standardized report is not available) and local factors that differ among patients according to their demographic, clinical, economic, and social characteristic and provenience (i.e., rural vs. urban area) [10,12,37]. The histological report and local factors should always be evaluated during postoperative disease assessment, and standardized and integrated into routine clinical care, as already reported [37].

Histological reports must always be accurately evaluated since, to date, a standardized report is not available and a poorly informative one is obtained in a not-negligible number of patients. Among local factors, the quality of pre- and postoperative nUS assessments, quality of Tg measurements (e.g., 1st vs. 2nd generation test), the skills and experience of the thyroid surgeon, and clinical concerns of the local disease management team must be considered in postoperative ^{131}I decision making [12,16,72–75].

Finally (*last but not least*), patients' will to maximize the intensity of care should always be considered before making a final decision about the pros and cons of using RIT [12,37].

Table 1 summarizes the ^{131}I activities suggested according to the risk-adapted approach.

Table 1. Suggested ^{131}I treatment activities in the context of therapeutic intent.

Clinical/Pathologic Context	Prescribed ^{131}I Activity	Strategy
Remnant ablation	1.11–1.85 GBq (30–50 mCi) ^{131}I *	Risk-adapted ^{131}I therapy
Adjuvant treatment	1.85–3.7 GBq (50–100 mCi) ^{131}I **	Risk-adapted ^{131}I therapy
Treatment of small-volume locoregional disease	3.7–5.6 GBq (100–150 mCi) ^{131}I	Risk-adapted ^{131}I therapy
Treatment of advanced locoregional disease and/or small-volume distant metastatic disease	5.6–7.4 GBq (150–200 mCi) ^{131}I	Risk-adapted ^{131}I therapy

* The FDA approved the use of rhTSH in combination with 100 mCi ^{131}I for remnant ablation in December 2007 [76,77]. ** Some committee members recommend up to 5.6 GBq (150 mCi) without extant data regarding the effectiveness and toxicity profiles of 1.85 GBq (100 mCi) vs. 5.6 GBq (150 mCi) for adjuvant treatment. Current guidelines advise that the frequency and severity of side effects are activity-dependent, with specifically an increased xerostomia risk for 3.7 GBq (100 mCi) and sialadenitis risk for 5.6 GBq (150 mCi) [78].

4.2. Postoperative Iodine-131 Therapy (p-RIT) Planning (Dosimetry Approach)

The dosimetric approach can be used in DTC patients whose p-RIT is performed for ablative or therapeutic purposes. Conversely, an empiric approach (functional image-guided or risk-adapted) should be preferred if p-RIT is performed with an adjuvant aim, since ^{131}I administration is linked to the will to irradiate suspected but unproved metastatic lesion(s) [18,37].

Two dosimetric approaches can be used to perform p-RIT, with ablative or therapeutic aims: (i) the blood or bone marrow dosimetry-based method approach and (ii) the lesion dosimetry-based method [16].

The *blood/bone marrow dosimetry-based method*, primarily targeting safety, is more broadly used, allowing the maximum tolerated activity (MTA) that can be administered to be calculated, and keeping the dose absorbed to the blood/bone marrow (*critical organ*) at $\leq$2 Gy. In addition, this approach permits preliminary verification that the administered ^{131}I activity does not exceed 4.44 GBq in whole-body retention at 48 h, or 3 Gy if pulmonary metastatic disease is present [16,79,80].

Noteworthily, the blood/bone marrow dosimetry-based method permits the avoidance of the risk related to the empiric approach of performing a p-RIT using a radioiodine activity over or under the MTA. Thus, the blood/bone marrow dosimetry-based method is able to avoid overtreatment (which may cause acute dose-related toxicities) [16].

The main limitation of the blood/bone marrow dosimetry-based method is due to the lack of information on the radiation-absorbed dose delivered to the target (i.e., thyroid remnant or loco-regional and/or distant metastases). Accordingly, the method can lead to over- or undertreatment of the target [16].

The goal of the *lesion dosimetry-based method* involves the personalization of ^{131}I activity, which would be able to deliver a sufficient radiation-absorbed dose to the target for achieving a therapeutic effect (i.e., ablation of thyroid remnant and/or treatment of metastases) [16]. However, there is no validated method to determine the target mass, either by morphological or functional imaging studies [16,18]. Accordingly, the reported absorbed dose thresholds for providing therapeutic effect change according to different literature data already published. Maxon et al. first proposed a value of 300 Gy to ablate the thyroid remnant and 80 Gy to treat loco-regional metastases. Conversely, Flux et al. proposed 49 Gy for thyroid remnant ablation, while Wierts et al. suggested at least 90 and 40 Gy to deliver treatments for thyroid remnant and loco-regional metastases, respectively [16,81–83].

In addition, the target size can be too little to be visualized (e.g., thyroid remnant and/or micro-lymph node metastasis), or metastasis may have loosened its functional ability to take up iodine (i.e., dedifferentiation) [18].

5. General Considerations on Patients' Preparation and Strategy to Deliver Postoperative Iodine-131 Therapy (p-RIT)

In general, a reduction in the daily intake or use of foods [low iodine diet (LID)] and/or products containing iodine should be suggested for two weeks before p-RIT with the aim to optimize ^{131}I uptake by normal and/or neoplastic cells (i.e., loco-regional and/or distant metastatic lesions). Similarly, the previous or current use of drugs and/or iodinated contrast media agents must be excluded to rule out an excess of stable iodine [12,84–88].

To date, the measurement of urinary stable iodine excretion is not recommended in all cases. Still, it should be considered in selected patients whose exposure to stable iodine is uncertain [12,89]. In preparation for p-RIT, iodine deprivation is considered adequate or optimal when spot urinary iodine is <100 or 50 µg/L, respectively [16,89,90].

Table 2 summarizes foods, drugs, and iodine-containing substances that reduce radioiodine uptake to thyroid remnants and/or metastatic lesions.

Table 2. Foods, drugs, and iodide-containing substances that can reduce radioiodine thyroid uptake.

Food and Products That Should Be *Avoided* or *Limited*	Type of Medication	Recommended Time of Withdrawal
Iodized salt **(avoided)**	Water-soluble intravenous radiographic contrast agents	6–8 wk *, assuming normal renal function
Any vitamins or supplements that contain iodine **(avoided)**	Lipophilic intravenous radiographic contrast agents	3–6 mo #
Foods from the sea **(avoided)**	Thyroxine	3–4 wk *
Herbal supplements **(avoided)**	Triiodothyronine	10–14 d §
Eggs **(avoided)**	Methimazole	2–5 d § before RAI therapy
Milk or other dairy products, including ice cream, cheese, yogurt, and butter **(avoided)**	Propylthiouracil	2–8 wk * if RAI therapy is performed by fixed-activity method (4–7 d § if RAI therapy is performed after personalized dosimetric approach)
Soy products **(avoided)**	Lugol solution	2–3 wk *, depending on iodide content
Grain products **(limited)**	Saturated solution of potassium iodide	2–3 wk *
Beef, chicken, and turkey **(limited)**	Topical iodine (e.g., surgical skin preparation)	2–3 wk *
	Amiodarone	3–6 mo # or longer

Note: § d, days; * wk, weeks; # mo, months.

There are two strategies for patients' preparation for p-RIT: (i) endogenous TSH stimulation by levothyroxine (L-T4) withdrawal (i.e., inducing hypothyroidism) or (ii) exogenous TSH stimulation by administering rhTSH according to the standard protocol (i.e., 0.9 mg/day intramuscularly administered on two consecutive days) [16]. The choice of strategy (i.e., L-T4 withdrawal or rhTSH-stimulation) must be personalized for each patient according to published data [16].

In low-risk DTC patients who underwent p-RIT with an ablative purpose (i.e., thyroid remnant ablation), rhTSH-stimulation proved to be as effective as L-T4 withdrawal. In addition, the use of rhTSH to avoid hypothyroidism can both maintain patients' quality of life and reduce radiation exposure [12,35,91–96]. Consequently, rhTSH-stimulation is the preferred strategy for p-RIT in such patients.

In DTC patients whose p-RIT is performed with an adjuvant purpose (i.e., intermediate-risk DTC), L-T4 withdrawal and rhTSH stimulation should both be considered. In such patients, the choice of stimulation strategy depends on several factors, such as histological features, clinical characteristics, and expected efficacy. In addition, economic feasibility and patients' quality of life must also be considered [12,16,37,94,97–106].

Finally, L-T4 withdrawal is currently the preferred strategy for p-RIT (and in case of further treatments) in DTC patients with morphological and/or functional imaging evidence of loco-regional and/or distant metastases. The evidence of iodine-avid metastases at functional imaging can be noted during (a) postoperative assessment according to the so-called *"functional imaging-guided approach"*, (b) at post-therapy whole-body scintigraphy, and (c) during follow-up.

In such patients, the choice of L-T4 withdrawal as the preferred strategy to perform RIT is based on the evidence that metastatic thyroid cells have lower density and poorer functionality of NIS. Accordingly, TSH elevation over time would be important to promote increased ^{131}I uptake and retention in tumor cells [10,18,107,108].

Conversely, the literature data recently published indicate that the stimulation strategy (i.e., L-T4 withdrawal vs. rhTSH-stimulation) used to deliver RIT has no significant impact on both RIT efficacy and (as per consequence) metastatic patients' outcome [12,109,110]. Noteworthily, Gomes-Lima and colleagues did not note any significant difference in terms of progression-free survival and overall survival among fifty-five metastatic DTC patients treated after L-T4 withdrawal (n = 28) or rhTSH-stimulation (n = 27) [109].

Accordingly, the use of L-T4 withdrawal or rhTSH-stimulation as the preferred strategy to deliver RIT in metastatic DTC patients should be deferred to clinical evaluations, taking into account patients' characteristics and comorbidities [111].

Finally, if a dosimetric approach is chosen instead of an empiric one (e.g., a functional imaging-guided approach or risk-adapted approach), p-RIT (or further treatments) has to be performed with the same functional status (e.g., hypothyroidism or euthyroidism) already used for dosimetric evaluation [12,16].

6. Conclusions

Radioiodine isotopes still play a fundamental role in the diagnostic and therapeutic management of most patients affected by benign or differentiated malignant thyroid disorders, representing an evergreen radiotracer family. Currently, the real-life related literature evidence confirms how a risk-orientated and personalized postoperative use of iodine isotopes can heavily impact (re)staging, the subsequent decision-making process (i.e., for or against RIT; the correct and tailored aim of RIT; and therapy modality: empiric vs. dosimetric approach), and the outcome of DTC patients. Additionally, diagnostic functional imaging represents the only diagnostic tool able to detect structural persistent disease in a not-negligible number of DTC patients, thus changing their subsequent assessment and management. Finally, the authors highlight the therapeutic and theragnostic role of iodine-131. It should always be considered as an oldie but goldie chance of definitive care for DTC patients who develop critical status when radioiodine-avid metastases are no longer noted. In conclusion, we wholly support the consideration of radioiodine isotopes as an oldie but goldie diagnostic, therapeutic, and theragnostic tool for the more correct and better-tailored management of patients with thyroid disorders.

Author Contributions: Conceptualization, A.C.; writing—original draft preparation, A.C.; review and editing, R.M.R., M.S. and A.C. All authors have read and agreed to the published version of the manuscript.

Funding: This research received no external funding.

Institutional Review Board Statement: Not applicable.

Informed Consent Statement: Informed consent was obtained from all subjects involved in the study.

Data Availability Statement: Data available on request.

Conflicts of Interest: The authors declare no conflicts of interest.

References

1. Campennì, A.; Giovanella, L. Nuclear medicine therapy of thyroid cancer post-thyroidectomy. In *Nuclear Medicine and Molecular Imaging*; Sathekge, M., Luster, M., Eds.; Elsevier: Amsterdam, The Netherlands, 2022; Volume 4, pp. 42–55. [CrossRef]
2. Chen, A.Y.; Jemal, A.; Ward, E.M. Increasing incidence of differentiated thyroid cancer in the United States, 1988–2005. *Cancer* **2009**, *115*, 3801–3807. [CrossRef] [PubMed]

3. Davies, L.; Welch, H.G. Increasing incidence of thyroid cancer in the United States, 1973–2002. *JAMA* **2006**, *295*, 2164–2167. [CrossRef] [PubMed]
4. Siegel, R.; Naishadham, D.; Jemal, A. Cancer statistics, 2013. *CA Cancer J. Clin.* **2013**, *63*, 11–30. [CrossRef] [PubMed]
5. Siegel, R.L.; Miller, K.D.; Fuchs, H.E.; Jemal, A. Cancer Statistics, 2021. *CA Cancer J. Clin.* **2021**, *71*, 7–33. [CrossRef]
6. Howlader, N.; Noone, A.M.; Krapcho, M.; Miller, D.; Bishop, K.; Kosary, C.L.; Yu, M.; Ruhl, J.; Tatalovich, Z.; Mariotto, A.; et al. (Eds.) *SEER Cancer Statistics Review, 1975–2014*; based on November 2016 SEER data submission, posted to the SEER web site, April 2017; National Cancer Institute: Bethesda, MD, USA; 2017. Available online: https://seer.cancer.gov/csr/1975_2014/ (accessed on 2 April 2018).
7. Gallicchio, R.; Giacomobono, S.; Capacchione, D.; Nardelli, A.; Barbato, F.; Nappi, A.; Pellegrino, T.; Storto, G. Should patients with remnants from thyroid microcarcinoma really not be treated with iodine-131 ablation? *Endocrine* **2013**, *44*, 426–433. [CrossRef]
8. Tuttle, R.M.; Tala, H.; Shah, J.; Leboeuf, R.; Ghossein, R.; Gonen, M.; Brokhin, M.; Omry, G.; Fagin, J.A.; Shaha, A. Estimating risk of recurrence in differentiated thyroid cancer after total thyroidectomy and radioactive iodine remnant ablation: Using response to therapy variables to modify the initial risk estimates predicted by the new American Thyroid Association staging system. *Thyroid Off. J. Am. Thyroid Assoc.* **2010**, *20*, 1341–1349. [CrossRef]
9. Lamartina, L.; Grani, G.; Durante, C.; Borget, I.; Filetti, S.; Schlumberger, M. Follow-up of differentiated thyroid cancer—What should (and what should not) be done. *Nat. Rev. Endocrinol.* **2018**, *14*, 538–551. [CrossRef]
10. Haugen, B.R.; Alexander, E.K.; Bible, K.C.; Doherty, G.M.; Mandel, S.J.; Nikiforov, Y.E.; Pacini, F.; Randolph, G.W.; Sawka, A.M.; Schlumberger, M.; et al. 2015 American Thyroid Association Management Guidelines for Adult Patients with Thyroid Nodules and Differentiated Thyroid Cancer: The American Thyroid Association Guidelines Task Force on Thyroid Nodules and Differentiated Thyroid Cancer. *Thyroid Off. J. Am. Thyroid Assoc.* **2016**, *26*, 1. [CrossRef]
11. Luster, M.; Clarke, S.E.; Dietlein, M.; Lassmann, M.; Lind, P.; Oyen, W.J.G.; Tennvall, J.; Bombardieri, E.; European Association of Nuclear Medicine (EANM). Guidelines for radioiodine therapy of differentiated thyroid cancer. *Eur. J. Nucl. Med. Mol. Imaging* **2008**, *35*, 1941–1959. [CrossRef]
12. Giovanella, L.; Tuncel, M.; Aghaee, A.; Campenni, A.; De Virgilio, A.; Ovčariček, P.P. Theranostics of Thyroid Cancer. *Semin. Nucl. Med.* **2024**, *54*, 470–487. [CrossRef]
13. Cooper, D.S.; Specker, B.; Ho, M.; Sperling, M.; Ladenson, P.W.; Ross, D.S.; Ain, K.B.; Bigos, S.T.; Brierley, J.D.; Haugen, B.R.; et al. Thyrotropin suppression and disease progression in patients with differentiated thyroid cancer: Results from the National Thyroid Cancer Treatment Cooperative Registry. *Thyroid Off. J. Am. Thyroid Assoc.* **1998**, *8*, 737–744. [CrossRef] [PubMed]
14. Bilimoria, K.Y.; Bentrem, D.J.; Ko, C.Y.; Stewart, A.K.; Winchester, D.P.; Talamonti, M.S.; Sturgeon, C. Extent of surgery affects survival for papillary thyroid cancer. *Ann. Surg.* **2007**, *246*, 375–384. [CrossRef] [PubMed]
15. Hay, I.D.; Bergstralh, E.J.; Grant, C.S.; McIver, B.; Thompson, G.B.; van Heerden, J.A.; Goellner, J.R. Impact of primary surgery on outcome in 300 patients with pathologic tumor-node-metastasis stage III papillary thyroid carcinoma treated at one institution from 1940 through 1989. *Surgery* **1999**, *126*, 1173–1182. [CrossRef] [PubMed]
16. Avram, A.M.; Giovanella, L.; Greenspan, B.; Lawson, S.A.; Luster, M.; Van Nostrand, D.; Peacock, J.G.; Ovčariček, P.P.; Silberstein, E.; Tulchinsky, M.; et al. SNMMI Procedure Standard/EANM Practice Guideline for Nuclear Medicine Evaluation and Therapy of Differentiated Thyroid Cancer: Abbreviated Version. *J. Nucl. Med. Off. Publ. Soc. Nucl. Med.* **2022**, *63*, 15N–35N.
17. Avram, A.M. Radioiodine scintigraphy with SPECT/CT: An important diagnostic tool for thyroid cancer staging and risk stratification. *J. Nucl. Med. Off. Publ. Soc. Nucl. Med.* **2012**, *53*, 754–764. [CrossRef]
18. Atkins, F.B.; Van Nostrand, D.; Wartofsky, L. *Dosimetrically Determined Prescribed Activity of ^{131}I for the Treatment of Metastatic Differentiated Thyroid Carcinoma*; Springer Science + Business Media: New York, NY, USA, 2016. [CrossRef]
19. Campennì, A.; Ruggeri, R.M.; Siracusa, M.; Comis, A.D.; Romano, D.; Vento, A.; Lanzafame, H.; Capoccetti, F.; Alibrandi, A.; Baldari, S.; et al. Early preablation rhTSH-stimulated thyroglobulin predicts outcome of differentiated thyroid cancer (DTC) patients. *Eur. J. Nucl. Med. Mol. Imaging* **2021**, *48*, 2466–2475. [CrossRef]
20. Campennì, A.; Vrachimis, A.; Siracusa, M.; Baldari, S.; Giovanella, L. Usefulness of ^{123}I-spect/ct to assess the response to initial therapy in differentiated thyroid cancer patients. *Endocrine* **2021**, *74*, 193–196. [CrossRef]
21. Barwick, T.; Murray, I.; Megadmi, H.; Drake, W.M.; Plowman, P.N.; Akker, S.A.; Chew, S.L.; Grossman, A.B.; Avril, N. Single photon emission computed tomography (SPECT)/computed tomography using Iodine-123 in patients with differentiated thyroid cancer: Additional value over whole body planar imaging and SPECT. *Eur. J. Endocrinol.* **2010**, *162*, 1131–1139. [CrossRef]
22. Alzahrani, A.S.; AlShaikh, O.; Tuli, M.; Al-Sugair, A.; Alamawi, R.; Al-Rasheed, M.M. Diagnostic value of recombinant human thyrotropin-stimulated ^{123}I whole-body scintigraphy in the follow-up of patients with differentiated thyroid cancer. *Clin. Nucl. Med.* **2012**, *37*, 229–234. [CrossRef]
23. Siddiqi, A.; Foley, R.R.; Britton, K.E.; Sibtain, A.; Plowman, P.N.; Grossman, A.B.; Monson, J.P.; Besser, G.M. The role of 123I-diagnostic imaging in the follow-up of patients with differentiated thyroid carcinoma as compared to 131I-scanning: Avoidance of negative therapeutic uptake due to stunning. *Clin. Endocrinol.* **2001**, *55*, 515–521. [CrossRef]
24. Avram, A.M.; Fig, L.M.; Frey, K.A.; Gross, M.D.; Wong, K.K. Preablation 131-I scans with SPECT/CT in postoperative thyroid cancer patients: What is the impact on staging? *J. Clin. Endocrinol. Metab.* **2013**, *98*, 1163–1171. [CrossRef] [PubMed]
25. Sisson, J.C.; Avram, A.M.; Lawson, S.A.; Gauger, P.G.; Doherty, G. The so-called stunning of thyroid tissue. *J. Nucl. Med. Off. Publ. Soc. Nucl. Med.* **2006**, *47*, 1406–1412.

26. Campennì, A.; Ruggeri, R.M.; Siracusa, M.; Giacoppo, G.; La Torre, F.; Saccomanno, A.; Alibrandi, A.; Dionigi, G.; Tuccari, G.; Baldari, S.; et al. Isthmus topography is a risk factor for persistent disease in patients with differentiated thyroid cancer. *Eur. J. Endocrinol.* **2021**, *185*, 397–404. [CrossRef] [PubMed]
27. Vasileiadis, I.; Boutzios, G.; Karalaki, M.; Misiakos, E.; Karatzas, T. Papillary thyroid carcinoma of the isthmus: Total thyroidectomy or isthmusectomy? *Am. J. Surg.* **2018**, *216*, 135–139. [CrossRef]
28. Wang, J.; Sun, H.; Gao, L.; Xie, L.; Cai, X. Evaluation of thyroid isthmusectomy as a potential treatment for papillary thyroid carcinoma limited to the isthmus: A clinical study of 73 patients. *Head Neck* **2016**, *38* (Suppl. S1), E1510–E1514. [CrossRef]
29. Karatzas, T.; Charitoudis, G.; Vasileiadis, D.; Kapetanakis, S.; Vasileiadis, I. Surgical treatment for dominant malignant nodules of the isthmus of the thyroid gland: A case control study. *Int. J. Surg.* **2015**, *18*, 64–68. [CrossRef]
30. Lee, Y.S.; Jeong, J.J.; Nam, K.; Chung, W.Y.; Chang, H.; Park, C.S. Papillary carcinoma located in the thyroid isthmus. *World J. Surg.* **2010**, *34*, 36–39. [CrossRef]
31. Song, C.M.; Lee, D.W.; Ji, Y.B.; Jeong, J.H.; Park, J.H.; Tae, K. Frequency and pattern of central lymph node metastasis in papillary carcinoma of the thyroid isthmus. *Head Neck* **2016**, *38* (Suppl. S1), E412–E416. [CrossRef]
32. Chai, Y.J.; Kim, S.; Choi, J.Y.; Koo, D.H.; Lee, K.E.; Youn, Y. Papillary thyroid carcinoma located in the isthmus or upper third is associated with Delphian lymph node metastasis. *World J. Surg.* **2014**, *38*, 1306–1311. [CrossRef]
33. Van Nostrand, D. Surveillance radioiodine whole body scans. In *Thyroid Cancer: A Comprehensive Guide to Clinical Management*, 3rd ed.; Wartofsky, L., Van Nostrand, D., Eds.; Springer: New York, NY, USA, 2016; pp. 471–474.
34. Ovčariček, P.P.; Campenni, A.; de Keizer, B.; Deandreis, D.; Kreissl, M.C.; Vrachimis, A.; Tuncel, M.; Giovanella, L. Molecular Theranostics in Radioiodine-Refractory Differentiated Thyroid Cancer. *Cancers* **2023**, *15*, 4290. [CrossRef]
35. Campennì, A.; Ruggeri, R.M.; Siracusa, M.; Romano, D.; Giacoppo, G.; Crocè, L.; Rosarno, H.; Russo, S.; Cardile, D.; Capoccetti, F.; et al. Thyroglobulin Value Predict Iodine-123 Imaging Result in Differentiated Thyroid Cancer Patients. *Cancers* **2023**, *15*, 2242. [CrossRef] [PubMed]
36. Spanu, A.; Solinas, M.E.; Chessa, F.; Sanna, D.; Nuvoli, S.; Madeddu, G. 131I SPECT/CT in the follow-up of differentiated thyroid carcinoma: Incremental value versus planar imaging. *J. Nucl. Med. Off. Publ. Soc. Nucl. Med.* **2009**, *50*, 184–190. [CrossRef] [PubMed]
37. Tuttle, R.M.; Ahuja, S.; Avram, A.M.; Bernet, V.J.; Bourguet, P.; Daniels, G.H.; Dillehay, G.; Draganescu, C.; Flux, G.; Fuehrer, D.; et al. Controversies, Consensus, and Collaboration in the Use of ^{131}I Therapy in Differentiated Thyroid Cancer: A Joint Statement from the American Thyroid Association, the European Association of Nuclear Medicine, the Society of Nuclear Medicine and Molecular Imaging, and the European Thyroid Association. *Thyroid Off. J. Am. Thyroid Assoc.* **2019**, *29*, 461–470. [CrossRef]
38. Giovanella, L.; D'aurizio, F.; Algeciras-Schimnich, A.; Görges, R.; Ovcaricek, P.P.; Tuttle, R.M.; Visser, W.E.; Verburg, F.A.; hsTg&TgAb Consensus Working Group; Borowczyk, M.; et al. Thyroglobulin and thyroglobulin antibody: An updated clinical and laboratory expert consensus. *Eur. J. Endocrinol.* **2023**, *189*, R11–R27. [CrossRef]
39. Rosario, P.W.; Xavier, A.C.M.; Calsolari, M.R. Value of postoperative thyroglobulin and ultrasonography for the indication of ablation and ^{131} activity in patients with thyroid cancer and low risk of recurrence. *Thyroid Off. J. Am. Thyroid Assoc.* **2011**, *21*, 49–53. [CrossRef]
40. Park, E.-K.; Chung, J.-K.; Lim, I.H.; Park, D.J.; Lee, D.S.; Lee, M.C.; Cho, B.Y. Recurrent/metastatic thyroid carcinomas false negative for serum thyroglobulin but positive by posttherapy I-131 whole body scans. *Eur. J. Nucl. Med. Mol. Imaging* **2009**, *36*, 172–179. [CrossRef]
41. RRobenshtok, E.; Grewal, R.K.; Fish, S.; Sabra, M.; Tuttle, R.M. A low postoperative nonstimulated serum thyroglobulin level does not exclude the presence of radioactive iodine avid metastatic foci in intermediate-risk differentiated thyroid cancer patients. *Thyroid Off. J. Am. Thyroid Assoc.* **2013**, *23*, 436–442. [CrossRef]
42. Mertens, I.J.R.; DE Klerk, J.M.H.; Zelissen, P.M.J.; Thijssen, J.H.H.; Sie-Go, D.M.D.S.; Han, S.H.; VAN Rijk, P.P. Undetectable serum thyroglobulin in a patient with metastatic follicular thyroid cancer. *Clin. Nucl. Med.* **1999**, *24*, 346–349. [CrossRef]
43. Brendel, A.J.; Lambert, B.; Guyot, M.; Jeandot, R.; Dubourg, H.; Roger, P.; Wynchauk, S.; Manciet, G.; Lefort, G. Low levels of serum thyroglobulin after withdrawal of thyroid suppression therapy in the follow up of differentiated thyroid carcinoma. *Eur. J. Nucl. Med.* **1990**, *16*, 35–38. [CrossRef]
44. Grant, S.; Luttrell, B.; Reeve, T.; Wiseman, J.; Wilmshurst, E.; Stiel, J.; Donohoe, D.; Cooper, R.; Bridgman, M. Thyroglobulin may be undetectable in the serum of patients with metastatic disease secondary to differentiated thyroid carcinoma. Follow-up of differentiated thyroid carcinoma. *Cancer* **1984**, *54*, 1625–1628. [CrossRef]
45. Rosário, P.W.S.; Guimarães, V.C.; Maia, F.F.R.; Fagundes, T.A.; Purisch, S.; Padrao, E.L.; Rezende, L.L.; Barroso, A.L. Thyroglobulin before ablation and correlation with posttreatment scanning. *Laryngoscope* **2005**, *115*, 264–267. [CrossRef] [PubMed]
46. Phan, H.T.T.; Jager, P.L.; van der Wal, J.E.; Sluiter, W.J.; Plukker, J.T.M.; Dierckx, R.A.J.O.; Wolffenbuttel, B.H.R.; Links, T.P. The follow-up of patients with differentiated thyroid cancer and undetectable thyroglobulin (Tg) and Tg antibodies during ablation. *Eur. J. Endocrinol.* **2008**, *158*, 77–83. [CrossRef] [PubMed]
47. Müller-Gärtner, H.-W.; Schneider, C. Clinical evaluation of tumor characteristics predisposing serum thyroglobulin to be undetectable in patients with differentiated thyroid cancer. *Cancer* **1988**, *61*, 976–981. [CrossRef] [PubMed]
48. Barbaro, D.; Campennì, A.; Forleo, R.; Lapi, P. False-positive radioiodine uptake after radioiodine treatment in differentiated thyroid cancer. *Endocrine* **2023**, *81*, 30–35. [CrossRef]

49. Triggiani, V.; Giagulli, V.A.; Iovino, M.; De Pergola, G.; Licchelli, B.; Varraso, A.; Dicembrino, F.; Valle, G.; Guastamacchia, E. False positive diagnosis on (131)iodine whole-body scintigraphy of differentiated thyroid cancers. *Endocrine* **2016**, *53*, 626–635. [CrossRef]
50. Gonzalez Carvalho, J.M.; Görlich, D.; Schober, O.; Wenning, C.; Riemann, B.; Verburg, F.A.; Vrachimis, A. Evaluation of ^{131}I scintigraphy and stimulated thyroglobulin levels in the follow up of patients with DTC: A retrospective analysis of 1420 patients. *Eur. J. Nucl. Med. Mol. Imaging* **2017**, *44*, 744–756. [CrossRef]
51. Filetti, S.; Durante, C.; Hartl, D.; Leboulleux, S.; Locati, L.; Newbold, K.; Papotti, M.; Berruti, A.; ESMO Guidelines Committee. Thyroid cancer: ESMO Clinical Practice Guidelines for diagnosis, treatment and follow-up. *Ann. Oncol. Off. J. Eur. Soc. Med. Oncol.* **2019**, *30*, 1856–1883. [CrossRef]
52. Leboulleux, S.; Bournaud, C.; Chougnet, C.N.; Zerdoud, S.; Al Ghuzlan, A.; Catargi, B.; Do Cao, C.; Kelly, A.; Barge, M.-L.; Lacroix, L.; et al. Thyroidectomy without Radioiodine in Patients with Low-Risk Thyroid Cancer. *N. Engl. J. Med.* **2022**, *386*, 923–932. [CrossRef]
53. Schvartz, C.; Bonnetain, F.; Dabakuyo, S.; Gauthier, M.; Cueff, A.; Fieffé, S.; Pochart, J.-M.; Cochet, I.; Crevisy, E.; Dalac, A.; et al. Impact on overall survival of radioactive iodine in low-risk differentiated thyroid cancer patients. *J. Clin. Endocrinol. Metab.* **2012**, *97*, 1526–1535. [CrossRef]
54. Padovani, R.D.P.; Chablani, S.V.; Tuttle, R.M. Radioactive iodine therapy: Multiple faces of the same polyhedron. *Arch. Endocrinol. Metab.* **2022**, *66*, 393–406, Advance online publication. [CrossRef]
55. Campennì, A.; Barbaro, D.; Guzzo, M.; Capoccetti, F.; Giovanella, L. Personalized management of differentiated thyroid cancer in real life—Practical guidance from a multidisciplinary panel of experts. *Endocrine* **2020**, *70*, 280–291. [CrossRef] [PubMed]
56. Verburg, F.A.; Flux, G.; Giovanella, L.; van Nostrand, D.; Muylle, K.; Luster, M. Differentiated thyroid cancer patients potentially benefitting from postoperative I-131 therapy: A review of the literature of the past decade. *Eur. J. Nucl. Med. Mol. Imaging* **2020**, *47*, 78–83. [CrossRef] [PubMed]
57. Campennì, A.; Giovanella, L.; Siracusa, M.; Stipo, M.E.; Alibrandi, A.; Cucinotta, M.; Ruggeri, R.M.; Baldari, S. Is malignant nodule topography an additional risk factor for metastatic disease in low-risk differentiated thyroid cancer? *Thyroid Off. J. Am. Thyroid Assoc.* **2014**, *24*, 1607–1611. [CrossRef] [PubMed]
58. Pacini, F.; Fuhrer, D.; Elisei, R.; Handkiewicz-Junak, D.; Leboulleux, S.; Luster, M.; Schlumberger, M.; Smit, J.W. 2022 ETA Consensus Statement: What are the indications for post-surgical radioiodine therapy in differentiated thyroid cancer? *Eur. Thyroid J.* **2022**, *11*, e210046. [CrossRef] [PubMed]
59. Filetti, S.; Durante, C.; Hartl, D.; Leboulleux, S.; Locati, L.; Newbold, K.; Papotti, M.; Berruti, A.; ESMO Guidelines Committee. ESMO Clinical Practice Guideline update on the use of systemic therapy in advanced thyroid cancer. *Ann. Oncol. Off. J. Eur. Soc. Med. Oncol.* **2022**, *33*, 674–684. [CrossRef]
60. Verburg, F.A.; Luster, M.; Cupini, C.; Chiovato, L.; Duntas, L.; Elisei, R.; Feldt-Rasmussen, U.; Rimmele, H.; Seregni, E.; Smit, J.W.; et al. Implications of thyroglobulin antibody positivity in patients with differentiated thyroid cancer: A clinical position statement. *Thyroid Off. J. Am. Thyroid Assoc.* **2013**, *23*, 1211–1225. [CrossRef]
61. D'Aurizio, F.; Metus, P.; Ferrari, A.; Caruso, B.; Castello, R.; Villalta, D.; Steffan, A.; Gaspardo, K.; Pesente, F.; Bizzaro, N.; et al. Definition of the upper reference limit for thyroglobulin antibodies according to the National Academy of Clinical Biochemistry guidelines: Comparison of eleven different automated methods. *Autoimmun. Highlights* **2017**, *8*, 8. [CrossRef]
62. Hänscheid, H.; Lassmann, M.; Luster, M.; Thomas, S.R.; Pacini, F.; Ceccarelli, C.; Ladenson, P.W.; Wahl, R.L.; Schlumberger, M.; Ricard, M.; et al. Iodine biokinetics and dosimetry in radioiodine therapy of thyroid cancer: Procedures and results of a prospective international controlled study of ablation after rhTSH or hormone withdrawal. *J. Nucl. Med. Off. Publ. Soc. Nucl. Med.* **2006**, *47*, 648–654.
63. Ruel, E.; Thomas, S.; Dinan, M.; Perkins, J.M.; Roman, S.A.; Sosa, J.A. Adjuvant radioactive iodine therapy is associated with improved survival for patients with intermediate-risk papillary thyroid cancer. *J. Clin. Endocrinol. Metab.* **2015**, *100*, 1529–1536. [CrossRef]
64. Reiners, C.; Biko, J.; Haenscheid, H.; Hebestreit, H.; Kirinjuk, S.; Baranowski, O.; Marlowe, R.J.; Demidchik, E.; Drozd, V.; Demidchik, Y. Twenty-five years after Chernobyl: Outcome of radioiodine treatment in children and adolescents with very high-risk radiation-induced differentiated thyroid carcinoma. *J. Clin. Endocrinol. Metab.* **2013**, *98*, 3039–3048. [CrossRef]
65. Tang, J.; Kong, D.; Cui, Q.; Wang, K.; Zhang, D.; Liao, X.; Gong, Y.; Wu, G. The role of radioactive iodine therapy in papillary thyroid cancer: An observational study based on SEER. *OncoTargets Ther.* **2018**, *11*, 3551–3560. [CrossRef] [PubMed]
66. Giovanella, L.; Deandreis, D.; Vrachimis, A.; Campenni, A.; Ovcaricek, P.P. Molecular Imaging and Theragnostics of Thyroid Cancers. *Cancers* **2022**, *14*, 1272. [CrossRef] [PubMed]
67. Shen, H.; Zhu, R.; Liu, Y.; Hong, Y.; Ge, J.; Xuan, J.; Niu, W.; Yu, X.; Qin, J.-J.; Li, Q. Radioiodine-refractory differentiated thyroid cancer: Molecular mechanisms and therapeutic strategies for radioiodine resistance. *Drug Resist. Updates Rev. Comment. Antimicrob. Anticancer. Chemother.* **2024**, *72*, 101013. [CrossRef] [PubMed]
68. Avram, A.M.; Dewaraja, Y.K. Thyroid Cancer Radiotheragnostics: The case for activity adjusted ^{131}I therapy. *Clin. Transl. Imaging* **2018**, *6*, 335–346. [CrossRef]
69. Chen, M.-K.; Yasrebi, M.; Samii, J.; Staib, L.H.; Doddamane, I.; Cheng, D.W. The utility of I-123 pretherapy scan in I-131 radioiodine therapy for thyroid cancer. *Thyroid Off. J. Am. Thyroid Assoc.* **2012**, *22*, 304–309. [CrossRef]

70. Gulec, S.A.; Kuker, R.A.; Goryawala, M.; Fernandez, C.; Perez, R.; Khan-Ghany, A.; Apaza, A.; Harja, E.; Harrell, M. ^{124}I PET/CT in Patients with Differentiated Thyroid Cancer: Clinical and Quantitative Image Analysis. *Thyroid Off. J. Am. Thyroid Assoc.* **2016**, *26*, 441–448. [CrossRef]
71. Santhanam, P.; Taieb, D.; Solnes, L.; Marashdeh, W.; Ladenson, P.W. Utility of I-124 PET/CT in identifying radioiodine avid lesions in differentiated thyroid cancer: A systematic review and meta-analysis. *Clin. Endocrinol.* **2017**, *86*, 645–651. [CrossRef]
72. Schneider, D.F.; Ojomo, K.A.; Chen, H.; Sippel, R.S. Remnant uptake as a postoperative oncologic quality indicator. *Thyroid Off. J. Am. Thyroid Assoc.* **2013**, *23*, 1269–1276. [CrossRef]
73. Adam, M.A.; Thomas, S.; Youngwirth, L.; Hyslop, T.; Reed, S.D.; Scheri, R.P.; Roman, S.A.; Sosa, J.A. Is There a Minimum Number of Thyroidectomies a Surgeon Should Perform to Optimize Patient Outcomes? *Ann. Surg.* **2017**, *265*, 402–407. [CrossRef]
74. Krajewska, J.; Chmielik, E.; Jarząb, B. Dynamic risk stratification in the follow-up of thyroid cancer: What is still to be discovered in 2017? *Endocr.-Relat. Cancer* **2017**, *24*, R387–R402. [CrossRef]
75. Cohen, O.; Blank, A.; Meiersdorf, S.; Hod, K.; Gabay, S.; Guindy, M.; Khafif, A. Impact of high-quality ultrasound following community ultrasound on surgical planning and active surveillance in patients with thyroid cancer. *Clin. Endocrinol.* **2021**, *94*, 990–997. [CrossRef] [PubMed]
76. Thyrogen Prescribing Information. Available online: https://www.accessdata.fda.gov/drugsatfda_docs/label/2014/020898s054 lbl.pdf (accessed on 21 April 2022).
77. Pacini, F.; Ladenson, P.W.; Schlumberger, M.; Driedger, A.; Luster, M.; Kloos, R.T.; Sherman, S.; Haugen, B.; Corone, C.; Molinaro, E.; et al. Radioiodine ablation of thyroid remnants after preparation with recombinant human thyrotropin in differentiated thyroid carcinoma: Results of an international, randomized, controlled study. *J. Clin. Endocrinol. Metab.* **2006**, *91*, 926–932. [CrossRef] [PubMed]
78. Singer, M.C.; Marchal, F.; Angelos, P.; Bernet, V.; Boucai, L.; Buchholzer, S.; Burkey, B.; Eisele, D.; Erkul, E.; Faure, F.; et al. Salivary and lacrimal dysfunction after radioactive iodine for differentiated thyroid cancer: American Head and Neck Society Endocrine Surgery Section and Salivary Gland Section joint multidisciplinary clinical consensus statement of otolaryngology, ophthalmology, nuclear medicine and endocrinology. *Head Neck* **2020**, *42*, 3446–3459. [CrossRef]
79. Diessl, S.; Holzberger, B.; Mäder, U.; Grelle, I.; Smit, J.W.A.; Buck, A.K.; Reiners, C.; Verburg, F.A. Impact of moderate vs stringent TSH suppression on survival in advanced differentiated thyroid carcinoma. *Clin. Endocrinol.* **2012**, *76*, 586–592. [CrossRef]
80. Brose, M.S.; Smit, J.; Capdevila, J.; Elisei, R.; Nutting, C.; Pitoia, F.; Robinson, B.; Schlumberger, M.; Shong, Y.K.; Takami, H. Regional approaches to the management of patients with advanced, radioactive iodine-refractory differentiated thyroid carcinoma. *Expert Rev. Anticancer Ther.* **2012**, *12*, 1137–1147. [CrossRef]
81. Schlumberger, M.; Brose, M.; Elisei, R.; Leboulleux, S.; Luster, M.; Pitoia, F.; Pacini, F. Definition and management of radioactive iodine-refractory differentiated thyroid cancer. *Lancet Diabetes Endocrinol.* **2014**, *2*, 356–358. [CrossRef]
82. Sacks, W.; Braunstein, G.D. Evolving approaches in managing radioactive iodine-refractory differentiated thyroid cancer. *Endocr. Pract. Off. J. Am. Coll. Endocrinol. Am. Assoc. Clin. Endocrinol.* **2014**, *20*, 263–275. [CrossRef]
83. Kiyota, N.; Robinson, B.; Shah, M.; Hoff, A.O.; Taylor, M.H.; Li, D.; Dutcus, C.E.; Lee, E.K.; Kim, S.-B.; Tahara, M. Defining Radioiodine-Refractory Differentiated Thyroid Cancer: Efficacy and Safety of Lenvatinib by Radioiodine-Refractory Criteria in the SELECT Trial. *Thyroid Off. J. Am. Thyroid Assoc.* **2017**, *27*, 1135–1141. [CrossRef]
84. Chung, J.H. Low iodine diet for preparation for radioactive iodine therapy in differentiated thyroid carcinoma in Korea. *Endocrinol. Metab.* **2013**, *28*, 157–163. [CrossRef]
85. Maxon, H.R.; Thomas, S.R.; Boehringer, A.; Drilling, J.; Sperling, M.I.; Sparks, J.C.; Chen, I.W. Low iodine diet in I-131 ablation of thyroid remnants. *Clin. Nucl. Med.* **1983**, *8*, 123–126. [CrossRef]
86. Park, J.T., 2nd; Hennessey, J.V. Two-week low iodine diet is necessary for adequate outpatient preparation for radioiodine rhTSH scanning in patients taking levothyroxine. *Thyroid Off. J. Am. Thyroid Assoc.* **2004**, *14*, 57–63. [CrossRef] [PubMed]
87. Tomoda, C.; Uruno, T.; Takamura, Y.; Ito, Y.; Miya, A.; Kobayashi, K.; Matsuzuka, F.; Amino, N.; Kuma, K.; Miyauchi, A. Reevaluation of stringent low iodine diet in outpatient preparation for radioiodine examination and therapy. *Endocr. J.* **2005**, *52*, 237–240. [CrossRef] [PubMed]
88. Barbaro, D.; Verburg, F.A.; Luster, M.; Reiners, C.; Rubello, D. ALARA in rhTSH-stimulated post-surgical thyroid remnant ablation: What is the lowest reasonably achievable activity? *Eur. J. Nucl. Med. Mol. Imaging* **2010**, *37*, 1251–1254. [CrossRef]
89. Sohn, S.Y.; Choi, J.Y.; Jang, H.W.; Kim, H.J.; Jin, S.M.; Kim, S.W.; Suh, S.; Hur, K.Y.; Kim, J.H.; Chung, J.H.; et al. Association between excessive urinary iodine excretion and failure of radioactive iodine thyroid ablation in patients with papillary thyroid cancer. *Thyroid Off. J. Am. Thyroid Assoc.* **2013**, *23*, 741–747. [CrossRef]
90. Bartel, T.B.; Magerefteh, S.; Avram, A.M.; Balon, H.R.; De Blanche, L.E.; Dadparvar, S.; Johnston, M.; Moreau, S. SNMMI Procedure Standard for Scintigraphy for Differentiated Thyroid Cancer. *J. Nucl. Med. Technol.* **2020**, *48*, 202–209. [CrossRef]
91. Schlumberger, M.; Catargi, B.; Borget, I.; Deandreis, D.; Zerdoud, S.; Bridji, B.; Bardet, S.; Leenhardt, L.; Bastie, D.; Schvartz, C.; et al. Strategies of radioiodine ablation in patients with low-risk thyroid cancer. *N. Engl. J. Med.* **2012**, *366*, 1663–1673. [CrossRef]
92. Mallick, U.; Harmer, C.; Yap, B.; Wadsley, J.; Clarke, S.; Moss, L.; Nicol, A.; Clark, P.M.; Farnell, K.; McCready, R.; et al. Ablation with low-dose radioiodine and thyrotropin alfa in thyroid cancer. *N. Engl. J. Med.* **2012**, *366*, 1674–1685. [CrossRef]

93. Elisei, R.; Schlumberger, M.; Driedger, A.; Reiners, C.; Kloos, R.T.; Sherman, S.I.; Haugen, B.; Corone, C.; Molinaro, E.; Grasso, L.; et al. Follow-up of low-risk differentiated thyroid cancer patients who underwent radioiodine ablation of postsurgical thyroid remnants after either recombinant human thyrotropin or thyroid hormone withdrawal. *J. Clin. Endocrinol. Metab.* **2009**, *94*, 4171–4179. [CrossRef]
94. Schroeder, P.R.; Haugen, B.R.; Pacini, F.; Reiners, C.; Schlumberger, M.; Sherman, S.I.; Cooper, D.S.; Schuff, K.G.; Braverman, L.E.; Skarulis, M.C.; et al. A comparison of short-term changes in health-related quality of life in thyroid carcinoma patients undergoing diagnostic evaluation with recombinant human thyrotropin compared with thyroid hormone withdrawal. *J. Clin. Endocrinol. Metab.* **2006**, *91*, 878–884. [CrossRef]
95. Dueren, C.; Dietlein, M.; Luster, M.; Plenzig, F.; Steinke, R.; Grimm, J.; Groth, P.; Eichhorn, W.; Reiners, C. The use of thyrogen in the treatment of differentiated thyroid carcinoma: An intraindividual comparison of clinical effects and implications of daily life. *Exp. Clin. Endocrinol. Diabetes Off. J. Ger. Soc. Endocrinol. Ger. Diabetes Assoc.* **2010**, *118*, 513–519. [CrossRef]
96. Tagay, S.; Herpertz, S.; Langkafel, M.; Erim, Y.; Bockisch, A.; Senf, W.; Görges, R. Health-related Quality of Life, depression and anxiety in thyroid cancer patients. *Qual. Life Res. Int. J. Qual. Life Asp. Treat. Care Rehabil.* **2006**, *15*, 695–703. [CrossRef] [PubMed]
97. Ovčariček, P.P.; Kreissl, M.C.; Campenni, A.; de Keizer, B.; Tuncel, M.; Vrachimis, A.; Deandreis, D.; Giovanella, L. SNMMI/EANM practice guideline vs. ETA Consensus Statement: Differences and similarities in approaching differentiated thyroid cancer management-the EANM perspective. *Eur. J. Nucl. Med. Mol. Imaging* **2022**, *49*, 3959–3963. [CrossRef] [PubMed]
98. Zanotti-Fregonara, P.; Hindié, E. On the effectiveness of recombinant human TSH as a stimulating agent for 131I treatment of metastatic differentiated thyroid cancer. *Eur. J. Nucl. Med. Mol. Imaging* **2010**, *37*, 2264–2266. [CrossRef] [PubMed]
99. Plyku, D.; Hobbs, R.F.; Huang, K.; Atkins, F.; Garcia, C.; Sgouros, G.; Van Nostrand, D. Recombinant Human Thyroid-Stimulating Hormone Versus Thyroid Hormone Withdrawal in ^{124}I PET/CT-Based Dosimetry for ^{131}I Therapy of Metastatic Differentiated Thyroid Cancer. *J. Nucl. Med. Off. Publ. Soc. Nucl. Med.* **2017**, *58*, 1146–1154. [CrossRef]
100. Botella-Carretero, J.I.; Galán, J.M.; Caballero, C.; Sancho, J.; Escobar-Morreale, H.F. Quality of life and psychometric functionality in patients with differentiated thyroid carcinoma. *Endocr.-Relat. Cancer* **2003**, *10*, 601–610. [CrossRef]
101. Tagay, S.; Herpertz, S.; Langkafel, M.; Erim, Y.; Freudenberg, L.; Schöpper, N.; Bockisch, A.; Senf, W.; Görges, R. Health-related quality of life, anxiety and depression in thyroid cancer patients under short-term hypothyroidism and TSH-suppressive levothyroxine treatment. *Eur. J. Endocrinol.* **2005**, *153*, 755–763. [CrossRef]
102. Taïeb, D.; Sebag, F.; Cherenko, M.; Baumstarck-Barrau, K.; Fortanier, C.; Farman-Ara, B.; De Micco, C.; Vaillant, J.; Thomas, S.; Conte-Devolx, B.; et al. Quality of life changes and clinical outcomes in thyroid cancer patients undergoing radioiodine remnant ablation (RRA) with recombinant human TSH (rhTSH): A randomized controlled study. *Clin. Endocrinol.* **2009**, *71*, 115–123. [CrossRef]
103. Badihian, S.; Jalalpour, P.; Mirdamadi, M.; Moslehi, M. Quality of Life, Anxiety and Depression in Patients with Differentiated Thyroid Cancer under Short Term Hypothyroidism Induced by Levothyroxine Withdrawal. Kvalita života, úzkost a deprese u pacientů s diferencovaným karcinomem štítné žlázy během krátkodobé hypotyreózy indukované vysazením levothyroxinu. *Klin. Onkol. Cas. Ceske A Slov. Onkol. Spol.* **2016**, *29*, 439–444.
104. Smith, C.D.; Grondin, R.; LeMaster, W.; Martin, B.; Gold, B.T.; Ain, K.B. Reversible cognitive, motor, and driving impairments in severe hypothyroidism. *Thyroid Off. J. Am. Thyroid Assoc.* **2015**, *25*, 28–36. [CrossRef]
105. Wu, S.-Q.; Feng, F.; Zou, R.-J.; Fu, H.-L.; Sun, J.-W.; Jia, X.-Z.; Yin, Y.-F.; Wang, H. Abnormal Brain Glucose Metabolism in Papillary Thyroid Cancer Patients 4 Weeks After Withdrawal of Levothyroxine: A Cross-Sectional Study Using ^{18}F-FDG PET/CT. *Front. Endocrinol.* **2021**, *12*, 595933. [CrossRef]
106. Duntas, L.H.; Biondi, B. Short-term hypothyroidism after Levothyroxine-withdrawal in patients with differentiated thyroid cancer: Clinical and quality of life consequences. *Eur. J. Endocrinol.* **2007**, *156*, 13–19. [CrossRef] [PubMed]
107. Münte, T.F.; Lill, C.; Ötting, G.; Brabant, G. Cognitive changes in short-term hypothyroidism assessed with event-related brain potentials. *Psychoneuroendocrinology* **2004**, *29*, 1109–1118. [CrossRef] [PubMed]
108. Pötzi, C.; Moameni, A.; Karanikas, G.; Preitfellner, J.; Becherer, A.; Pirich, C.; Dudczak, R. Comparison of iodine uptake in tumour and nontumour tissue under thyroid hormone deprivation and with recombinant human thyrotropin in thyroid cancer patients. *Clin. Endocrinol.* **2006**, *65*, 519–523. [CrossRef] [PubMed]
109. Freudenberg, L.S.; Jentzen, W.; Petrich, T.; Frömke, C.; Marlowe, R.J.; Heusner, T.; Brandau, W.; Knapp, W.H.; Bockisch, A. Lesion dose in differentiated thyroid carcinoma metastases after rhTSH or thyroid hormone withdrawal: 124I PET/CT dosimetric comparisons. *Eur. J. Nucl. Med. Mol. Imaging* **2010**, *37*, 2267–2276. [CrossRef] [PubMed]
110. Gomes-Lima, C.J.; Chittimoju, S.; Wehbeh, L.; Dia, S.; Pagadala, P.; Al-Jundi, M.; Jhawar, S.; Tefera, E.; Mete, M.; Klubo-Gwiezdzinska, J.; et al. Metastatic Differentiated Thyroid Cancer Survival Is Unaffected by Mode of Preparation for ^{131}I Administration. *J. Endocr. Soc.* **2022**, *6*, bvac032. [CrossRef]
111. Giovanella, L.; Garo, M.L.; Campenní, A.; Ovčariček, P.P.; Görges, R. Thyroid Hormone Withdrawal versus Recombinant Human TSH as Preparation for I-131 Therapy in Patients with Metastatic Thyroid Cancer: A Systematic Review and Meta-Analysis. *Cancers* **2023**, *15*, 2510. [CrossRef]

Journal of
Clinical Medicine

MDPI

Review

Redifferentiation Therapies in Thyroid Oncology: Molecular and Clinical Aspects

Petra Petranović Ovčariček [1,2,*], Murat Tuncel [3], Atena Aghaee [4], Alfredo Campennì [5] and Luca Giovanella [6,7]

1 Department of Oncology and Nuclear Medicine, University Hospital Center Sestre Milosrdnice, 10 000 Zagreb, Croatia
2 School of Medicine, University of Zagreb, 10 000 Zagreb, Croatia
3 Department of Nuclear Medicine, Hacettepe University, 06230 Ankara, Turkey; murat.tuncel@hacettepe.edu.tr
4 Nuclear Medicine Research Center, Mashhad University of Medical Sciences, Mashhad 9177948564, Iran; aghaeeat@gmail.com
5 Unit of Nuclear Medicine, Department of Biomedical and Dental Sciences and Morpho-Functional Imaging, University of Messina, 98100 Messina, Italy; acampenni@unime.it
6 Department of Nuclear Medicine, Gruppo Ospedaliero Moncucco, 6900 Lugano, Switzerland; luca.giovanella.md@gmail.com
7 Clinic for Nuclear Medicine, University Hospital and University of Zurich, 8004 Zurich, Switzerland
* Correspondence: p.petranovic@gmail.com; Tel.: +385-958311107

Abstract: Since the 1940s, 131-I radioiodine therapy (RIT) has been the primary treatment for metastatic differentiated thyroid cancer (DTC). Approximately half of these patients respond favorably to RIT, achieving partial or complete remission or maintaining long-term stable disease, while the other half develop radioiodine-refractory DTC (RAI-R DTC). The main genomic alteration involved in radioiodine resistance is the activated mitogen-activated protein kinase (MAPK) pathway, which results in the loss of sodium iodide symporters (NIS). Therefore, RAI-R DTC requires alternative treatment options such as tyrosine kinase inhibitors. Over the past decade, several studies have investigated pharmacological induction or enhancement of NIS expression through "redifferentiation" therapies, mainly targeting the MAPK pathway. These novel approaches can restore radioiodine sensitivity in previously refractory patients and, therefore, potentially reestablish the efficacy of RIT. This review discusses various redifferentiation strategies, including their molecular mechanisms and clinical implications.

Keywords: differentiated thyroid cancer; radioactive iodine refractory; redifferentiation; tyrosine kinase inhibitors; BRAF; MEK; NTRK; RET

1. Introduction

The management of RAI-R DTC represents a clinical challenge, demanding a balance between timely intervention and avoiding premature cessation of potentially beneficial treatments. RAI-R DTC presents as clinically heterogeneous, ranging from stable to rapidly progressing disease. This variability underlines the importance of accurately identifying radioiodine refractoriness, a key to initiating appropriate therapy at the optimal time. Given the limited treatment options, it is crucial to avoid prematurely discontinuing 131-I therapy without proper justification.

The definition of RAI-R DTC has been debated within the medical community. The inhibition of NIS expression impairs the ability of DTC cells to accumulate radioiodine, making them refractory to this standard radioiodine treatment. The loss of radioiodine avidity is often associated with other features of dedifferentiation, such as changes in cell morphology and altered expression of thyroid-specific genes. Various criteria have been proposed to identify RAI-R disease. Ten years ago, Schlumberger et al. suggested discontinuing RIT when at least one DTC lesion becomes radioiodine-negative and progresses in size [1]. In the same year, Sacks and Braunstein proposed ceasing RIT in case of negative diagnostic radioiodine scintigraphy in the presence of known structural disease, [^{18}F]FDG-positive lesions, or cumulative 131-I activities > 22 GBq [2]. The first and third criteria are highly controversial and largely debated in the literature. Radioiodine uptake on diagnostic radioiodine scan is often considered inadequate since some lesions may show uptake only with high radioiodine activities applied, i.e., on a post-therapy radioiodine scan [3]. Furthermore, in addition to radioiodine uptake in DTC lesions, its response to previous radioiodine treatments and time to progression should be considered when another radioiodine therapy is indicated rather than just cumulative activity applied, especially during a long-term period. Progression is commonly considered if it develops during 6–12 months following RIT [3]. [^{18}F]FDG uptake is considered useful in classifying disease as RAI-R. According to a prospective study by Li et al., the FDG SUVmax cut-off of four predicts RAI-R disease with sensitivity, specificity, positive predictive value, and negative predictive value of 75.3%, 56.7%, 76.1%, and 54.8%, respectively [4] (Figure 1).

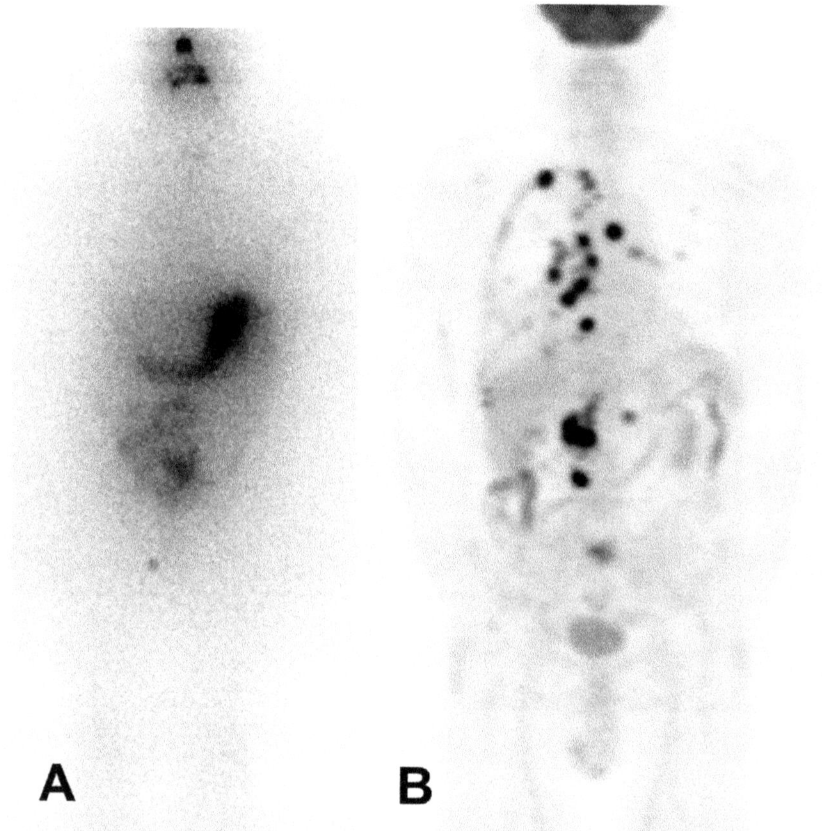

Figure 1. Patient with negative post-treatment whole-body radioiodine scintigraphy (**A**) and multiple [^{18}F]FDG-avid lesions (**B**). Legend: male, 67 years, affected by papillary thyroid carcinoma with increasing thyroglobulin level 2 years after thyroidectomy and radioiodine therapy [4.4 GBq]. (**A**) Post-treatment whole-body scintigraphy [7.4 GBq] showing no radioiodine-avid lesions. (**B**) [^{18}F]FDG PET/CT: multiple [^{18}F]FDG-avid lesions in the mediastinum and lung, with an associated [^{18}F]FDG-active pleural effusion (right side), and [^{18}F]FDG-avid lesions in the retroperitoneal region. A biopsy on an abdominal lesion confirmed metastasis of papillary thyroid carcinoma.

In 2015, the American Thyroid Association defined RAI-R disease as DTC lesions outside the thyroid bed not accumulating radioiodine on the first post-therapeutic whole-body scan (WBS), lesions that previously accumulated radioiodine but subsequently lost uptake, mixed radioiodine uptake (some lesions radioiodine-positive, others radioiodine-negative), and disease progression despite significant radioiodine uptake [5]. Aggressive variants of papillary thyroid carcinoma (e.g., tall cell, diffuse sclerosing, and hobnail) and mutations such as BRAF V600E and TERT promoter are also associated with increased tumor aggressiveness and RAI-R disease [6,7].

It is important to note that standardization in preparation for radioiodine scans, administered activity, and imaging protocols, including single-photon emission computed tomography/computed tomography (SPECT/CT), is crucial to avoid false-negative scans and ensure the continuation of potentially beneficial RIT [8].

In a joint statement, the American Thyroid Association, European Association of Nuclear Medicine, Society of Nuclear Medicine and Molecular Imaging, and European Thyroid Association acknowledged that the current criteria for defining RAI-R disease are inadequate and should not be considered absolute determinants for recommending or withholding RIT [9].

RIT is stopped once RAI-R disease is confirmed and alternative therapeutic options are considered. However, it is crucial to note that RAI-R disease can remain asymptomatic and indolent for years, not always requiring immediate therapy. These patients typically undergo thyroid-stimulating hormone (TSH) suppression and active surveillance that includes measurement of serum thyroglobulin (Tg) and Tg antibodies, conventional cross-sectional imaging (i.e., computed tomography, CT, magnetic resonance imaging, MRI, and [^{18}F]FDG positron emission tomography/computed tomography, PET/CT) every 3–6 months [5,6,10]. During surveillance, disease progression may show heterogeneous patterns, with some lesions progressing while others remain stable or have mixed metabolic features at molecular imaging (Figure 2).

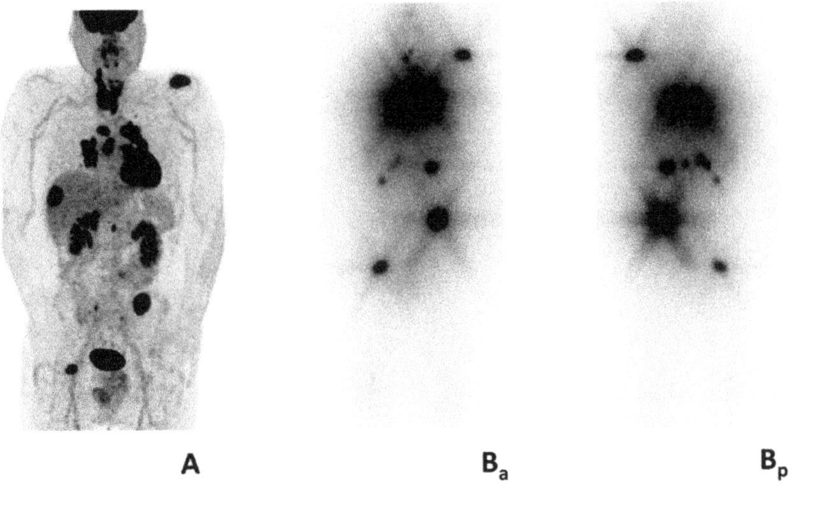

Figure 2. Mixed metabolic features in patient with metastatic follicular thyroid carcinoma. Multiple [^{18}F]FDG avid (**A**) and radioiodine avid lesions (**Ba**, anterior; **Bp** posterior). Legend: male, 48 years, referred to the emergency room for intense pain corresponding to the right scapula. Multiple bone, lymph node, lung, liver, and renal metastasis at computed tomography. Bone biopsy (right scapula): follicular thyroid carcinoma. (**A**) preoperative [^{18}F]FDG PET/CT: gross involvement of the thyroid gland and multiple intensely [^{18}F]FDG-avid metastasis. Post-treatment whole body scan (**Ba**, anterior; **Bp**, posterior): intense radioiodine-avidity of most [^{18}F]FDG-avid metastases.

At this point, localized treatments such as surgery, external beam radiation therapy, thermal ablation, or stereotactic radiosurgery may be employed. In cases of significant, multi-lesional progression that cannot be managed with localized therapies, systemic treatment with tyrosine kinase inhibitors is usually initiated [10].

Several studies have focused on strategies to reinduce or enhance radioiodine uptake in RAI-R disease, potentially reestablishing radioiodine sensitivity and enabling the de novo application of radioiodine in previously RAI-R DTC patients (Figure 3).

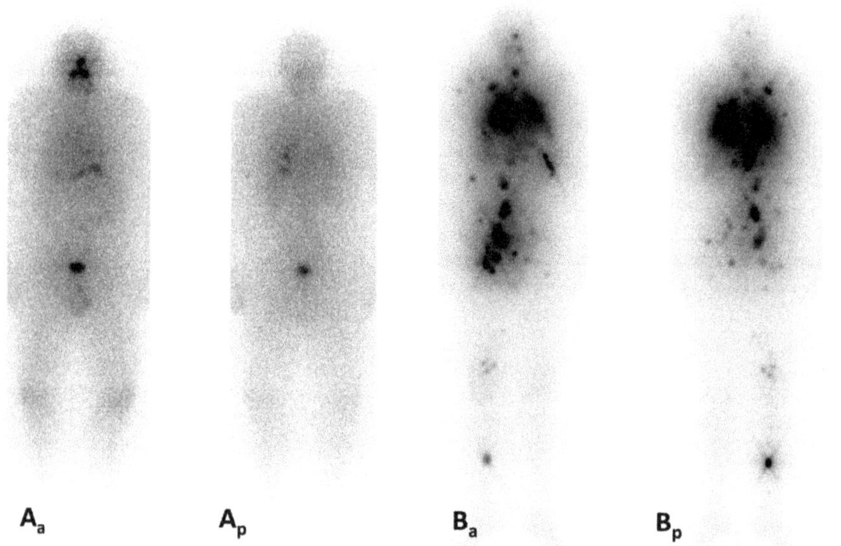

Figure 3. Redifferentiation of radioiodine-refractory disease. **Legend:** Male, 63 years, affected by a papillary thyroid carcinoma [pT3a(m), pN1b, pMx] developed multiple lung and bone metastasis without iodine-uptake whole-body scintigraphy 5 days after administration of 7.4 GBq I-131 (**Aa**, anterior; **Ap**, posterior). An off-label treatment with dabrafenib (150 mg/2xday) and trametinib (2 mg/day) was started after approval from the insurance company. Two months later, 7.4 GBq of I-131 were administered, and the post-treatment whole-body scintigraphy (**Ba**, anterior, **Bp**, posterior) showed multiple, intensely radioiodine-avid lesions at the level of the lymph nodes, lungs, and musculoskeletal metastases. Six months after treatment, a partial biochemical response was recorded with a thyroglobulin decrease from 2276 to 825 µg/L.

2. Redifferentiation Concepts

The concept of reinducing or enhancing NIS expression for RIT is in line with personalized therapeutic principles that offer a tailored approach to treating RAI-R DTC. Early attempts to redifferentiate metastatic RAI-R DTC using retinoic acid and PPAR-γ agonists, for example, demonstrated low efficacy. However, more recent advances in understanding the molecular pathways of RAI-R disease have enabled more focused research with promising results [7].

In vitro studies have shown a crucial relationship between the MAPK pathway and NIS expression [11,12]. The MAPK pathway, which is also known as the RAS-RAF-MEK-ERK pathway, is a signaling molecular cascade involved in cell proliferation and differentiation. Stimulation of the MAPK pathway via MEK and ERK activation is associated with reduced NIS expression at transcriptional and post-transcriptional levels. The activated MAPK pathway is commonly noted in DTC harboring mutations in BRAF, RAS, or RET genes, which links genetic alterations and radioiodine refractoriness. BRAF mutations are present in approximately 50% of papillary thyroid cancers (PTC) and are strongly associated with the inhibition of NIS expression and the development of RAI-R disease [13]. RET mutations, which are commonly detected in PTC, and RAS mutations, frequently noted in follicular thyroid cancer (FTC), are also involved in MAPK pathway activation [7]. Moreover, a positive correlation has been demonstrated between the degree of DTC dedifferentiation and its loss of NIS expression with the level of MAPK pathway activation. This relationship seems to be hierarchical, with BRAF V600E mutations associated with more enhanced effects than RAS or RET mutations [14]. This hierarchy may result from varying degrees of MAPK pathway activation linked with each mutation. The loss of NIS expression and radioiodine avidity often occurs continuously during a certain period rather than instantly, which correlates with the progressive activation of the MAPK pathway. It may explain why some DTCs retain partial radioiodine sensitivity while others become entirely refractory. Even within a single patient, different metastatic lesions may have varying degrees of MAPK pathway activation and, consequently, different levels of radioiodine avidity. Understanding this molecular basis of RAI-R DTC provides a solid basis to targeting the MAPK pathway as a potential strategy for redifferentiation [15].

Preclinical studies using animal models demonstrated that inhibiting activated intracellular signaling pathways could lead to the re-expression of NIS on the DTC cell membrane [16,17]. By reactivating the cellular mechanisms responsible for iodine uptake, redifferentiation therapy has the potential to reestablish the effectiveness of RIT in patients who have become unresponsive.

Recently, Aghaee and colleagues reported a case of a RAI-R patient with lung and bone metastases that restored RAI-avidity after treatment with receptor radioactive therapy (PRRT) with [^{177}Lu]Lu- DOTA-TATE [18].

The biological basis of this phenomenon is not known, but the possibility of sequential nuclear medical therapy introduces a fascinating perspective. Naturally, the phenomenon will have to be replicated, and currently, no clinical studies are available.

3. Clinical Studies

The first clinical trial conducted at Memorial Sloan Kettering Cancer Center, published in 2013, was a significant step forward in redifferentiation treatments [19]. This study demonstrated that targeted MEK inhibitor therapy could effectively reinduce 131-I uptake in previously RAI-R tumors. The trial enrolled 24 patients with RAI-R DTC, each presenting with at least one radioiodine-negative lesion on 124-I PET/CT scans and radiographically progressive disease within the previous 12 months. Participants received selumetinib, a MEK1/2 inhibitor, at 75 mg twice daily for four weeks. Following treatment, 20 patients underwent follow-up 124-I PET/CT scans after recombinant human TSH (rhTSH) administration. The study demonstrated that 60% of evaluated patients (12 out of 20) showed restored radioiodine uptake. Subsequent lesion-specific dosimetry identified eight patients who met the threshold for RIT, defined as a dose of $\geq$20 Gy with a 131-I administered activity $\leq$ 11.1 GBq. These patients received RIT, resulting in five partial responses (PR) and three cases of stable disease (SD) over a six-month follow-up period. Notably, all treated patients showed a reduction in DTC lesion size. The treatment was mainly well-tolerated, with rash, fatigue, and edema being the most common side effects. More severe adverse events were rare, with one case each of grade 3 pain and increased liver enzymes, and no grade 4 or 5 events reported. Interestingly, the study revealed a potential correlation between genetic mutations and treatment response. Patients with NRAS mutations demonstrated a higher response rate compared to those with BRAF mutations, i.e., all five patients with NRAS mutations showed restored radioiodine uptake and received RIT. On the other hand, only four out of nine patients with BRAF mutations restored radioiodine uptake, with just one reaching the dosimetry threshold for RIT. The remaining two treated patients had RET-rearrangements and wild-type PTC, respectively. This study provided the first prospective evidence that targeted therapy could restore radioiodine avidity in RAI-R DTC. It also underlined the importance of tumor genotype in predicting response to redifferentiation therapy, particularly the high response rate observed in NRAS-mutant tumors. The differential response between NRAS and BRAF mutant tumors was suggested to be due to insufficient blockade of the MAPK pathway with MEK inhibitors in BRAF-mutant tumors. This finding encouraged further investigation with specific BRAF inhibitors such as dabrafenib and vemurafenib. These therapies were subsequently evaluated as monotherapies or in combination with MEK inhibitors in additional clinical trials focused on BRAF-mutated RAI-R disease.

Rothenberg and colleagues published a study on the efficacy of BRAF inhibition in patients with BRAF V600E-mutant RAI-R DTC two years later [20]. This targeted approach addressed the previously observed findings related to BRAF-mutant tumors. The study enrolled ten patients, each receiving a four-week course of the BRAF inhibitor dabrafenib at a dose of 150 mg twice daily. Following this initial treatment period, patients underwent a 131-I WBS after rhTSH stimulation to assess changes in radioiodine uptake. Six out of ten patients exhibited new sites of radioiodine uptake on diagnostic 131-I WBS. For these responders, the dabrafenib therapy was extended for an additional two weeks, followed by a fixed empiric activity of 5.5 GBq of 131-I. Two patients demonstrated PR at the three-month follow-up, while four maintained SD. Importantly, the treatment regimen was generally well-tolerated. Most detected adverse events were mild to moderate (grade 1 or 2). However, one patient developed a grade 3 squamous cell carcinoma of the skin, a well-known side effect associated with BRAF inhibitors. This lesion was successfully managed through excision with clear margins, underlining the importance of careful patient monitoring during redifferentiation therapies.

The results of this study were encouraging, regarding the restored radioiodine uptake and clinical outcomes in BRAF-mutated RAI-R DTC. The findings suggested a potential advantage of BRAF inhibitors over MEK inhibitors in BRAF-mutated tumors.

Jaber et al. conducted a retrospective study of 13 patients with RAI-R thyroid cancer who were treated with either single-agent or combination MEK/BRAF inhibitors and underwent 131-I diagnostic WBS during treatment [21]. Among the study population, nine patients harbored BRAF V600E mutations, three had NRAS mutations, and one patient had wild-type thyroid cancer. The median duration of targeted therapy before diagnostic WBS was 14.4 months, ranging from 0.9 to 76.4 months. Initial evaluation revealed that eight patients demonstrated restored 131-I uptake and subsequently received a median activity of 7.4 GBq of 131-I. One additional patient was treated empirically despite no clear evidence of restored 131-I uptake. Of note, only three patients underwent dosimetric pre-therapeutic evaluation, while the remaining patients received empirically determined 131-I activities. Prior to 131-I treatment, eight patients had SD disease, and one patient showed progressive disease (PD). Following 131-I treatment, with a median follow-up of 14.3 months, three patients achieved PR while six maintained SD, including the empirically treated patient.

In another study at Memorial Sloan Kettering Cancer Center, Dunn and colleagues further evaluated the potential of BRAF inhibition in RAI-R DTC [22]. This research focused on vemurafenib, another BRAF inhibitor, as a redifferentiation therapy for patients with BRAF-mutated RAI-R DTC. The study enrolled 12 patients, administering vemurafenib (960 mg twice daily) for four weeks. Of the initial cohort, ten patients completed the whole treatment cycle. Following the vemurafenib regimen, patients underwent a 124-I PET/CT scan with rhTSH stimulation to assess changes in radioiodine uptake and perform lesional dosimetry. The criterion for subsequent RIT was at least one radioiodine-negative lesion $\geq$ 5 mm in diameter, achieving a target dose of $\geq$20 Gy with calculated administered 131-I activity of $\leq$11.1 GBq. After redifferentiation therapy, the 124-I PET/CT demonstrated new or increased radioiodine uptake in six out of ten patients. Four out of six patients met the dosimetry threshold criteria and underwent RIT. At the six-month follow-up, two patients achieved PR, while two maintained SD. In general, the treatment was well-tolerated, with common side effects including rash, fatigue, nausea, and arthralgia. Importantly, no grade 4 or 5 adverse effects were observed.

Interestingly, molecular studies conducted on tumor biopsies from three patients provided valuable findings into the mechanism of action. The data revealed an increased thyroid differentiation score, a lower mitotic index, and higher NIS mRNA levels. These molecular changes corroborated the clinical findings and suggested that vemurafenib promoted redifferentiation of the RAI-R cancer cells.

Weber et al. conducted another prospective study (ERRITI) investigating the efficacy of genotype-guided MAPK inhibition redifferentiation therapy in RAI-R DTC [23]. The study included twenty patients: six with BRAF-mutated tumors that received a combination of dabrafenib in a dose of 75 mg twice daily and trametinib 2 mg daily, while fourteen with BRAF wild-type tumors received trametinib alone (2 mg daily) for 21 days. Post-treatment, patients underwent 123-I SPECT/CT imaging. Redifferentiation was considered successful if a target-to-background ratio > 4, and a 2-fold higher uptake than mean liver uptake was detected in at least one tumor lesion. This criterion was met in seven patients (two BRAF-mutated, five BRAF wild-type), indicating similar redifferentiation rates regardless of BRAF mutation status. All responding patients received personalized, dosimetry-guided RIT, taking into account activity in the lungs, blood, and individual tumor lesions. Patients received a mean (range) activity of 300.0 (273.0–421.6) mCi of 131-I therapy. Any thyroglobulin decline was seen in 57% (4/7) of the patients. Peak standardized uptake value (SUVpeak) < 10 on [^{18}F] FDG PET was linked with successful redifferentiation ($p = 0.01$). One-year follow-up revealed RECIST 1.1 PR in one patient, SD in five, and PD in one case. The treatment was mainly well-tolerated, with most adverse events (38/40) graded 1 or 2. Common side effects included rash and diarrhea. More severe reactions were rare: one BRAF-mutated patient experienced grade 3 pyrexia, which resolved after a 2-day treatment interruption, and one BRAF wild-type patient developed a transient grade 4 skin rash three days post-therapy completion.

Leboulleux conducted a MERAIODE multicentric prospective phase II trial in patients with RAI-R DTC, with two independent cohorts, one for BRAF V600E and one for RAS mutated DTC. From one of these cohorts, Leboulleux et al. published a prospective phase II multicenter trial focusing on patients with BRAF-mutated RAI-R DTC [24]. The study included twenty-four patients who had experienced RECIST progression within 18 months and had lesions < 3 cm. The treatment protocol consisted of dabrafenib in a dose of 150 mg twice daily and trametinib 2 mg once daily for five weeks, followed by an empiric activity of 5.5 GBq RIT after rhTSH stimulation, regardless of diagnostic 131-I WBS results. Twenty-one patients were evaluated for treatment efficacy at six months. Post-therapeutic WBS showed uptake in twenty patients. The 6-month follow-up revealed PR in eight patients (38%), SD in eleven (52%), and PD in two (10%), with no complete responses (CR). Patients achieving PR at 6 or 12 months were eligible for a second course of targeted therapy. Of the eleven patients undergoing it, there was one CR, six PR, two SD, and one PD at the 6-month follow-up, with one patient not evaluable. The progression-free survival (PFS) rate was 82% at one year and 68% at two years. One patient died due to PD at two years. Most detected adverse events were mild to moderate, with 25% grade 1 and 42% grade 2. Six patients experienced nine grade 3 adverse events (infectious syndrome, psoas hematoma), and there was one grade 4 event (anicteric cholestasis). Common side effects included asthenia, nausea, lymphopenia, fever, diarrhea, fatigue, and skin-related issues. The higher response rates in this study compared to Weber's may be due to the longer duration of redifferentiation therapy, higher dabrafenib dosage, small tumor foci, and more limited tumor volume. In many patients, a decreased tumor size was already significant at one month of dabrafenib-trametinib treatment, and this clearly raises the question of whether benefits from the treatment are related to the dabrafenib-trametinib treatment or to the addition of 131-I to dabrafenib-trametinib. However, due to the long PFS, and because the 6-month response was independent of the 1-month tumor response, the treatment efficacy was believed to be not only due to dabrafenib-trametinib treatment during the 6 weeks but also to its association with 131-I. As this is a similar issue with other redifferentiation agents, a comparative randomized trial comparing kinase inhibition $\pm$ RIT would be the only way to answer this specific question.

In another patient cohort, Leboulleux et al. conducted another study focusing on metastatic RAI-R RAS-mutated DTC [25]. The study investigated the efficacy of trametinib treatment followed by 131-I administration after rhTSH stimulation. Eleven patients were initially enrolled, with ten evaluated six months after the first treatment course. The protocol consisted of daily 2 mg trametinib for seven weeks, with a fixed 131-I activity of 5.5 GBq administered on day 35 ($\pm$2 days), regardless of diagnostic 131-I WBS results. Six months after the initial treatment, there were two PR (20%), seven cases of SD (70%), and one PD. Patients achieving PR at 6 or 12 months were eligible for a second course of trametinib and 131-I therapy. Of the three patients who received this second course, one maintained PR for 18 months, while two experienced PD at 3- and 6-months post-treatment. The median progression-free survival was one year. Adverse events occurred in nine out of eleven patients (82%), predominantly grade 1 (36%) and grade 2 (27%). Two patients experienced grade 3 adverse events, with no grade 4 events reported. Treatment discontinuation was necessary in two cases due to grade 3 erythematous colitis and grade 2 decrease in left ventricular ejection fraction. The six-week trametinib therapy increased 131-I uptake in two-thirds of RAI-R RAS-mutated DTC patients. However, the treatment's efficacy was limited, with only a 20% response rate at six months. These results suggest that while the approach shows some promise in restoring radioiodine uptake, its overall effectiveness in managing this specific subtype of thyroid cancer is suboptimal.

Iravani et al. treated patients with tumors harboring an NRAS mutation with a MEK inhibitor (trametinib) and tumors with a BRAF V600E mutation with combined BRAF and MEK inhibition (dabrafenib and trametinib; or vemurafenib and cobimetinib) for four weeks. Six patients received redifferentiation therapy. Three patients had an NRAS mutation, two with FTC and one with a poorly differentiated thyroid carcinoma, and three patients had a BRAF V600E mutation and PTC. One NRAS and all BRAF V600E mutation cases demonstrated restoration of RAI uptake and proceeded to RAI therapy with a median follow-up of 16.6 months (range 13.5–42.3 months). The patient with an NRAS mutation and two of three patients with a BRAF V600E demonstrated partial imaging response beyond a three-month follow-up [26].

Burman et al. conducted a phase 2 trial evaluating trametinib's efficacy in RAI-R DTC patients with RAS mutations and wild-type RAS [27]. If the post-therapy 124-I PET/CT demonstrated increased radioiodine uptake, allowing a target dose of $\geq$20 Gy with a calculated 131-I activity of $\leq$11.1 GBq, patients received RIT according to whole body and blood dosimetry. In the RAS-mutant group of twenty-five patients, fifteen met the dosimetry threshold for RIT based on 124-I PET/CT imaging. Fourteen of these patients received RIT. The 6-month follow-up revealed PR in eight patients (57%), SD in three patients (21%), and PD in three patients (21%). The PFS rate at 6 months was 44% for the RAS-mutant group. The RAS wild-type group consisted of nine patients, including those with BRAF mutations, RET alterations, and one case of STK11 mutation. In this cohort, three out of four patients with BRAF mutations and one out of four patients with RET alterations met the dosimetry threshold for RIT. Treatment outcomes for the RAS wild-type group showed three cases of SD and one PR, with the PR observed in a patient with a BRAF-mutated tumor.

This study again demonstrates varying degrees of treatment efficacy across different genetic profiles in RAI-R DTC, with RAS-mutant patients showing a significant response to the trametinib-RIT combination therapy. Redifferentiation therapy has shown promising results beyond tumors with BRAF and RAS mutations, demonstrating potential efficacy in thyroid cancers with various other genetic alterations.

Groussin et al. reported a successful case of redifferentiation therapy using larotrectinib in a patient with RAI-R DTC characterized by an EML4–NTRK3 gene fusion [28]. However, similar to BRAF mutations, the co-occurrence of TERT mutations and NTRK fusions may also contribute to re-sensitization failure [29].

Similarly, encouraging results have been observed in patients with RET rearrangement RAI-R DTC. Specifically, two RET inhibitors, pralsetinib [30] and selpercatinib [31], have both been reported to re-sensitize RET rearrangement-positive tumors to RIT. Recently, Werner et al. used a successful combination of selpercatinib and radioiodine after pretherapeutic dose estimation in RET-altered RAI-R DTC. Upon disease progression, the patient received the selpercatinib. A diagnostic 131-I WBS was conducted after 15.5 months of RET inhibitor therapy, showing intense radiotracer accumulation in sites of disease. After RIT (9.4 GBq), previously negative lung nodules showed intense radiotracer accumulation on post-therapeutic scans, followed by a decrease in Tg levels and nodule size on CT. This individualized approach allowed the administration of substantially higher activities (achieving tumor doses of 197 Gy) [32].

Similar to BRAF inhibitors, as the RET inhibitors induce redifferentiation, I-131 uptake increases, and [^{18}F]FDG uptake decreases [30].

In two distinct cases, comprehensive genomic profiling revealed the presence of specific fusion oncogenes: TPR-NTRK1 and CCDC6-RET [31]. Considering these gene alterations, a combined approach using two targeted therapies (larotrectinib, an NTRK inhibitor, and selpercatinib, a RET inhibitor) was implemented, which resulted in decreased tumor size and reinduced RAI uptake.

Toro-Tobon et al., in a retrospective study, evaluated thirty-three patients with progressive metastatic RAIR-DTC who underwent redifferentiation therapy at Mayo Clinic between 2017–2022 [33]. Depending on genetic alterations, patients received MEK, RET, or ALK inhibitors alone or BRAF-MEK inhibitor combinations for four weeks, with high-activity 131-I therapy administered to those showing increased RAI avidity at week three. Radioiodine uptake was restored in 57.6% of patients. Among PTCs, 42.1% showed restoration, while all invasive encapsulated follicular variant PTCs and FTCs demonstrated restored uptake. Notably, all RAS mutant tumors responded to redifferentiation, compared to 38.9% of BRAF mutant cases. Both redifferentiated and non-redifferentiated groups showed similar clinical outcomes, with approximately 12% tumor shrinkage at three weeks. The redifferentiated group achieved an additional 20% tumor reduction at six months follow-up. No significant differences were observed in PFS or time to additional therapy between groups. Among observed adverse outcomes, anaplastic transformation occurred in 6.1% (2/33) of patients. Five patients (15.1%) died during follow-up, with all deaths occurring in patients who had undergone both redifferentiation and subsequent 131-I therapy. Redifferentiation therapy showed particular promise in RAS-driven follicular phenotypes, though further research is needed to evaluate survival outcomes and potential risks of anaplastic transformation following high-activity RIT.

Table 1 summarizes different redifferentiation studies and their protocols.

Table 1. Redifferentiation studies and their protocols.

Study	Type of the Study	Number of Patients	Redifferentiation Agent	Mechanism of Action	Protocol
Ho et al. [19]	Clinical trial	20	Selumetinib	MEK inhibitor	Selumetinib 75 mg p.o. bid for 4 weeks. If the 124-I PET scan indicated increased iodine uptake and delivered a projected absorbed dose of 2000 cGy or more to the lesion, then selumetinib continued to perform dosimetry and was subsequently discontinued 2 days after 131-I therapy with rhTSH stimulation.

Table 1. *Cont.*

Study	Type of the Study	Number of Patients	Redifferentiation Agent	Mechanism of Action	Protocol
Rothenberg et al. [20]	Clinical trial	10	Dabrafenib	BRAF inhibitor	Dabrafenib 150 mg p.o. q.d. for 25 days before the 131-I scan. If positive, dabrafenib was continued for 17 days, therapy with 150 mCi of 131-I was applied, and dabrafenib was continued for five more days.
Jaber et al. [21]	Retrospective	13	Selective trametinib, dabrafenib, and/or vemurafenib	MEK inhibitor, BRAF inhibitor	Patients with BRAF mutation were treated with BRAF inhibitors (7 with dabrafenib, 1 with vemurafenib, and 1 with a combination of dabrafenib/trametinib). Three patients with RAS mutation were treated with MEK inhibitors (two with trametinib and one with an investigational MEK inhibitor). The patient without identified somatic mutations was treated with trametinib
Dunn et al. [22]	Clinical trial	10	Vemurafenib	BRAF inhibitor	124-I PET scan performed before and after Vemurafenib 960 mg p.o. bid for approximately 4 weeks. Those with increased 131-I concentration exceeding a predefined lesional dosimetry threshold were treated with I-131. Vemurafenib was discontinued 2 days after 131-I therapy.
Weber et al. [23]	Prospective study	20	Dabrafenib and Trametinib	BRAF inhibitor and MEK inhibitor	Trametinib 2 mg daily in BRAF-WT for 21 $\pm$ 3 days. Trametinib 2 mg trametinib daily + dabrafenib 75 mg twice daily in BRAF-MUT for 21 $\pm$ 3 days. Patients in whom the posttreatment 123-I SPECT/CT demonstrated a regional target/background ratio of more than 4 and a 2-fold higher iodine uptake than the mean uptake in liver parenchyma (in at least one tumor lesion) by visual assessment were considered responders, and 131-I therapy was performed
Leboulleux et al. [24]	Clinical trial	21	Dabrafenib trametinib	BRAF inhibitor and MEK inhibitor	Dabrafenib 150 mg p.o. bid and trametinib 2 mg po q.d. for 42 days. On day 28, a radioiodine scan was performed. After 35 days, a therapy of 131-I was administered.
Leboulleux et al. [25]	Clinical trial	10	Trametinib	MEK inhibitor	Trametinib 2 mg po q.d. for 42 days. On day 28, a radioiodine scan was performed. After 35 days, a therapy of 131-I was administered.
Iravani et al. [26]	Retrospective	6	Dabrafenib and Trametinib	BRAF inhibitor and MEK inhibitor	For NRAS: trametinib 2 mg p.o. q.d. 4 weeks For BRAF V600E: combination of dabrafenib 150 mg p.o. q.d. and trametinib 2 mg p.o. q.d. 4 weeks.

Table 1. *Cont.*

Study	Type of the Study	Number of Patients	Redifferentiation Agent	Mechanism of Action	Protocol
Groussin et al. [28]	Case report	1	Larotrectinib	Tropomyosin receptor kinase (TRK) inhibitor	Larotrectinib 100 mg p.o. bid (6 months).
Lee et al. [31]	Two cases	2	Larotrectinib; Selpercatinib	Tropomyosin receptor kinase (TRK) inhibitor; RET inhibitor	Larotrectinib 100 mg p.o. bid; Selpercatinib 80 mg bid.
Werner et al. [32]	Case report	1	Selpercatinib	RET inhibitor	Selpercatinib 160 mg p.o. bid for 3 weeks
Toro-Tobon et al. [33]	Retrospective	33	Trametinib, Selpercatinib, Pralsetinib, Alectinib, Dabrafenib + Trametinib	MEK, RET, or ALK inhibitors alone, or combination BRAF-MEK inhibitors	Redifferentiation therapy for 4 weeks. At the end of week 3, all patients underwent rhTSH-stimulated 123-I WBS. At week 4, those who redifferentiated (any uptake of at least one lesion based on a qualitative assessment) received high-activity 131I therapy.

Legend: PET, positron emission tomography; BRAF-WT, BRAF-wild type; BRAF-MUT, BRAF-mutated; TSH, thyroid stimulating hormone; p.o., per os; q.d. quaque die; bid, *bis in die*.

An example of the clinical flowchart in redifferentiation therapies is shown in Figure 4.

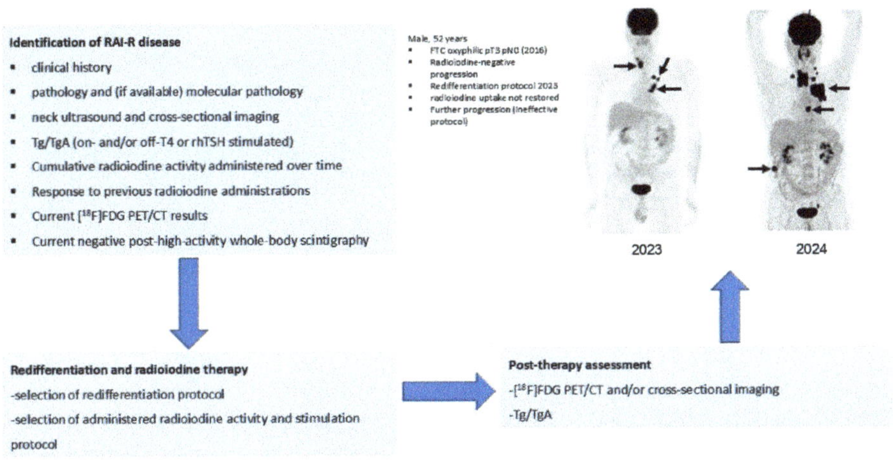

Figure 4. Clinical flowchart in redifferentiation therapies. **Legend**: FTC, follicular thyroid carcinoma; Tg, thyroglobulin; TgA, thyroglobulin antibodies; T4, thyroxine, rhTSH, recombinant human thyroid-stimulating hormone; PET/CT, positron-emission tomography.

4. Second-Line TKI-Related Adverse Effects

The side effects related to the use of first-line TKI drugs are well known since they are widely reported in the literature, also highlighting their different prevalence according to the use of lenvatinib or sorafenib [34,35].

However, the use of second-line TKI drugs, either BRAF or MEK inhibitors or both (e.g., dabrafenib or trametinib), is also associated with numerous adverse effects having a negative impact on patients' quality of life, necessitating dosage reductions in nearly two-thirds of patients or treatment withdrawal in up to 20% of patients, while therapy-related death was reported in 1.5–2% [26].

Recently, some authors reported on the most common treatment-related adverse effects due to the use of a BRAF inhibitor alone or in combination with a MEK inhibitor, highlighting their different prevalence [36].

Table 2 summarizes the most common adverse effects due to the use of second-line TKI agents either as single-line therapy (i.e., using BRAF or MEK inhibitors) or in combination (i.e., using BRAF and MEK inhibitors)

Table 2. Tyrosine kinase inhibitors' adverse effects.

Adverse Event	*Dabrafenib Alone (n = 26) Any Grade (%)* *	*Dabrafenib + Trametinib (n = 27) Any Grade (%)* *	*Selumetinib + RAI (n = 154) Any Grade (%)* **	*Dabrafenib + Trametinib (n = 24) Any Grade (%)* ***
Skin/subcutaneous disorders	17 (65)	9 (33)	69 (45)	-
Fever	13 (50)	16 (59)	-	5 (21)
Hyperglycemia	12 (46)	5 (19)	-	-
Anemia	11 (42)	8 (30)	-	-
Palmar-plantar erythrodysesthesia syndrome	11 (42)	6 (22)	-	-
Nausea	11 (42)	14 (52)	44 (29)	10 (42)
Alopecia	11 (42)	0 (0)	-	-
Chills	11 (42)	14 (52)	-	-
Fatigue	10 (38)	14 (52)	44 (29)	2 (8)
Hypophosphatemia	9 (35)	11 (41)	-	-
Vomiting	7 (27)	6 (22)	-	2 (8)
Rash maculo-papular	7 (27)	4 (15)	19 (12)	5 (21)
Weight loss	7 (27)	0 (0)	-	-
Anorexia	6 (23)	9 (33)	-	3 (13)
Pruritus	6 (23)	3 (11)	21 (14)	-
Arthralgia	6 (23)	0 (0)	-	1 (4)
Myalgia	5 (19)	6 (22)	-	-
Lymphocyte count decreased	5 (19)	0 (0)	-	3 (13)
Headache	5 (19)	0 (0)	8 (5)	2 (8)
Diarrhea	4 (15)	7 (26)	68 (44)	5 (21)
Edema limbs	3 (12)	5 (19)	30 (19)	-
Aspartate aminotransferase increased	0 (0)	10 (37)	-	1 (4)
Alanine aminotransferase increased	0 (0)	8 (30)	-	1 (4)
Alkaline phosphatase increased	0 (0)	5 (19)	-	-
Generalized muscle weakness	0 (0)	5 (19)	-	10 (42)
Blood creatine phosphokinase increased	-	-	31 (20)	-
Hypertension	-	-	20 (13)	3 (13)
Stomatitis	-	-	17 (11)	2 (8)
Vision blurred	-	-	16 (10)	-
Constipation	-	-	-	2 (8)
Cough	-	-	-	1 (4)
Abdominal pain	-	-	-	1 (4)
Bronchitis	-	-	-	0 (0)

Table 2. *Cont.*

Adverse Event	*Dabrafenib Alone (n = 26) Any Grade (%)* *	*Dabrafenib + Trametinib (n = 27) Any Grade (%)* *	*Selumetinib + RAI (n = 154) Any Grade (%)* **	*Dabrafenib + Trametinib (n = 24) Any Grade (%)* ***
Hyposialia	-	-	-	2 (8)
Leukopenia	-	-	-	1 (4)
Neutropenia	-	-	-	1 (4)
Thrombopenia	-	-	-	0
Vertigo	-	-	-	1 (4)
Urinary infection	-	-	-	0

Legend: RIT, radioiodine therapy; * [36]; ** [37]; *** [24].

Finally, it is important to consider in the clinical management of RAI-R disease that some patients can develop TKI resistance, thus worsening their outcome [26].

Accordingly, the ability of these agents to restore or enhance radioiodine uptake in such patients, offering the possibility of a de novo application of radioiodine therapy, should always be taken into account as soon as possible, also to reduce the risk of adverse effects (especially if severe) that could cause discontinuation (temporarily or permanently) of their use.

5. Current Paradigms and Future Perspectives

Current evidence suggests that specific targeted therapies have the potential to modulate the iodine-handling mechanisms of thyroid cancer cells, effectively restoring or enhancing their ability to accumulate 131-I.

These targeted therapies, based on gene profiling, demonstrate efficacy in two main scenarios [38]:

1. *Re-establishing 131-I uptake*: Targeted therapies can re-induce the expression of radioiodine uptake and retention. This "redifferentiation" effect could potentially convert RAI-R tumors back to a radioiodine-treatable state.
2. *Enhancing existing uptake*: These agents may increase the uptake of 131-I in DTC lesions that still demonstrate some degree of iodine accumulation. Optimizing the cellular pathways responsible for iodine processing could significantly increase the amount of radioiodine concentrated within tumor tissues.

The implications of these effects on treatment outcomes are multifactorial:

1. *Increased tumor radiation absorbed dose*: Enhanced 131-I uptake translates to a higher absorbed radiation dose per unit of administered 131-I activity (Gy/GBq or rad/mCi.
2. *Improved treatment efficacy*: The increased radiation dose to tumor tissues may lead to better clinical outcomes, including partial tumor regression or stabilization of disease.
3. *Potential for dose reduction*: The enhanced uptake efficiency might allow the same therapeutic effect with a lower administered activity of 131-I. This strategy may be especially valuable for patients at higher risk of radioiodine-associated side effects.
4. *Minimization of side effects*: By potentially reducing the total activity of 131-I needed for effective treatment, these agents may help reduce the risk of adverse effects associated with high 131-I activity. These side effects can include salivary gland dysfunction, bone marrow suppression, and a small but non-zero risk of secondary malignancies.
5. *Expanded treatment options*: The redifferentiation therapies could reopen new treatment options for patients previously deemed unsuitable for further 131-I therapy.

These preliminary findings of redifferentiation therapy effectiveness are encouraging. However, further studies are essential to:

1. *Validate uptake restoration and enhancement in different clinical and genomic scenarios*: Larger, well-designed studies are needed to confirm the initial observations on the

ability of these agents to modulate radioiodine uptake in diverse patient populations and different tumor types based on gene profiling.

2. *Evaluate long-term safety*: As with any new therapeutic approach, it is important to thoroughly investigate these agents' long-term safety profile, particularly considering their effects on iodine-concentrating organs.
3. *Optimize treatment protocols*: Research should focus on determining the ideal timing, imaging, dosing, and duration of the therapy in relation to 131-I administration to maximize their beneficial effects while minimizing any potential risks.
4. *Identify predictive biomarkers*: Developing reliable methods to predict which patients are most likely to benefit from redifferentiation therapies could help personalize treatment approaches and avoid unnecessary interventions in non-responders.
5. Compare redifferentiation vs. tyrosine kinase inhibitors.
6. Criteria of therapeutic outcomes for consideration of redifferentiation and 131-I re-treatment (Tg response, RECIST response, etc.).
7. Cost-effectiveness.

As this field progresses, it holds the potential to significantly reshape the treatment options in RAI-R DTC.

In addition to these specific redifferentiation therapies, several SPECT and PET radiopharmaceuticals offer promising fields for research. Tracers targeting prostate-specific membrane antigens, somatostatin receptors, or fibroblast activation proteins can help determine different molecular features of RAI-R disease. Novel theranostic strategies that extend beyond traditional radioiodine-guided therapies may potentially broaden the therapeutic options for patients with RAI-R thyroid cancer [39]. The application of these diverse radiopharmaceuticals enables a more comprehensive molecular profiling of RAI-R thyroid cancer. This multi-factorial approach can reveal:

1. Heterogeneity within and between primary and metastatic tumors
2. Identify previously unrecognized targets for therapy
3. Guide the selection of the most appropriate treatment strategy for each patient
4. Monitor treatment response at a molecular level.

6. Conclusions

Current data suggest that the redifferentiation approach may be adaptable to various genetic profiles in RAI-R DTC, potentially offering new treatment options for patients with diverse molecular subtypes of the disease. Available evidence demonstrates that MAPK pathway blockage is an efficient strategy to redifferentiate some types of RAI-R DTC. This approach is effective both as a single therapy and, more promisingly, as part of a combination treatment regimen. However, several other targets are also available according to gene profiling, with promising results in small studies.

Still, available studies are very heterogeneous in multiple aspects, i.e., definition of RAI-R DTC, the duration of redifferentiation therapy, the imaging modality used to determine restoration of RAI uptake (I-131/I-123/I-124), the applied radioiodine activity, and the method of choice for applied activity—dosimetry-guided or empiric fixed activity. It also remains unclear whether the increase in uptake on diagnostic WBS performed after redifferentiation therapy can serve as a reliable criterion for selecting patients for RAI therapy. To address these uncertainties, additional large-scale multicenter studies are necessary. These studies should aim to identify the optimal choice and duration of redifferentiation therapy, selection criteria for redifferentiation therapy based on genetic testing, characteristics of patients who are the best candidates for this treatment, the risk-benefit ratio of the therapy, and its impact on patient's quality of life.

Author Contributions: Conceptualization, P.P.O. and L.G.; methodology, P.P.O.; data curation, P.P.O., M.T., A.A., A.C., and L.G.; writing—original draft preparation, P.P.O.; writing—review and editing, P.P.O., M.T, A.C, A.A., and L.G.; supervision, P.P.O. and L.G. All authors have read and agreed to the published version of the manuscript.

Funding: This research received no external funding.

Institutional Review Board Statement: Not applicable.

Informed Consent Statement: Not applicable.

Data Availability Statement: Not applicable.

Conflicts of Interest: The authors declare no conflicts of interest.

References

1. Schlumberger, M.; Brose, M.; Elisei, R.; Leboulleux, S.; Luster, M.; Pitoia, F.; Pacini, F. Definition and Management of Radioactive Iodine-Refractory Differentiated Thyroid Cancer. *Lancet Diabetes Endocrinol.* **2014**, *2*, 356–358. [CrossRef] [PubMed]
2. Sacks, W.; Braunstein, G.D. Evolving Approaches in Managing Radioactive Iodine-Refractory Differentiated Thyroid Cancer. *Endocr. Pract.* **2014**, *20*, 263–275. [CrossRef] [PubMed]
3. Giovanella, L.; Van Nostrand, D. Advanced Differentiated Thyroid Cancer: When to Stop Radioiodine? *Q. J. Nucl. Med. Mol. Imaging* **2019**, *63*, 267–270. [CrossRef] [PubMed]
4. Liu, M.; Cheng, L.; Jin, Y.; Ruan, M.; Sheng, S.; Chen, L. Predicting 131I-Avidity of Metastases from Differentiated Thyroid Cancer Using 18F-FDG PET/CT in Postoperative Patients with Elevated Thyroglobulin. *Sci. Rep.* **2018**, *8*, 4352. [CrossRef] [PubMed]
5. Haugen, B.R.; Alexander, E.K.; Bible, K.C.; Doherty, G.M.; Mandel, S.J.; Nikiforov, Y.E.; Pacini, F.; Randolph, G.W.; Sawka, A.M.; Schlumberger, M.; et al. 2015 American Thyroid Association Management Guidelines for Adult Patients with Thyroid Nodules and Differentiated Thyroid Cancer: The American Thyroid Association Guidelines Task Force on Thyroid Nodules and Differentiated Thyroid Cancer. *Thyroid* **2016**, *26*, 1–133. [CrossRef]
6. Fugazzola, L.; Elisei, R.; Fuhrer, D.; Jarzab, B.; Leboulleux, S.; Newbold, K.; Smit, J. 2019 European Thyroid Association Guidelines for the Treatment and Follow-Up of Advanced Radioiodine-Refractory Thyroid Cancer. *Eur. Thyroid. J.* **2019**, *8*, 227–245. [CrossRef]
7. Deandreis, D.; Ovčariček, P.P.; Campenni, A.; Vrachimis, A.; Giovanella, L. A Spotlight on Redifferentiation Strategies and Target Modulation in Differentiated Thyroid Cancer. *Clin. Transl. Imaging* **2021**, *9*, 405–408. [CrossRef]
8. Van Nostrand, D. Radioiodine Refractory Differentiated Thyroid Cancer: Time to Update the Classifications. *Thyroid* **2018**, *28*, 1083–1093. [CrossRef]
9. Michael Tuttle, R.; Ahuja, S.; Avram, A.M.; Bernet, V.J.; Bourguet, P.; Daniels, G.H.; Dillehay, G.; Draganescu, C.; Flux, G.; Führer, D.; et al. Controversies, Consensus, and Collaboration in the Use of 131I Therapy in Differentiated Thyroid Cancer: A Joint Statement from the American Thyroid Association, the European Association of Nuclear Medicine, the Society of Nuclear Medicine and Molecular Imaging, and the European Thyroid Association. *Thyroid* **2019**, *29*, 461–470. [CrossRef]
10. Filetti, S.; Durante, C.; Hartl, D.M.; Leboulleux, S.; Locati, L.D.; Newbold, K.; Papotti, M.G.; Berruti, A. ESMO Clinical Practice Guideline Update on the Use of Systemic Therapy in Advanced Thyroid Cancer. *Ann. Oncol.* **2022**, *33*, 674–684. [CrossRef]
11. Aashiq, M.; Silverman, D.A.; Na'ara, S.; Takahashi, H.; Amit, M. Radioiodine-Refractory Thyroid Cancer: Molecular Basis of Redifferentiation Therapies, Management, and Novel Therapies. *Cancers* **2019**, *11*, 1382. [CrossRef] [PubMed]
12. Landa, I.; Pozdeyev, N.; Korch, C.; Marlow, L.A.; Smallridge, R.C.; Copland, J.A.; Henderson, Y.C.; Lai, S.Y.; Clayman, G.L.; Onoda, N.; et al. Comprehensive Genetic Characterization of Human Thyroid Cancer Cell Lines: A Validated Panel for Preclinical Studies. *Clin. Cancer Res.* **2019**, *25*, 3141–3151. [CrossRef] [PubMed]
13. Kebebew, E.; Weng, J.; Bauer, J.; Ranvier, G.; Clark, O.H.; Duh, Q.Y.; Shibru, D.; Bastian, B.; Griffin, A. The Prevalence and Prognostic Value of BRAF Mutation in Thyroid Cancer. *Ann. Surg.* **2007**, *246*, 466–470. [CrossRef] [PubMed]
14. Fagin, J.A.; Wells, S.A. Biologic and Clinical Perspectives on Thyroid Cancer. *N. Engl. J. Med.* **2016**, *375*, 1054–1067. [CrossRef] [PubMed]
15. Gild, M.L.; Bullock, M.; Tsang, V.; Clifton-Bligh, R.J.; Robinson, B.G.; Wirth, L.J. Challenges and Strategies to Combat Resistance Mechanisms in Thyroid Cancer Therapeutics. *Thyroid* **2023**, *33*, 682–690. [CrossRef]
16. Nagarajah, J.; Le, M.; Knauf, J.A.; Ferrandino, G.; Montero-Conde, C.; Pillarsetty, N.; Bolaender, A.; Irwin, C.; Krishnamoorthy, G.P.; Saqcena, M.; et al. Sustained ERK Inhibition Maximizes Responses of BrafV600E Thyroid Cancers to Radioiodine. *J. Clin. Investig.* **2016**, *126*, 4119–4124. [CrossRef]
17. Chakravarty, D.; Santos, E.; Ryder, M.; Knauf, J.A.; Liao, X.H.; West, B.L.; Bollag, G.; Kolesnick, R.; Thin, T.H.; Rosen, N.; et al. Small-Molecule MAPK Inhibitors Restore Radioiodine Incorporation in Mouse Thyroid Cancers with Conditional BRAF Activation. *J. Clin. Investig.* **2011**, *121*, 4700–4711. [CrossRef]
18. Hadad, B.; Askari, E.; Zakavi, S.R.; Aryana, K.; Erfani, S.; Sahafi, P.; Nabavi, N.; Aghaee, A. Case Report: Regaining Radioiodine Uptake Following PRRT in Radioiodine-Refractory Thyroid Cancer: A New Re-Differentiation Strategy? *Front. Nucl. Med.* **2022**, *2*, 1071022. [CrossRef]
19. Ho, A.L.; Grewal, R.K.; Leboeuf, R.; Sherman, E.J.; Pfister, D.G.; Deandreis, D.; Pentlow, K.S.; Zanzonico, P.B.; Haque, S.; Gavane, S.; et al. Selumetinib-Enhanced Radioiodine Uptake in Advanced Thyroid Cancer. *N. Engl. J. Med.* **2013**, *368*, 623–632. [CrossRef]
20. Rothenberg, S.M.; McFadden, D.G.; Palmer, E.L.; Daniels, G.H.; Wirth, L.J. Redifferentiation of Iodine-Refractory BRAF V600E-Mutant Metastatic Papillary Thyroid Cancer with Dabrafenib. *Clin. Cancer Res.* **2015**, *21*, 1028–1035. [CrossRef]

21. Jaber, T.; Waguespack, S.G.; Cabanillas, M.E.; Elbanan, M.; Vu, T.; Dadu, R.; Sherman, S.I.; Amit, M.; Santos, E.B.; Zafereo, M.; et al. Targeted Therapy in Advanced Thyroid Cancer to Resensitize Tumors to Radioactive Iodine. *J. Clin. Endocrinol. Metab.* **2018**, *103*, 3698–3705. [CrossRef]
22. Dunn, L.A.; Sherman, E.J.; Baxi, S.S.; Tchekmedyian, V.; Grewal, R.K.; Larson, S.M.; Pentlow, K.S.; Haque, S.; Tuttle, R.M.; Sabra, M.M.; et al. Vemurafenib Redifferentiation of BRAF Mutant, Rai-Refractory Thyroid Cancers. *J. Clin. Endocrinol. Metab.* **2019**, *104*, 1417–1428. [CrossRef]
23. Weber, M.; Kersting, D.; Riemann, B.; Brandenburg, T.; Führer-Sakel, D.; Grünwald, F.; Kreissl, M.C.; Dralle, H.; Weber, F.; Schmid, K.W.; et al. Enhancing Radioiodine Incorporation into Radioiodine-Refractory Thyroid Cancer with MAPK Inhibition (ERRITI): A Single-Center Prospective Two-Arm Study. *Clin. Cancer Res.* **2022**, *28*, 4194–4202. [CrossRef]
24. Leboulleux, S.; Do Cao, C.; Zerdoud, S.; Attard, M.; Bournaud, C.; Lacroix, L.; Benisvy, D.; Taïeb, D.; Bardet, S.; Terroir-Cassou-Mounat, M.; et al. A Phase II Redifferentiation Trial with Dabrafenib-Trametinib and 131I in Metastatic Radioactive Iodine Refractory BRAF p.V600E-Mutated Differentiated Thyroid Cancer. *Clin. Cancer Res.* **2023**, *29*, 2401–2409. [CrossRef]
25. Leboulleux, S.; Benisvy, D.; Taieb, D.; Attard, M.; Bournaud, C.; Terroir-Cassou-Mounat, M.; Lacroix, L.; Anizan, N.; Schiazza, A.; Garcia, M.E.; et al. MERAIODE: A Phase II Redifferentiation Trial with Trametinib and 131I in Metastatic Radioactive Iodine Refractory RAS Mutated Differentiated Thyroid Cancer. *Thyroid* **2023**, *33*, 1124–1129. [CrossRef]
26. Iravani, A.; Solomon, B.; Pattison, D.A.; Jackson, P.; Ravi Kumar, A.; Kong, G.; Hofman, M.S.; Akhurst, T.; Hicks, R.J. Mitogen-Activated Protein Kinase Pathway Inhibition for Redifferentiation of Radioiodine Refractory Differentiated Thyroid Cancer: An Evolving Protocol. *Thyroid* **2019**, *29*, 1634–1645. [CrossRef]
27. Burman, B.; Tuttle, R.M.; Grewal, R.K.; Sherman, E.J.; Baxi, S.S.; Boucai, L.; Sabra, M.; Fish, S.; Pentlow, K.S.; Haque, S.; et al. Phase 2 of Trametinib plus Radioiodine in RAS-Mutant and Wild-Type, Radioiodine-Refractory Thyroid Cancer (ETCTN9446). *J. Clin. Oncol.* **2022**, *40*, 6089. [CrossRef]
28. Groussin, L.; Clerc, J.; Huillard, O. Larotrectinib-Enhanced Radioactive Iodine Uptake in Advanced Thyroid Cancer. *N. Engl. J. Med.* **2020**, *383*, 1686–1687. [CrossRef]
29. Syed, A.R.; Gorana, A.; Nohr, E.; Yuan, X.K.; Masc, P.A.; Ghaznavi, S.; Lamb, D.; McIntyre, J.; Eszlinger, M.; Paschke, R. Predictors of Radioiodine (RAI)-Avidity Restoration for NTRK Fusion-Positive RAI-Resistant Metastatic Thyroid Cancers. *Eur. Thyroid J.* **2024**, *13*, e230227. [CrossRef]
30. Chan, H.P.; Chen, I.F.; Tsai, F.R.; Kao, C.H.; Shen, D.H.Y. Reversing "Flip-Flop" Phenomenon of 131 I and Glucose Avidity in RET-Fusion Positive Radioiodine-Refractory Thyroid Cancer Lesions After Treatment of Pralsetinib. *Clin. Nucl. Med.* **2023**, *48*, E147–E148. [CrossRef]
31. Lee, Y.A.; Lee, H.; Im, S.-W.; Song, Y.S.; Oh, D.-Y.; Kang, H.J.; Won, J.-K.; Jung, K.C.; Kwon, D.; Chung, E.-J.; et al. NTRK and RET Fusion–Directed Therapy in Pediatric Thyroid Cancer Yields a Tumor Response and Radioiodine Uptake. *J. Clin. Investig.* **2021**, *131*, e144847. [CrossRef]
32. Werner, R.A.; Sayehli, C.; Hänscheid, H.; Higuchi, T.; Serfling, S.E.; Fassnacht, M.; Goebeler, M.E.; Buck, A.K.; Kroiss, M. Successful Combination of Selpercatinib and Radioiodine after Pretherapeutic Dose Estimation in RET-Altered Thyroid Carcinoma. *Eur. J. Nucl. Med. Mol. Imaging* **2023**, *50*, 1833–1834. [CrossRef] [PubMed]
33. Toro-Tobon, D.; Morris, J.C.; Hilger, C.; Peskey, C.; Durski, J.M.; Ryder, M. Clinical Outcomes of Radioactive Iodine Redifferentiation Therapy in Previously Iodine Refractory Differentiated Thyroid Cancers. *Thyroid* **2024**, *34*, 70–81. [CrossRef] [PubMed]
34. Verburg, F.A.; Amthauer, H.; Binse, I.; Brink, I.; Buck, A.; Darr, A.; Dierks, C.; Koch, C.; König, U.; Kreissl, M.C.; et al. Questions and Controversies in the Clinical Application of Tyrosine Kinase Inhibitors to Treat Patients with Radioiodine-Refractory Differentiated Thyroid Carcinoma: Expert Perspectives. *Horm. Metab. Res.* **2021**, *53*, 149–160. [CrossRef]
35. Yu, S.T.; Ge, J.N.; Luo, J.Y.; Wei, Z.G.; Sun, B.H.; Lei, S.T. Treatment-Related Adverse Effects with TKIs in Patients with Advanced or Radioiodine Refractory Differentiated Thyroid Carcinoma: A Systematic Review and Meta-Analysis. *Cancer Manag. Res.* **2019**, *11*, 1525–1532. [CrossRef] [PubMed]
36. Busaidy, N.L.; Konda, B.; Wei, L.; Wirth, L.J.; Devine, C.; Daniels, G.A.; Desouza, J.A.; Poi, M.; Seligson, N.D.; Cabanillas, M.E.; et al. Dabrafenib Versus Dabrafenib + Trametinib in BRAF-Mutated Radioactive Iodine Refractory Differentiated Thyroid Cancer: Results of a Randomized, Phase 2, Open-Label Multicenter Trial. *Thyroid* **2022**, *32*, 1184–1192. [CrossRef]
37. Ho, A.L.; Dedecjus, M.; Wirth, L.J.; Tuttle, R.M.; Inabnet, W.B.; Tennvall, J.; Vaisman, F.; Bastholt, L.; Gianoukakis, A.G.; Rodien, P.; et al. Selumetinib Plus Adjuvant Radioactive Iodine in Patients With High-Risk Differentiated Thyroid Cancer: A Phase III, Randomized, Placebo-Controlled Trial (ASTRA). *J. Clin. Oncol.* **2022**, *40*, 1870–1878. [CrossRef]
38. Van Nostrand, D.; Veytsman, I.; Kulkarni, K.; Heimlich, L.; Burman, K.D. Redifferentiation of Differentiated Thyroid Cancer: Clinical Insights from a Narrative Review of Literature. *Thyroid* **2023**, *33*, 674–681. [CrossRef]
39. Petranović Ovčariček, P.; Campenni, A.; de Keizer, B.; Deandreis, D.; Kreissl, M.C.; Vrachimis, A.; Tuncel, M.; Giovanella, L. Molecular Theranostics in Radioiodine-Refractory Differentiated Thyroid Cancer. *Cancers* **2023**, *15*, 4290. [CrossRef]

Journal of
Clinical Medicine

MDPI

Article

Does Radioactive Iodine Treatment Affect Thyroid Size and Tracheal Diameter?

Kadriye Yazici Demir [1], Zulkuf Kaya [1], Ramazan Dayanan [2], Tolga Mercantepe [3,*] and Filiz Mercantepe [4,*]

1 Department of Otorhinolaryngology, Faculty of Medicine, University of Ataturk, Erzurum 25240, Türkiye; dr.kadriyeyazicidemir@kapadokyahastanesi.com.tr (K.Y.D.); zulkuf.kaya@atauni.edu.tr (Z.K.)
2 Department of Endocrinology and Metabolism, Batman Training and Research Hospital, Batman 72070, Türkiye; ramazan.dayanan@saglik.gov.tr
3 Department of Histology, Faculty of Medicine, Recep Tayyip Erdogan University, Rize 53100, Türkiye
4 Department of Endocrinology and Metabolism, Faculty of Medicine, Recep Tayyip Erdogan University, Rize 53100, Türkiye
* Correspondence: tolga.mercantepe@erdogan.edu.tr (T.M.); filiz.mercantepe@saglik.gov.tr (F.M.)

Abstract: Background/Objectives: There exist three principal treatment modalities employed in the management of hyperthyroidism attributable to excessive hormone secretion by the thyroid gland: antithyroid pharmacotherapy, surgical intervention, and radioactive iodine (RAI) therapy. Surgical intervention is typically indicated for markedly enlarged thyroid glands that exert pressure on the trachea. The objective of this investigation was to ascertain the influence of RAI on thyroid volume and tracheal diameter. **Methods:** This study included 20 patients, six females and 14 males, who received 20 mCi radioactive iodine treatment for toxic nodular goiter at a tertiary university hospital between March 2019 and February 2020. Pre-treatment and six-month post-treatment neck MRI scans were conducted on the cohort. Thyroid and tracheal volumes were quantified using the Cavalieri method based on MRI sections, and comparisons were conducted pre-and post-treatment. Statistical analysis of the comparative values was performed using the dependent samples t-test. **Results:** A statistically significant reduction in thyroid volume was observed among the 20 patients, averaging a decrease of 36.06% following RAI treatment compared to baseline measurements ($p < 0.001$). Additionally, an average increase of 12.76% in tracheal volume was noted post-treatment in comparison to initial measurements, which was also statistically significant ($p < 0.05$). None of the patients exhibited respiratory distress in the immediate postoperative period. **Conclusions:** The findings indicate that RAI therapy leads to a reduction in thyroid size, accompanied by an increase in tracheal diameters subsequent to treatment. Given the potential complications and risks associated with surgical intervention, it may be prudent to consider large thyroids for RAI therapy as an alternative to surgery.

Keywords: radioactive iodine; hyperthyroidism; tracheal diameter; thyroid size; Cavalieri method

1. Introduction

Hyperthyroidism represents a prevalent endocrine disorder, afflicting approximately 0.2 to 1.4% of the population globally, typically occurring between the ages of 20 and 40. This condition exhibits a higher prevalence in females, with a female-to-male ratio approximating 5:1 [1,2]. The predominant etiology of hyperthyroidism is Graves' disease, which arises from an autoimmune mechanism [3]. In geographic areas characterized by iodine deficiency and among the geriatric population, toxic nodular goiter is encountered more frequently [4].

While three therapeutic modalities exist for the management of Graves' disease—namely pharmacotherapy, surgical intervention, and radioactive iodine (RAI)—pharmacotherapy demonstrates limited efficacy in cases of toxic nodular goiter [5]. In such instances, RAI or surgical intervention is generally employed [6]. Antithyroid medications encompass compounds such as methimazole and propylthiouracil, which are extensively utilized in the management of Graves' disease and toxic multinodular goiter. These pharmacological agents may elicit a spectrum of adverse effects, ranging from mild manifestations such as dermal reactions, alterations in taste perception, and arthralgia to more severe complications including agranulocytosis, hepatotoxicity, and ANCA-positive vasculitis [7,8]. Propylthiouracil is linked with the potential for hepatotoxicity and vasculitis, while methimazole is correlated with cholestatic adverse effects and teratogenicity [9,10]. Routine monitoring of hematological parameters and hepatic function tests is advised to mitigate the incidence of adverse effects [11].

Surgical intervention is regarded as a more efficacious approach for both thyrotoxicosis and symptoms related to compression. Nevertheless, it necessitates lifelong hormone replacement therapy, and there exists a risk for complications such as hypoparathyroidism and permanent recurrent laryngeal nerve paralysis [12]. I131 therapy is recognized as an effective and safe treatment modality in both primary management and secondary treatment in cases where a pharmacological response is inadequate [13,14]. In several European and Latin American nations, RAI therapy has supplanted surgical options in the management of hyperthyroidism [15], a transition that is also endorsed by contemporary clinical guidelines [16]. In scenarios involving hyperthyroidism with an enlarged thyroid gland, the prevailing clinical strategy is to recommend surgical intervention for the patient. This recommendation is predicated on the observation that RAI does not achieve sufficient volumetric reduction and may exacerbate compression symptoms through the potential induction of tracheal stenosis. The objective of this study was to elucidate the possible ramifications of RAI treatment on patients presenting with substantial thyroid volumes by assessing its impact on thyroid size and tracheal diameter utilizing the Cavalieri method, an objective measurement technique.

2. Participants and Methods

The present investigation received endorsement from the Ethics Committee at Atatürk University Faculty of Medicine (dated 13 March 2019 and numbered B.30.2.ATA.0.01.00/225). The research was executed in alignment with the principles outlined in the Declaration of Helsinki. Informed voluntary consent was duly acquired from every participant involved.

2.1. Study Design and Data Collections

The current investigation encompassed 20 patients who sought treatment at the Department of Endocrinology, Atatürk University Faculty of Medicine, and underwent 20 mCi radioactive iodine therapy due to toxic nodular goiter at the Department of Nuclear Medicine, Atatürk University Faculty of Medicine between March 2019 and February 2020. Prior to the administration of RAI, malignancy was systematically excluded in all participants. Magnetic Resonance Imaging (MRI) of the neck was conducted on the subjects both prior to and six months subsequent to the treatment. The peak efficacy of RAI treatment is typically observed within a timeframe of 4–8 weeks, with enhancements in thyroid function potentially persisting for as long as six months. Consequently, follow-up MRIs were executed on the subjects six months following the treatment. Thyroid and tracheal volumes were quantitatively assessed in the neck MRIs of the subjects utilizing the Cavalieri method, a recognized stereological approach, and comparative analyses were conducted before and after RAI. All calculations were performed by the same specialist on each occasion while remaining blinded to the treatment cohorts.

2.2. Calculation of Total Volume of Thyroid and Trachea

The Cavalieri method constitutes a non-invasive and highly accurate technique for volume measurement, grounded in fundamental stereological principles [17]. This methodology facilitates the estimation of the three-dimensional volume of any object by aggregating its two-dimensional cross-sectional areas [18]. Named in honor of the renowned Italian mathematician Bonaventura Cavalieri, this approach is extensively employed in the biomedical sciences for the accurate and reliable quantification of tissue volume or organ dimensions [18–21]. In the current investigation, a sophisticated instrument system known as Stereo-Investigator (version 7.0, Microbrightfield, Colchester, VT, USA) was employed, incorporating specialized software equipped with a dotted area ruler that facilitates area calculations via the Cavalieri method [18–21]. This instrument system comprises a microscope integrated with a digital camera, a motorized apparatus that facilitates the movement of the microscope stage, and a high-performance computer equipped with software that governs their operational parameters (Figure 1). In the context of this study, the computational component of this instrument system was exclusively utilized.

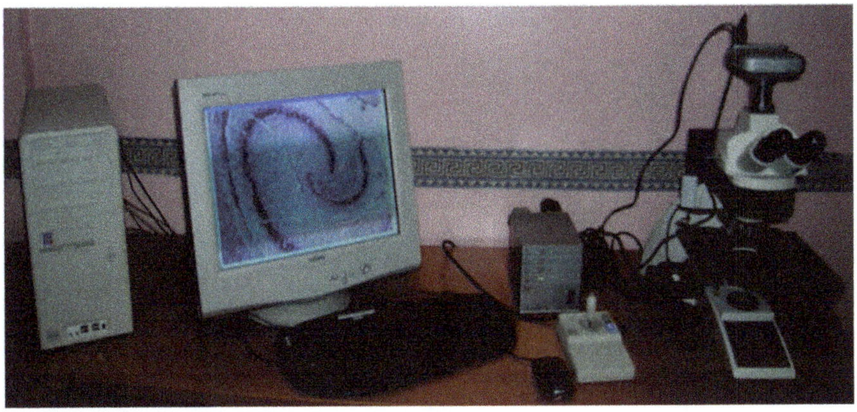

Figure 1. Stereo-Investigator (version 7.0, Microbrightfield, Colchester, VT, USA).

All participants in the study underwent an MRI of the cervical region with 5 mm slice thickness both prior to and six months subsequent to RAI treatment. Thyroid sections within the MR images were meticulously selected for analysis. The delineation of the thyroid and trachea contours in the selected sections was performed (Figure 2). Subsequently, a dotted area ruler featuring a systematic arrangement of evenly spaced points was superimposed onto the section on the computer (Figure 3). The frequency of this dotted area ruler was determined in accordance with a suitable error coefficient value. In the subsequent phases of the study, the points corresponding to the thyroid and trachea were separately marked with distinct colored indicators (Figure 4).

According to the reference volume formula given below, in each section:

$$\text{Reference V} = t \times a/p \times \Sigma P$$

Expressions in the formula;

V: reference volume,

t: section thickness or distance between corresponding surfaces, a/p is the area represented by a point,

Σ P: is the total number of points falling on the marked thyroid and trachea in a section.

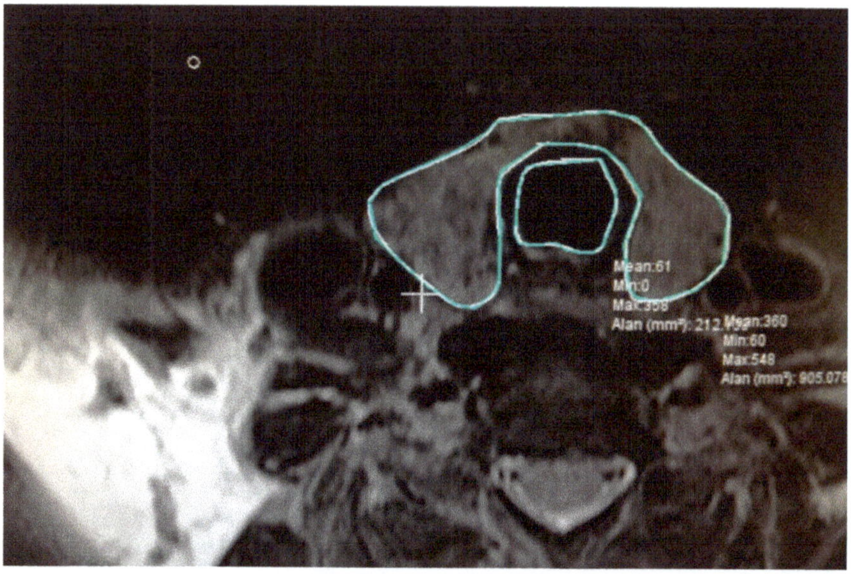

Figure 2. Marked image of the thyroid and trachea outlines in MRI slices.

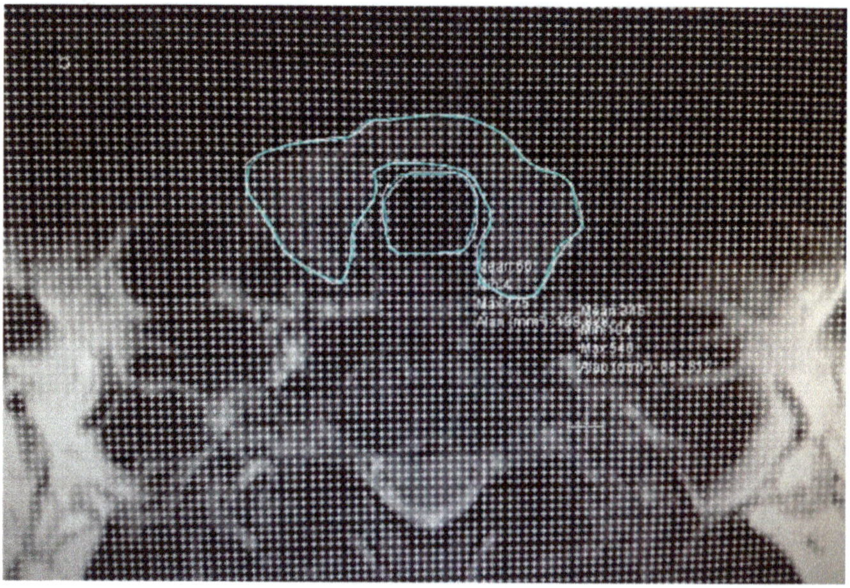

Figure 3. The dotted area ruler is placed on the section on the screen.

The same procedures were applied for all sections containing the thyroid for all patients. Finally, in accordance with the Cavalieri principle, the software automatically calculated the total volume for the thyroid and trachea separately according to the following total volume formula [18–21].

$$\text{Vtotal} = \text{V1} + \text{V2} + \ldots + \text{Vn}$$

Symbols of the formula:
Vtotal: total volume
V1: thyroid/trachea volume in the first section
V2: thyroid/trachea volume in the second section
Vn: thyroid/trachea volume in the last section

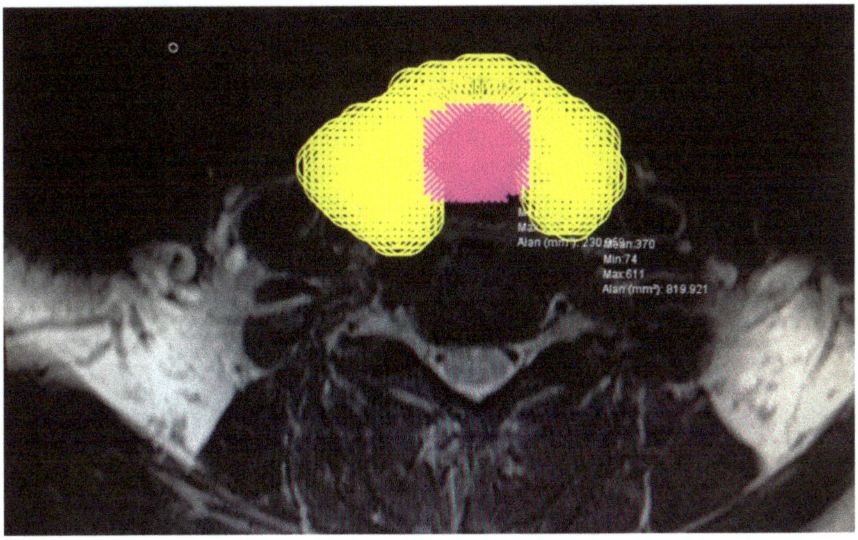

Figure 4. The points on the thyroid and trachea are marked with separate-colored markers.

2.3. Statistical Analysis

Data were analyzed using Windows SPSS 20 package program. Pearson correlation coefficient was used to analyze the relationship between pre-treatment thyroid volume, the difference between pre- and post-treatment thyroid volumes, and the ratio parameters of pre- and post-treatment thyroid/trachea volume values. A comparison of pre- and post-treatment thyroid and trachea volume values was made with a dependent sample *t* test. A *p* value of less than 0.05 was considered statistically significant.

3. Results

The present study encompassed a cohort of 20 patients who underwent a 20 mCi RAI treatment for toxic multinodular goiter [22,23] during the period extending from March 2019 to February 2020. The data delineating the demographic characteristics of the patients, stratified by age and gender, are elucidated in Table 1. Upon examination of the gender distribution among the patients, it is observed that 6 (30%) were male and 14 (70%) were female. The predominance of female patients regarding thyroid disease aligns with the existing literature.

The comparative analysis of thyroid and tracheal volumes among the participants, conducted prior to and subsequent to RAI treatment, is illustrated in Table 2. The results of the study revealed a statistically significant difference in the volume measurements of the thyroid and trachea pre- and post-treatment ($p < 0.001$, $p < 0.05$, respectively). When evaluating the thyroid volumes before and after treatment in terms of percentage change, it was found that the thyroid volume exhibited a reduction of 36.06% (Figure 5). The p-value determined through the dependent sample t-test was $p < 0.001$, indicating a statistically significant decrease. A little increase in volume was noted in three patients; however, this change did not reach statistical significance.

Table 1. Age and gender distribution of participants.

Variables		N = 20
Age, years (min-max)		61 (36–84)
Gender	Male, n (%)	6 (30)
	Female, n (%)	14 (70)

Table 2. Thyroid and tracheal volumes of participants pre- and post-RAI treatment.

Volume	Minimum Volume (μm³)	Maximum Volume (μm³)	Mean Volume (μm³)
Pre-RAI Thyroid volume	59,625,000,000	586,440,000,000	331,940,725,000
Post-RAI Thyroid volume	67,612,500,000	571,275,000,000	216,330,725,000
Pre-RAI Trachea volume	16,920,000,000	71,662,500,000	42,768,375,000
Post-RAI Trachea volume	17,010,000,000	99,450,000,000	48,594,875,000

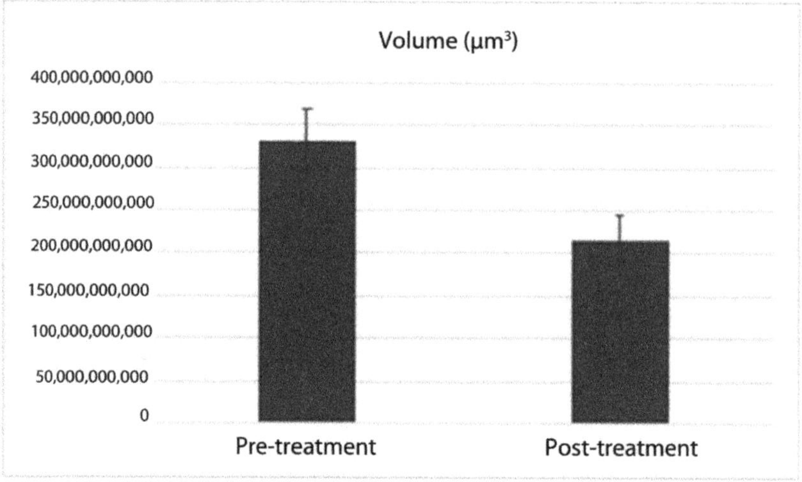

Figure 5. Pre- and post-treatment thyroid volume means.

In the comparison of tracheal volumes before and after treatment, expressed as a percentage, it was observed that the tracheal volume increased by 12.76% (Figure 6). The p-value derived from the dependent sample t-test was $p < 0.05$, indicating a statistically significant increase. A reduction in tracheal volume was noted in four patients, while no volume alteration occurred in three patients. Nonetheless, these changes were statistically insignificant, and no instances of respiratory distress were recorded in the acute post-treatment phase among any of the patients.

According to the statistical evaluations conducted, a positive correlation was identified between the pre-treatment thyroid volume and the differential between the pre-treatment and post-treatment thyroid volumes (Figure 7, rp = 0.653, $p = 0.002$). Consequently, it was ascertained that larger pre-treatment thyroid volumes were associated with a more substantial decrease in volume following treatment. Furthermore, a positive correlation was established between the pre-treatment and post-treatment thyroid/tracheal volume ratios (Figure 8, rp = 0.770, $p < 0.001$). Thus, it was concluded that the ratios of pre-treatment thyroid/trachea volumes were directly proportional to those observed post-treatment.

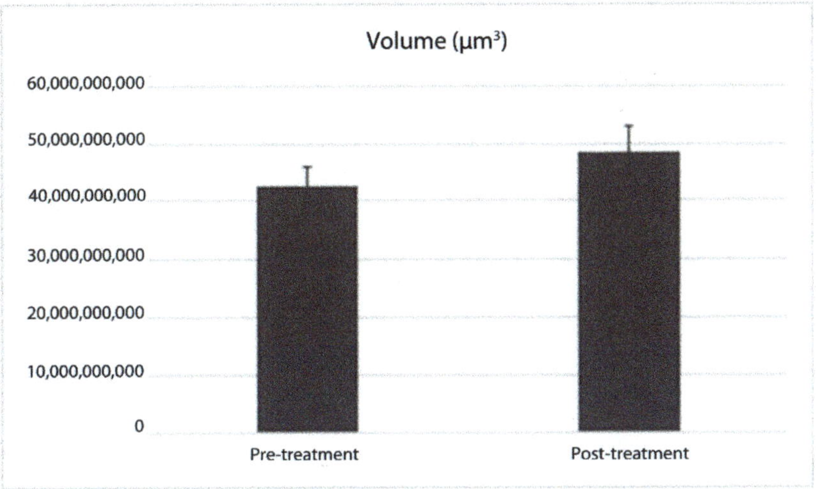

Figure 6. Pre- and post-treatment trachea volume means.

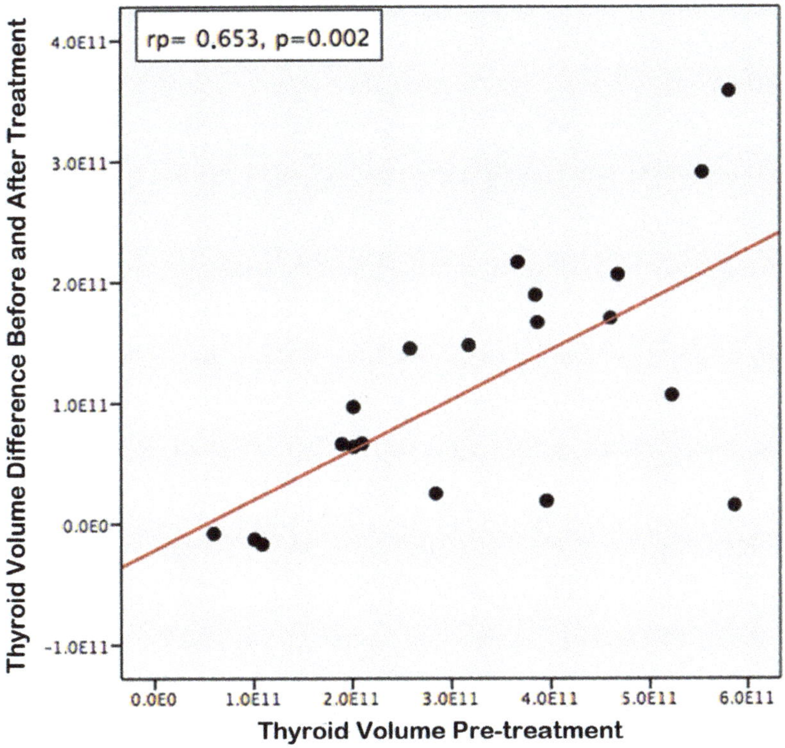

Figure 7. Correlation of pre-treatment thyroid volume and difference between pre- and post-treatment thyroid volumes.

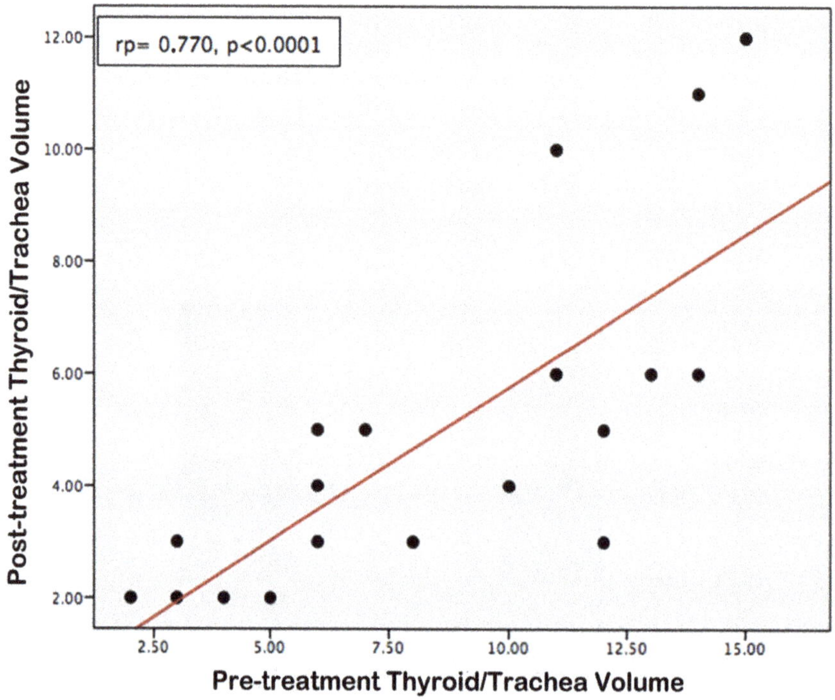

Figure 8. Correlation between pre-treatment thyroid/trachea volume ratio and post-treatment thyroid/trachea volume ratio.

4. Discussion

In the current investigation, thyroid volumes and tracheal diameters derived from MRI images obtained prior to and six months subsequent to the administration of treatment in 20 patients who underwent 20 mCi RAI therapy for hyperthyroidism were meticulously analyzed. Based on this analysis, it was determined that RAI treatment did not yield a statistically significant increase in thyroid volume; however, a notable increase in tracheal diameter was observed. This finding indicates that RAI treatment resulted in a reduction in thyroid diameter by approximately one-third when assessed after an extended duration, such as six months, and did not induce tracheal stenosis by causing an increase in tracheal diameter.

Hyperthyroidism represents a prevalent endocrine disorder within the population [24]. While some individuals with hyperthyroidism may remain asymptomatic, others may experience severe symptoms that markedly disrupt daily functioning [25]. Thyroid hormones serve as the primary regulators of basal metabolic rate. The most critical physiological effects of thyroid hormones include the elevation of heart rate, the enhancement of ventilation, and the reduction in peripheral resistance [26]. Furthermore, in the majority of hyperthyroid patients, the thyroid gland may hypertrophy to two to three times its standard size. The proliferation of cells is significantly augmented due to hyperplasia and follicular expansion. Additionally, the secretion rate per cell may increase several-fold [1].

As a consequence of the enlargement of the thyroid gland, certain patients may encounter cosmetic concerns, while others may suffer from respiratory distress attributable to the close anatomical relationship between the thyroid and trachea. Three principal modalities are employed in the management of hyperthyroidism: antithyroid drug therapy, surgical intervention, and RAI therapy [1,27]. The selection of the treatment modality is contingent upon the individual patient's condition. There exists a lack of global consensus regarding the optimal initial treatment approach. Antithyroid medications are typically favored for the management of newly diagnosed hyperthyroid patients exhibiting mild symptoms [28]. Nevertheless, prolonged pharmacological therapy is generally discouraged due to the potential for adverse effects [11]. I-131 therapy has been utilized for over 70 years in the treatment of Graves' disease and for 30 years in cases of benign nodular goiter. I-131 therapy not only addresses hyperthyroidism but also contributes to the reduction in thyroid volume [23,29–32]. Surgical intervention is predominantly indicated for the management of substantial goiters, as I-131 may be less efficacious and often necessitates a secondary RAI treatment [33–35]. Surgical options represent a more effective resolution for both thyrotoxicosis and compressive symptoms; however, they necessitate lifelong hormone replacement therapy and carry risks of complications such as hypoparathyroidism and permanent recurrent nerve paralysis [36]. In comparison, I-131 treatment is a more economical alternative to surgical intervention [37]. It can also be administered orally and offers the advantage of treatment in a single dose. I-131 therapy induces radiation exposure to thyroid follicle cells via beta particle radiation [32]. Consequently, cellular necrosis ensues, followed by inflammation and fibrosis. This cascade ultimately diminishes the capacity for hormone synthesis, thereby providing an efficacious treatment avenue for hyperthyroidism [38].

Particularly, patients diagnosed with toxic nodular goiter represent a cohort particularly well-suited for RAI therapy. In the context of toxic nodular goiter, the isotope I-131 demonstrates preferential accumulation in hyperfunctioning autonomous nodules, while the surrounding paranodular thyroid tissue experiences reduced exposure to radiation. Consequently, a significant proportion, specifically 80% or more, of individuals with toxic nodules attain a state of euthyroidism within a 12-month period, and the incidence of enduring permanent hypothyroidism is markedly lower in comparison with those with Graves' disease [28]. The previous investigations into I-131 treatment have indicated that thyroid volume diminishes by 35–50% over the course of one year [39]. In the current study, a reduction in thyroid volume of 36.06% was noted six months post-treatment, aligning with the existing literature. A more pronounced decrease is anticipated with extended follow-up periods associated with RAI therapy. While individual responses to RAI treatment exhibit variability, there is often an amelioration of symptoms accompanied by a high level of patient satisfaction (63, 65, 67). Vereist et al. reported that optimal outcomes were typically observed within a timeframe of less than one year; however, the maximal therapeutic effect was reached between 24 and 30 months [40]. Bonnema et al. conducted measurements of thyroid volume via ultrasonography prior to, and at one year and three years subsequent to, I-131 treatment in a cohort of 43 patients. Their findings revealed that thyroid volume diminished by nearly 50% after one year, and no statistically significant difference was observed at the three-year mark compared to the one-year assessment [32]. Should symptoms of thyrotoxicosis persist due to inadequate volume reduction, a secondary I-131 treatment may be administered [41]. The existence of a substernal goiter does not negate the favorable outcomes associated with I-131 treatment [42]. Nonetheless, such goiters tend to be considerably large, and despite the administration of equivalent radiation doses, the relative reduction in goiter size resulting from I-131 treatment is inversely correlated with the initial goiter volume [23]. In contrast to the findings presented in this study, we observed that larger baseline thyroid volumes corresponded with greater reductions in thyroid volume. Massaro et al. conducted research involving 75 patients, measuring thyroid volumes via ultrasonography before and after I-131 treatment in subgroups comprising 27 patients with multinodular goiter (MNG), 32 with Graves' disease, and 16 with uninodular goiter. They documented a volume reduction of 28.6% in the

Graves' cohort, 53.3% in the MNG group, and 57.8% in patients with uninodular goiter 12 months post-treatment [43]. The extent of thyroid volume reduction is contingent upon both the initial thyroid volume and the uptake of RAI [44]. In instances of significantly enlarged goiters, the insufficiency of adequate thyroid volume reduction constrains the application of I 131 therapies. Although the dosage of I 131 can be escalated to facilitate enhanced volume reduction, this adjustment concomitantly leads to an elevation in the radiation exposure experienced by the organism [22]. Furthermore, the efficacy of I 131 is diminished in goiters characterized by low radioactive iodine uptake (RAIU). Should the thyroid RAIU be augmented to enhance thyroid irradiation, the likelihood of successful I 131 interventions may be improved. Over the years, numerous strategies have been implemented, including the adoption of a low iodine diet, the administration of lithium, and the use of diuretics. Nevertheless, the most potent agent identified to date in this context is recombinant human TSH (rhTSH). RhTSH has been demonstrated to elevate 24 h RAIU by 100% or greater without impacting the half-life of I 131 [45–48].

Despite the long-standing application of I 131, it is not extensively favored for patients presenting with exceedingly large goiters. The rationale for this apprehension stems from the belief that the already enlarged thyroid gland may undergo further enlargement during the acute phase under the influence of I 131, potentially exacerbating tracheal compression [22,33]. Nonetheless, this anticipated complication has not manifested in clinical practice and remains undocumented [23]. In our investigation, no patient reported experiencing respiratory distress during the acute phase.

Numerous investigations within the existing literature have sought to ascertain the impact of RAI treatment on the diameter of the trachea. Bonnema et al. administered a high-dose mean of 61 mCi (ranging from 26 to 124 mCi) of I-131 to a cohort of 23 patients diagnosed with MNG whose thyroid volume exceeded 150 mL. A pre-treatment neck MRI was conducted on the subjects with 8 mm slices, followed by subsequent scans at 1 week and 1-year post-treatment. The dimensions of the thyroid and trachea were quantified in axial sections. Notably, the minimum cross-sectional area of the trachea exhibited a reduction of 9.2% within one week following treatment, while the tracheal area demonstrated a subsequent increase of 17.9% by the conclusion of the one-year period. Furthermore, it was documented that the thyroid volume diminished by 15% after one week and by 34% after one year. Importantly, no patient experienced acute respiratory distress during the treatment interval [23].

In our investigation, we observed that the tracheal volume expanded by 12.76% for six months subsequent to treatment. Albino et al. conducted neck MRI evaluations on 22 patients prior to I-131 treatment and at intervals of 2-, 7-, 180-, and 360 days post-treatment to assess tracheal diameter and thyroid volume. An indirect estimation of tracheal compression was achieved by analyzing the tracheal cross-sectional area (TCA). While no alterations in thyroid volume were noted on the 2nd and 7th days, a gradual decline was recorded at the 6th and 12th months. No statistically significant differences in TCA were identified following treatment [49].

The primary objective of our study was to elucidate the effects of RAI treatment on thyroid size and tracheal diameter employing an objective methodology. In our findings, it was determined that the trachea experienced an expansion of 12.76% and the thyroid volume demonstrated a decrease of 36.06% six months post-treatment. Acute tracheal compression and respiratory distress are frequently cited as justifications for discontinuing RAI treatment in cases of enlarged thyroids; however, acute respiratory distress did not manifest in any of the patients in the current study. Additionally, there exist scholarly articles in the literature that corroborate the absence of respiratory distress. In our cohort, the pressure subsided, and symptoms were alleviated six months following treatment.

We posit that RAI treatment does not induce acute respiratory distress as previously apprehended and ultimately offers long-term relief to patients in a safe manner.

Our investigation undoubtedly possesses certain constraints, and these constraints should be regarded with prudence. Primarily, our investigation was characterized by a relatively modest sample size. Owing to the financial implications associated with MRI, longitudinal imaging could not be conducted on patients, particularly during the initial phase of post-RAI treatment. Nevertheless, patients were subjected to rigorous monitoring, particularly concerning the potential emergence of respiratory distress. Subsequent investigations that incorporate serial assessments of thyroid volume and tracheal diameters in a larger cohort and during the initial period will serve to mitigate these limitations.

5. Conclusions

The findings of the present investigation indicate that radioactive iodine therapy does not lead to an increase in thyroid volume, nor does it result in tracheal stenosis; consequently, patients may be appropriately referred for radioactive iodine therapy as an alternative to surgical intervention. Therefore, the likelihood of encountering surgical complications is mitigated. To thoroughly assess the initial effects of radioactive iodine treatment, it is imperative that future studies involve a larger cohort of patients and employ a standardized methodology for quantifying tracheal volume during the early stages of treatment.

Author Contributions: All the authors contributed to the study of conception and design. Material preparation, data collection and laboratory analyses were performed by K.Y.D., Z.K., R.D. and F.M. Statistical analysis was performed by K.Y.D., Z.K. and T.M. The first draft of the manuscript was written by K.Y.D., Z.K., F.M. and T.M., and all the authors commented on previous versions of the manuscript. All authors have read and agreed to the published version of the manuscript.

Funding: The Recep Tayyip Erdogan University Development Foundation provided funding for the open-access publishing of this study (Grant number: 02024012009211).

Institutional Review Board Statement: The study was conducted in accordance with the Declaration of Helsinki, and approved by the Ethics Committee at Atatürk University Faculty of Medicine (Approval date: 13 March 2019 and approval number: B.30.2.ATA.0.01.00/225).

Informed Consent Statement: Written informed consent has been obtained from the patients to publish this paper.

Data Availability Statement: All data generated or analyzed during this study are included in this article. The data will be available upon reasonable request (contact persons: filiz.mercantepe@saglik.gov.tr).

Conflicts of Interest: The authors declare that they have no known competing financial interests or personal relationships that could have appeared to influence the work reported in this paper.

References

1. Lee, S.Y.; Pearce, E.N. Hyperthyroidism: A Review. *JAMA* **2023**, *330*, 1472–1483. [CrossRef] [PubMed]
2. Taylor, P.N.; Albrecht, D.; Scholz, A.; Gutierrez-Buey, G.; Lazarus, J.H.; Dayan, C.M.; Okosieme, O.E. Global Epidemiology of Hyperthyroidism and Hypothyroidism. *Nat. Rev. Endocrinol.* **2018**, *14*, 301–316. [CrossRef] [PubMed]
3. Brent, G.A. Clinical practice. Graves' disease. *N. Engl. J. Med.* **2008**, *358*, 2594–2605. [CrossRef] [PubMed]
4. Derwahl, M.; Studer, H. Multinodular Goitre: "Much More to It than Simply Iodine Deficiency". *Best Pract. Res. Clin. Endocrinol. Metab.* **2000**, *14*, 577–600. [CrossRef]
5. Şakı, H.; Cengiz, A.; Yürekli, Y. Effectiveness of Radioiodine Treatment for Toxic Nodular Goiter. *Mol. Imaging Radionucl. Ther.* **2015**, *24*, 100–104. [CrossRef] [PubMed]
6. Burch, H.B.; Cooper, D.S.; Ross, D.S.; Greenlee, M.C.; Laurberg, P.; Maia, A.L.; Rivkees, S.A.; Samuels, M.; Sosa, J.A.; Stan, M.N. 2016 American Thyroid Association Guidelines for Diagnosis and Management of Hyperthyroidism and Other Causes of Thyrotoxicosis. *Thyroid* **2016**, *26*, 1343–1421. [CrossRef]

7. Kut, E.; Atmaca, H. Tirotoksikoz. *J. Exp. Clin. Med.* **2013**, *29*, 309–314. [CrossRef]
8. Karaşahin, Ö.; İba-Yılmaz, S. Soft Tissue Infection after Antithyroid Drug-Associated Agranulocytosis. *Klimik Derg.* **2018**, *31*, 235–237. [CrossRef]
9. Abdi, H.; Amouzegar, A.; Azizi, F. Antithyroid Drugs. *Iran. J. Pharm. Res.* **2019**, *18*, 1–12. [CrossRef]
10. Romeo, A.N.; Običan, S.G. Teratogen Update: Antithyroid Medications. *Birth Defects Res.* **2020**, *112*, 1150–1170. [CrossRef]
11. Dayanan, R.; Bilen, A.; Demirci, T.; Ciftel, S.; Ciftel, E.; Mercantepe, F.; Onalan, E.; Capoglu; Bilen, H. Investigation on the Prevalence of Thyroid Cancer in Graves' Patients in Northeastern Part of Turkey: Is Surgery a Better Option for Patients with Graves' Disease Who Develop Antithyroid Drug-Related Major Adverse Events? *Eur. Rev. Med. Pharmacol. Sci.* **2022**, *26*, 3562–3569. [CrossRef]
12. Darr, E.A.; Randolph, G.W. Management of Laryngeal Nerves and Parathyroid Glands at Thyroidectomy. *Oral Oncol.* **2013**, *49*, 665–670. [CrossRef] [PubMed]
13. Burch, H.B.; Burman, K.D.; Cooper, D.S. A 2011 Survey of Clinical Practice Patterns in the Management of Graves' Disease. *J. Clin. Endocrinol. Metab.* **2012**, *97*, 4549–4558. [CrossRef] [PubMed]
14. Liu, B.; Tian, R.; Peng, W.; He, Y.; Huang, R.; Kuang, A. Radiation Safety Precautions in 131I Therapy of Graves' Disease Based on Actual Biokinetic Measurements. *J. Clin. Endocrinol. Metab.* **2015**, *100*, 2934–2941. [CrossRef] [PubMed]
15. Diehl, L.A.; Garcia, V.; Bonnema, S.J.; Hegedüs, L.; Albino, C.C.; Graf, H. Management of the Nontoxic Multinodular Goiter in Latin America: Comparison with North America and Europe, an Electronic Survey. *J. Clin. Endocrinol. Metab.* **2005**, *90*, 117–123. [CrossRef]
16. Paschke, R.; Hegedüs, L.; Alexander, E.; Valcavi, R.; Papini, E.; Gharib, H. Thyroid Nodule Guidelines: Agreement, Disagreement and Need for Future Research. *Nat. Rev. Endocrinol.* **2011**, *7*, 354–361. [CrossRef]
17. Mayhew, T.M.; Olsen, D.R. Magnetic Resonance Imaging (MRI) and Model-Free Estimates of Brain Volume Determined Using the Cavalieri Principle. *J. Anat.* **1991**, *178*, 133–144. [PubMed]
18. Stehr, M.; Kiderlen, M.; Dorph-Petersen, K.A. Improving Cavalieri Volume Estimation Based on Non-Equidistant Planar Sections: The Trapezoidal Estimator. *J. Microsc.* **2022**, *288*, 40–53. [CrossRef]
19. Heidari, Z.; Mahmoudzadeh-Sagheb, H.; Shakiba, M.; Gorgich, E.A.C. Brain Structural Changes in Schizophrenia Patients Compared to the Control: A MRI-Based Cavalieri's Method. *Basic Clin. Neurosci.* **2023**, *14*, 355–364. [CrossRef] [PubMed]
20. Mohammed, W.; Ismail, N.; Zidan, M.; Elgyoum, A.; Hassan, H.; Abdelrahman, O. Estimation of Spleen Volume Using MRI Segmentation: Would One Slice Be Enough? *Cureus* **2022**, *14*, 3–9. [CrossRef] [PubMed]
21. Karaca, O.; Buyukmert, A.; Tepe, N.; Ozcan, E.; Kus, I. Volume Estimation of Brain Ventricles Using Cavalieri's Principle and Atlas-Based Methods in Alzheimer Disease: Consistency between Methods. *J. Clin. Neurosci.* **2020**, *78*, 333–338. [CrossRef] [PubMed]
22. Huysmans, D.A.K.C.; Hermus, A.R.M.M.; Corstens, F.H.M.; Barentsz, J.O.; Kloppenborg, P.W.C. Large, Compressive Goiters Treated with Radioiodine. *Ann. Intern. Med.* **1994**, *121*, 757–762. [CrossRef]
23. Bonnema, S.J.; Bertelsen, H.; Mortensen, J.; Andersen, P.B.; Knudsen, D.U.; Bastholt, L.; Hegedüs, L. The Feasibility of High Dose Iodine 131 Treatment as an Alternative to Surgery in Patients with a Very Large Goiter: Effect on Thyroid Function and Size and Pulmonary Function. *J. Clin. Endocrinol. Metab.* **1999**, *84*, 3636–3641. [CrossRef] [PubMed]
24. Gabriele, R.; Letizia, C.; Borghese, M.; De Toma, G.; Celi, M.; Izzo, L.; Cavallaro, A. Hyperthyroidism. *Horm. Res.* **2003**, *60*, 79–83. [CrossRef]
25. Elbers, L.P.B.; Fliers, E.; Cannegieter, S.C. The Influence of Thyroid Function on the Coagulation System and Its Clinical Consequences. *J. Thromb. Haemost.* **2018**, *16*, 634–645. [CrossRef] [PubMed]
26. Yuan, S.; Liu, C.; Liu, Z.; Wang, J.; Xu, Y.; Shi, J. Correlation between Thyroid Function Indices and Urine Iodine Levels in Patients with Nodular Goiter. *Am. J. Transl. Res.* **2023**, *15*, 4147–4154. [PubMed]
27. Kahaly, G.J. Management of Graves Thyroidal and Extrathyroidal Disease: An Update. *J. Clin. Endocrinol. Metab.* **2020**, *105*, 3704–3720. [CrossRef] [PubMed]
28. Metso, S.; Jaatinen, P.; Huhtala, H.; Luukkaala, T.; Oksala, H.; Salmi, J. Long-Term Follow-up Study of Radioiodine Treatment of Hyperthyroidism. *Clin. Endocrinol. (Oxf.)* **2004**, *61*, 641–648. [CrossRef] [PubMed]
29. Hegedus, L.; Molholm Hansen, B.; Knudsen, N.; Molholm Hansen, J. Reduction of Size of Thyroid with Radioactive Iodine in Multinodular Non-Toxic Goitre. *Br. Med. J.* **1988**, *297*, 661–662. [CrossRef] [PubMed]
30. Nygaard, B.; Hegedüs, L.; Ulriksen, P.; Nielsen, K.G.; Hansen, J.M. Radioiodine Therapy for Multinodular Toxic Goiter. *Arch. Intern. Med.* **1999**, *159*, 1364–1368. [CrossRef] [PubMed]
31. Nygaard, B.; Hegedüs, L.; Nielsen, K.G.; Ulriksen, P.; Hansen, J.M. Long-Term Effect of Radioactive Iodine on Thyroid Function and Size in Patients with Solitary Autonomously Functioning Toxic Thyroid Nodules. *Clin. Endocrinol. (Oxf.)* **1999**, *50*, 197–202. [CrossRef] [PubMed]
32. Bonnema, S.J.; Nielsen, V.E.; Hegedüs, L. Long-Term Effects of Radioiodine on Thyroid Function, Size and Patient Satisfaction in Non-Toxic Diffuse Goitre. *Eur. J. Endocrinol.* **2004**, *150*, 439–445. [CrossRef] [PubMed]

33. Sorensen, J.R.; Lauridsen, J.F.; Døssing, H.; Nguyen, N.; Hegedüs, L.; Bonnema, S.J.; Godballe, C. Thyroidectomy Improves Tracheal Anatomy and Airflow in Patients with Nodular Goiter: A Prospective Cohort Study. *Eur. Thyroid J.* **2017**, *6*, 307–314. [CrossRef]
34. Weetman, A.P. Radioiodine Treatment for Benign Thyroid Diseases. *Clin. Endocrinol. (Oxf.)* **2007**, *66*, 757–764. [CrossRef] [PubMed]
35. Tasche, K.K.; Dorneden, A.M.; Swift, W.M.; Boyd, N.H.; Shonka, D.C.; Pagedar, N.A. Airway Management in Substernal Goiter Surgery. *Ann. Otol. Rhinol. Laryngol.* **2022**, *131*, 225–228. [CrossRef] [PubMed]
36. Bible, K.C.; Kebebew, E.; Brierley, J.; Brito, J.P.; Cabanillas, M.E.; Clark, T.J.; Di Cristofano, A.; Foote, R.; Giordano, T.; Kasperbauer, J.; et al. 2021 American Thyroid Association Guidelines for Management of Patients with Anaplastic Thyroid Cancer. *Thyroid* **2021**, *31*, 337–386. [CrossRef] [PubMed]
37. Bachmann, J.; Kobe, C.; Bor, S.; Rahlff, I.; Dietlein, M.; Schicha, H.; Schmidt, M. Radioiodine Therapy for Thyroid Volume Reduction of Large Goitres. *Nucl. Med. Commun.* **2009**, *30*, 466–471. [CrossRef]
38. Vargas-Uricoechea, H.; Bonelo-Perdomo, A.; Sierra-Torres, C.H.; Meza-Cabrera, I. Autoimmune Thyroid Disease (Flajani-Parry-Graves-von Basedow Disease): An Overview of Treatment BT—Thyroid Disorders: Basic Science and Clinical Practice. In *Thyroid Disorders*; Imam, S.K., Ahmad, S.I., Eds.; Springer International Publishing: Cham, Switzerland, 2016; pp. 169–184. ISBN 978-3-319-25871-3.
39. Kaniuka-Jakubowska, S.; Lewczuk, A.; Mizan-Gross, K.; Piskunowicz, M.; Zapaśnik, A.; Lass, P.; Sworczak, K. Large Multinodular Goitre—Outpatient Radioiodine Treatment. *Endokrynol. Pol.* **2015**, *66*, 301–307. [CrossRef] [PubMed]
40. Maurer, A.H.; Charkes, N.D. Radioiodine treatment for nontoxic multinodular goiter. *J. Nucl. Med.* **1999**, *40*, 1313–1316. [PubMed]
41. Nygaard, B.; Hegedus, L.; Gervil, M.; Hjalgrim, H.; Soe-Jensen, P.; Molholm Hansen, J. Radioiodine Treatment of Multinodular Non-Toxic Goitre. *Br. Med. J.* **1993**, *307*, 828–832. [CrossRef] [PubMed]
42. Hegedüs, L.; Bonnema, S.J. Approach to Management of the Patient with Primary or Secondary Intrathoracic Goiter. *J. Clin. Endocrinol. Metab.* **2010**, *95*, 5155–5162. [CrossRef] [PubMed]
43. Massaro, F.; Vera, L.; Schiavo, M.; Lagasio, C.; Caputo, M.; Bagnasco, M.; Minuto, F.; Giusti, M. Ultrasonography Thyroid Volume Estimation in Hyperthyroid Patients Treated with Individual Radioiodine Dose. *J. Endocrinol. Investig.* **2007**, *30*, 318–322. [CrossRef] [PubMed]
44. Bonnema, S.J.; Hegedüs, L. A 30-Year Perspective on Radioiodine Therapy of Benign Nontoxic Multinodular Goiter. *Curr. Opin. Endocrinol. Diabetes Obes.* **2009**, *16*, 379–384. [CrossRef]
45. Nielsen, V.E.; Bonnema, S.J.; Boel-Jørgensen, H.; Veje, A.; Hegedüs, L. Recombinant Human Thyrotropin Markedly Changes the 131I Kinetics during 131I Therapy of Patients with Nodular Goiter: An Evaluation by a Randomized Double-Blinded Trial. *J. Clin. Endocrinol. Metab.* **2005**, *90*, 79–83. [CrossRef]
46. Fast, S.; Nielsen, V.E.; Bonnema, S.J.; Hegegüs, L. Time to Reconsider Nonsurgical Therapy of Benign Non-Toxic Multinodular Goitre: Focus on Recombinant Human TSH Augmented Radioiodine Therapy. *Eur. J. Endocrinol.* **2009**, *160*, 517–528. [CrossRef] [PubMed]
47. Braverman, L.; Kloos, R.T.; Law, B.; Kipnes, M.; Dionne, M.; Magner, J. Evaluation of Various Doses of Recombinant Human Thyrotropin in Patients with Multinodular Goiters. *Endocr. Pract.* **2008**, *14*, 832–839. [CrossRef] [PubMed]
48. Albino, C.C.; Mesa, C.O.; Olandoski, M.; Ueda, C.E.; Woellner, L.C.; Goedert, C.A.; Souza, A.M.; Graf, H. Recombinant Human Thyrotropin as Adjuvant in the Treatment of Multinodular Goiters with Radioiodine. *J. Clin. Endocrinol. Metab.* **2005**, *90*, 2775–2780. [CrossRef] [PubMed]
49. Albino, C.C.; Graf, H.; Paz-Filho, G.; Diehl, L.A.; Olandoski, M.; Sabbag, A.; Buchpiguel, C. Radioiodine plus Recombinant Human Thyrotropin Do Not Cause Acute Airway Compression and Are Effective in Reducing Multinodular Goiter. *Braz. J. Med. Biol. Res.* **2010**, *43*, 303–309. [CrossRef]

Journal of
Clinical Medicine

MDPI

Review

Autoimmune Thyroid Disease and Pregnancy: The Interaction Between Genetics, Epigenetics and Environmental Factors

Tatjana Bogović Crnčić [1,†], Božena Ćurko-Cofek [2,†], Lara Batičić [3,*], Neva Girotto [4], Maja Ilić Tomaš [1], Antea Kršek [5], Ines Krištofić [6], Tea Štimac [6], Ivona Perić [7], Vlatka Sotošek [8,9,*] and Sanja Klobučar [7,10]

1 Department of Nuclear Medicine, Faculty of Medicine, University of Rijeka, Braće Branchetta 20, 51000 Rijeka, Croatia; tatjanabc@medri.uniri.hr (T.B.C.); maja.ilic.tomas@uniri.hr (M.I.T.)
2 Department of Physiology, Immunology and Pathophysiology, Faculty of Medicine, University of Rijeka, Braće Branchetta 20, 51000 Rijeka, Croatia; bozena.curko.cofek@uniri.hr
3 Department of Medical Chemistry, Biochemistry and Clinical Chemistry, Faculty of Medicine, University of Rijeka, Braće Branchetta 20, 51000 Rijeka, Croatia
4 Department of Radiology Diagnostics, Faculty of Health Studies, University of Rijeka, Viktora Cara Emina 2, 51000 Rijeka, Croatia; neva.girotto@uniri.hr
5 Faculty of Medicine, University of Rijeka, Braće Branchetta 20, 51000 Rijeka, Croatia; antea.krsek@uniri.hr
6 Department of Obstetrics and Gynecology, Faculty of Medicine, University of Rijeka, Braće Branchetta 20, 51000 Rijeka, Croatia; ines.kristofic@uniri.hr (I.K.); tea.stimac@uniri.hr (T.Š.)
7 Department of Endocrinology, Diabetes and Metabolic Diseases, Clinical Hospital Centre Rijeka, 51000 Rijeka, Croatia; ivona.peric@uniri.hr (I.P.); sanja.klobucar@uniri.hr (S.K.)
8 Department of Anesthesiology, Reanimatology, Emergency and Intensive Care Medicine, University of Rijeka, Braće Branchetta 20, 51000 Rijeka, Croatia
9 Department of Clinical Medical Sciences II, Faculty of Health Studies, University of Rijeka, Viktora Cara Emina 2, 51000 Rijeka, Croatia
10 Department of Internal Medicine, Faculty of Medicine, University of Rijeka, Braće Branchetta 20, 51000 Rijeka, Croatia
* Correspondence: lara.baticic@uniri.hr (L.B.); vlatkast@uniri.hr (V.S.)
† These authors contributed equally to this work.

Abstract: Autoimmune thyroid disease (AITD) is the leading cause of thyroid dysfunction globally, characterized primarily by two distinct clinical manifestations: Hashimoto's thyroiditis (HT) and Graves' disease (GD). The prevalence of AITD is approximately twice as high in women compared to men, with a particularly pronounced risk during the reproductive years. Pregnancy exerts profound effects on thyroid physiology and immune regulation due to hormonal fluctuations and immune adaptations aimed at fostering maternal–fetal tolerance, potentially triggering or exacerbating AITD. The impact of AITD on pregnancy outcomes is multifaceted. Both HT and GD have been associated with adverse obstetric and neonatal outcomes, including miscarriage, preterm delivery, preeclampsia and fetal growth restriction. Inadequately managed AITD can also affect fetal neurodevelopment due to disrupted maternal thyroid hormone availability during critical periods of brain maturation. This review explores the complex interplay between the genetic, epigenetic and environmental factors that drive AITD during pregnancy, highlighting their roles in disease development and impacts on pregnancy outcomes. Gaining a deeper understanding of these mechanisms is crucial for improving diagnostic tools, treatment options and preventive measures to enhance the health and well-being of both the mother and the newborn.

Keywords: autoimmune thyroid disease; Graves' disease; Hashimoto's thyroiditis; maternal-fetal health; pregnancy; thyroid dysfunction

1. Introduction

Autoimmune thyroid disease (AITD) is caused by dysregulation of the immune system which results in an autoimmune attack on the thyroid gland. Hypothyroidism and hyperthyroidism are the two clinical faces of AITD, the most common cause of thyroid dysfunction involving various cellular and humoral interactions within thyroid tissue, mainly categorized as Hashimoto's thyroiditis (HT) and Graves' disease (GD). The global prevalence of AITD has increased and now affects approximately 5% of the world's population. However, despite having a history more than a century long, the pathogenesis of both entities is still not fully understood [1].

The development of AITD is believed to result from a complex interplay of genetic predisposition and environmental factors that lead to a breakdown in immune tolerance and trigger an autoimmune response against the thyroid gland. Central to this process is the disruption of tolerance to self-antigens involving a complex network of interactions between thyroid follicular cells (TFCs), stromal cells and immune cells [2].

In patients with AITD, cellular and humoral immunity play a role. As a result, lymphocytes infiltrate the thyroid parenchyma, targeting thyroid antigens such as the sodium iodide symporter, thyroglobulin (Tg), thyroid-stimulating hormone receptor (TSH-R) and the enzyme thyroid peroxidase (TPO) [3,4]. One of the components that have an immunomodulatory effect is thyroid hormone status, as immune cells contain receptors for thyroid hormones [5]. In AITD, other factors such as genetic susceptibility through the polymorphism of human leukocyte antigen (HLA) system genes and thyroid-specific AITD susceptibility genes also appear to play a role, together with epigenetic and environmental factors including excessive iodine consumption, selenium [6,7] and vitamin D deficiency [8], infectious agents [9] and gut microbiota dysbiosis [10,11]. A link between HT and interferon (IFN)-α, lithium or amiodarone therapy has also been recognized [12,13], and even a possible connection with climate factors, with an increased incidence in colder regions of the world, has been suggested [14]. Smoking and stress are also associated with the risk of GD [15,16]. Thyroid hormones play an important role in both innate immunity and the adaptive immune response. Both disorders, GD and HT, are defined by circulating thyroid-specific antibodies and the infiltration of autoreactive lymphocytes into the thyroid gland and are of great concern during pregnancy as they can greatly affect both maternal and fetal outcomes [2,9,15]. The involvement of environmental factors in the development and expression of AITD is important in terms of disease progression and pregnancy outcome. Therefore, lifestyle intervention with the above modifiable risk factors could help to maintain low AITD risk and improve pregnancy outcomes.

The prevalence of AITD in the general population is estimated to be approximately 5–10%, with variations depending on demographic and geographic factors. AITD is a common endocrine disorder among pregnant women, with a prevalence ranging from 2% to 5% [1–4]. Its clinical significance during pregnancy is substantial, as thyroid dysfunction can impact both maternal and fetal health. For instance, maternal hypothyroidism is associated with adverse pregnancy outcomes, including preterm birth, low birth weight and impaired neurodevelopment in the newborn [3,5]. On the other hand, untreated maternal hyperthyroidism induces risks such as preeclampsia, preterm delivery and fetal growth restriction [4,5,14]. Therefore, the early identification and management of AITD in pregnancy are critical to optimizing outcomes for both the mother and the child. The aim of this review is to describe the main genetic, epigenetic and environmental factors involved in the pathogenesis of AITD, focusing on their role in pregnancy in patients with thyroid autoimmunity.

2. Clinical Forms of Autoimmune Thyroid Diseases

The clinical presentations of AITD are diverse and can manifest as hyperthyroidism (e.g., GD), hypothyroidism (e.g., HT) or a combination of thyrotoxicosis and hypothyroidism, as seen in postpartum thyroiditis (PPT). Importantly, while GD is commonly associated with hyperthyroidism, it can also present with hypothyroidism in cases involving blocking thyroid receptor antibodies (TRAb). Furthermore, in GD, phases of hyperthyroidism and hypothyroidism may alternate or overlap, which is also a common feature of this condition.

2.1. Autoimmune Hyperthyroidism

GD was named after Robert Graves, an Irish physician, who first described this form of hyperthyroidism in 1835. There are differences in incidence between genders (women 5–15% and men 1–5%) [17], especially during the reproductive period [18]. GD includes a range of symptoms including hyperthyroidism, diffuse goiter, Graves' orbitopathy (GO) and dermopathy [19,20] and is the most common cause of hyperthyroidism, representing 60% to 80% of cases of hyperthyroidism [21]. It is most common between the ages of 40 and 60 [22]. GD is characterized by a hypoechoic and inhomogeneous parenchyma, often accompanied by thyroid gland enlargement, as seen on ultrasound. A family history of thyroid disease, especially in maternal relatives, is associated with an increased risk of GD [23]. GD occurs due to the presence of stimulatory anti-TSH-R autoantibodies (TRAbs), which bind to and activate the TSH-R. Activation of the receptor leads to cell hyperplasia and hypertrophy of the thyroid follicles and, consequently, to the increased synthesis of thyroid hormones. TRAbs are mainly synthesized by B lymphocytes in the thyroid gland but can also be produced in lymph nodes and bone marrow. After the sensitization of T lymphocytes with thyroid antigens, B lymphocytes are activated [23].

The pathology of thyroid diseases lies in the interaction between thyroid hormones, the immune system and minerals. The minerals that are mostly involved in this interaction are magnesium, selenium, calcium, zinc, iron and copper [24]. Zinc participates in the immune system as an immunomodulator, and its deficiency suppresses the innate and adaptive response [24]. In hyperthyroidism, the impaired mitochondrial function in hyperthyroidism is likely related to deficiencies in magnesium, selenium and the antioxidant coenzyme Q10. [24]. Clinically, hyperthyroidism manifests itself through general signs of metabolic acceleration: nervousness, hyperactivity, mood swings, sleep disorders, sensitivity to heat, muscle weakness and diarrhea.

2.2. Autoimmune Hypothyroidism

In his report, from 1912, Hakaru Hashimoto was the first to describe the lymphocytic infiltration of the enlarged thyroid gland and, thus, introduced the term lymphomatous goiter [25]. It is now considered the most common autoimmune disease characterized by the cellular immune response and lymphocytic infiltration resulting in the gradual destruction of thyroid tissue, and often leading to hypothyroidism [26,27].

The incidence of HT is estimated at 0.3–1.5 cases per 1000 people [28], with a higher prevalence in women (5–15% vs. 1–5% in men), especially those middle aged and living in iodine-sufficient areas [29]. Recent data also suggest a higher incidence in the same geographical areas compared to prior studies, and an overall increase in the incidence of AITD in recent years [30].

Typical ultrasonography findings include enlargement of the thyroid gland with hypoechoic and inhomogeneous parenchyma [31]. The risk of HT is higher in relatives, especially those with other autoimmune diseases. Although thyroid autoantibody titers do not seem to play a significant role in the pathogenesis of this disease, thyroid peroxidase antibodies (TPOAbs) are present in almost 90% of cases and 5–20% of women of reproductive age are considered positive for thyroid autoimmunity [32].

Subclinical cases of HT are defined by elevated thyroid-stimulating hormone (TSH) and normal thyroid hormone levels, without typical symptoms, but with an increased rate of cardiovascular morbidity [33]. It is estimated that hypothyroidism develops in approximately 20–30% of patients with HT. Interestingly, some large population studies suggest that subclinical hypothyroidism in the elderly population may be associated with reduced morbidity [34].

When it occurs clinically, hypothyroidism is manifested by general signs of a metabolic slowdown (weight gain, slowed heart rate and bowel movements, edema, fatigue, normocytic anemia, skin changes with hair and body hair loss and anovulatory cycles with menorrhagia) and memory impairment [35]. In an early stage, symptoms and signs of thyrotoxicosis, due to a massive release of thyroid hormones from damaged thyroid cells, may also occur [36].

The diagnosis of HT is based on clinical symptoms, the presence of circulating antibodies to thyroid antigens (mainly TPOAbs and TgAbs) and / or a typical sonographic appearance of the thyroid gland. Ultrasonography is particularly important in establishing the diagnosis in patients with seronegative HT, which occurs in 5–10% of cases [28].

3. Pregnancy and Autoimmune Thyroid Disease

A healthy pregnancy and proper fetal development are of the utmost importance. During pregnancy, maintaining optimal thyroid function is crucial for the health of the mother and the development of the fetus. Pregnancy places increased demands on the thyroid gland as thyroid hormones play a critical role in fetal growth and neurological development, especially in the first trimester when the fetus is completely dependent on maternal thyroid hormones. Thyroid hormones are critical for fetal brain development, and the disruption of thyroid function due to AITD can have detrimental effects on the child's neurological outcomes [37].

The course and progression of AITD can vary during pregnancy and may change after delivery. This is because the mother's immune system undergoes significant changes during pregnancy, with metabolic adaptations that help maintain immune tolerance to the fetus, which carries paternal antigens on its cells [38]. Therefore, despite transient immunosuppression, maternal immunity must be able to maintain effective protection of both the mother and the fetus against infection while protecting the fetus from the maternal immune system. It is, therefore, assumed that cellular immunity is reduced during pregnancy in order not to reject the fetus. However, these changes in the immune status of the pregnant woman appear to influence the course of the autoimmune disease itself [39]. The natural history of GD includes improvement in the second half of the pregnancy and worsening or recurrence after delivery, which is partly explained by the immunomodulation of the maternal immune response during pregnancy [40]. However, the pathophysiology and mechanisms underlying these changes are unknown and require further research.

3.1. Autoimmune Hyperthyroidism in Pregnancy

Hyperthyroidism during pregnancy is rare, occurring in 1–3/1000 pregnancies (its prevalence is 0.1–0.3%), depending on whether overt or subclinical forms are considered [41,42]. The most common cause is GD, which is estimated to account for 85–95% of clinically significant cases of hyperthyroidism [43]. Since some authors have shown that the functional activity of TRAbs changes from stimulation to inhibition [44–46], this means that GD should be well monitored during pregnancy. The symptoms of GD in pregnancy are no different from those in non-pregnant women but can be confused with the symptoms of pregnancy [47].

Since maternal thyroid function undergoes significant changes during pregnancy, different approaches are needed when interpreting thyroid function tests in pregnant women compared to non-pregnant women [47]. The evaluation begins with the TSH level, which is often lowered during pregnancy due to human chorionic gonadotropin (hCG) stimulation. TSH levels are trimester-specific, and the disease is characterized by an elevated thyroxine (T4) and triiodothyronine (T3) level and suppressed serum TSH [48]. Free T4 (FT4) and free T3 (FT3) levels are evaluated, and total T4, T3 and thyroxin-binding globulin (TBG) levels may be clinically useful when available [41,43,49–53]. In GD, (stimulating) TRAbs are usually measurable and can be used to confirm the diagnosis and differentiate it from transient gestational thyrotoxicosis [50] (Figure 1). Uncontrolled GD during pregnancy can lead to significant maternal, fetal and neonatal complications [49].

Since the fetal thyroid gland is mature from 20 weeks onwards, it could respond to the influence of both antithyroid drugs (ATDs) and TRAbs [47]. Fetal hyperthyroidism could be caused by the transplacental passage of excess thyroid hormone or by the activation of the thyroid gland with stimulating TRAbs [54–56]. Autoimmune hyperthyroidism has even been documented in babies born to mothers who were treated for GD several years earlier but who still had detectable circulating thyroid receptor antibodies [57]. Serious complications are usually due to fetal hyperthyroidism, which can even lead to fetal death [58]. Obstetric ultrasound offers the possibility of screening for thyroid dysfunction. The findings may include an enlarged thyroid gland, intrauterine growth restriction, hydrops, advanced bone maturity, heart failure, goiter and oligohydramnios [43,51,53,54]. In addition, thyroid hormones have an impact on neurodevelopmental abnormalities by regulating the migration, growth and differentiation of fetal neurons [54]. The guidelines of the American Thyroid Association (2017) and the European Thyroid Association (2018) recommend monitoring TRAb levels in maternal blood during pregnancy and the additional testing of fetal thyroid function in newborns shortly after birth [58–60].

Significant thyroid enlargement can lead to difficulties in fetal head mobility and, possibly, abnormal presentation at birth, dysphagia leading to polyhydramnios and, consequently, premature birth, or the compression of immature tracheal cartilage leading to airway obstruction. Polyhydramnios can trigger and promote premature birth, the leading cause of neonatal morbidity and mortality [47].

Neonatal hyperthyroidism because of the persistence of maternal TRAb (half-life about 2 weeks) can occur in 1–5% of infants. After the disappearance of maternal TRAbs, neonatal central hypothyroidism may occur due to the persistent suppression of fetal pituitary TSH production [41].

Maternal complications of hyperthyroidism include hypertension, preeclampsia and placental abruption [50]. Two other serious complications are thyroid storm, which is characterized by altered mental status, hyperthermia, tachycardia, left dentate dysfunction, multiorgan failure and congestive heart failure [41], which can be diagnosed in 10% of untreated severe hyperthyroidism cases due to the increased cardiac workload. The much higher rate in pregnant women compared with non-pregnant women could be explained by co-existing pregnancy complications (severe preeclampsia, anemia, hemorrhage, etc.) [61].

Hyperthyroidism in pregnancy is treated with drugs that inhibit the excessive synthesis of thyroid hormones [50]. All ATDs cross the placenta and can, therefore, affect the fetal thyroid gland, so the lowest dose should be used to maintain FT4 levels [62]. Treatment with ATDs is necessary despite the potential teratogenicity due to the negative impact on maternal health and the risk of fetal loss in untreated overt hyperthyroidism [48,52].

Hypothyroidism caused by ATDs is usually transient and corrects itself when the drug is metabolized after birth, although this requires close monitoring [58].

Due to the immunosuppressive effect of pregnancy, GD is in remission in many women towards the end of pregnancy [52]. As with other autoimmune diseases, GD typically improves due to immune tolerance during pregnancy, which aims to prevent the fetus from being rejected as a foreign body by immunologic molecules of trophoblastic origin and T-cell subsets [T-regulatory cells (T-reg)] that arise in the decidua [41,42,63]. T-reg cells induce transient immunosuppression in the maternal circulation, which can attenuate the onset of GD [41]. After delivery, the abrupt drop in T-reg cells is the reason for the postpartum resurgence of autoimmunity and the exacerbation of GD [41]. In some cases, TRAbs may have an inhibitory effect instead of stimulating the thyroid gland. After delivery, there is a risk of exacerbation or relapse due to the rebound of the maternal immune system, usually 7–9 months after pregnancy [64].

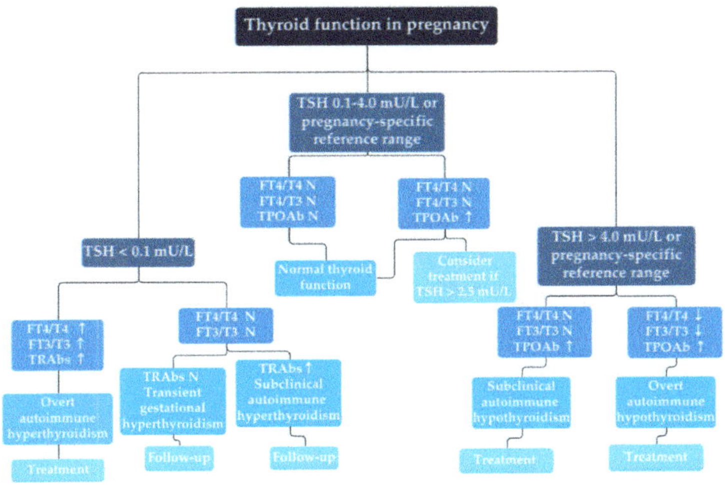

Figure 1. Assessment of thyroid function during pregnancy. The figure shows a schematic representation of thyroid function tests during pregnancy according to the American Thyroid Association (2017) [58]. Overt autoimmune hyperthyroidism is characterized by a thyroid stimulating hormone (TSH) level of less than 0.1 mU/L and elevated thyroid hormones and thyroid receptor antibodies (TRAbs), indicating the need for treatment. Transient gestational thyrotoxicosis is suspected when normal thyroid hormone levels are observed while TSH is suppressed and TRAb levels are in the reference range. If TRAb levels are elevated, subclinical autoimmune hyperthyroidism should be considered. In both cases, a follow-up examination is required. (Abbreviations: TSH—thyroid stimulating hormone, T4—thyroxine, FT4—free thyroxine, T3—triiodothyronine, FT3—free triiodothyronine, TRAbs—thyroid receptor antibodies, TPOAb—thyroid peroxidase antibody, and N—normal, ↑—elevated, ↓—decreased).

Maternal overt or subclinical hypothyroidism is defined when the TSH level is above the population-based pregnancy-specific reference range; if this is not available, a TSH cut-off value of 4.0 mU/L is recommended. A TSH value between 0.1 and 4.0 mU/L or a population-based pregnancy-specific reference range with normal thyroid hormone and TPOAb indicates normal thyroid function and requires no further testing. However, if the TSH level is above 2.5 mU/L and the TPOAbs are elevated, levothyroxine therapy could be considered. On the other hand, if TSH is above 4.0 mU/L or the population-based pregnancy-specific reference range and TPOAbs are elevated, subclinical (normal thyroid hormone levels) or overt (reduced thyroid hormone levels) autoimmune hypothyroidism is diagnosed and supplementation with levothyroxine is recommended.

3.2. Autoimmune Hypothyroidism in Pregnancy

It is estimated that 5–15% of healthy women of reproductive age are affected by HT [65]. In addition, approximately 2–17% of pregnant women have increased levels of TPOAb and TgAb. These antibodies have been shown to gradually decrease during pregnancy, reaching their lowest levels in the third trimester, then rising again as early as 6 weeks post-partum and returning to pre-pregnancy levels approximately 12 weeks later [66].

The inability of the thyroid gland to cope with increased hormonal demands during pregnancy often results in subclinical or overt hypothyroidism, which has significant implications for maternal and fetal health, including an increased risk of miscarriage, preterm labor, placental abruption, preeclampsia and gestational hypertension, postpartum thyroid dysfunction and other risks [67]. In developing fetuses, an association between low birth weight, prematurity, developmental delays and stillbirths with maternal hypothyroidism has been confirmed [68]. Maternal hypothyroidism can also have serious effects on the child's cognitive development, as optimal levels of thyroid hormones are necessary to regulate certain processes in the fetal brain, such as neuronal migration and myelination [69,70]. Maternal hypothyroidism is defined as a TSH level that is above the pregnancy-specific reference range. In areas where a pregnancy-specific reference range is not available, a TSH cut-off value of 4.0 mU/L should be used (Figure 1) [58,68]. Women who are euthyroid but tested positive for TPOAb prior to pregnancy are at increased risk of developing elevated TSH during pregnancy and require regular TSH monitoring [69]. In addition, the presence of thyroid autoantibodies in women is associated with a two- to threefold increased risk of pregnancy loss, although the mechanism of action is unknown [71,72]. Even in euthyroid pregnant women, an increased risk of preterm delivery has been found in the presence of thyroid autoantibodies [73].

While overt hypothyroidism affects about 0.2–0.6% of pregnant women [74], subclinical hypothyroidism (SH) is more common and occurs in 3.5–18% of pregnancies [75]. It is characterized by normal levels of free thyroid hormones and TSH levels above the pregnancy reference range [59]. Korevaar et al., in a meta-analysis of 19 cohort studies, found an increased risk of preterm delivery in pregnant women with SH, with an odds ratio 1.04 (95%CI, 1.00–1.09) for each one standard deviation increase in TSH. The risk was also increased in the presence of TPO antibodies [76].

There is a broad consensus on the treatment of overt hypothyroidism in pregnancy. In SH, levothyroxine (LT4) treatment is indicated in TPOAb-positive pregnant women with TSH values above the pregnancy-specific reference range and in TPOAb-negative pregnant women with TSH values above 10.0 mU/L. The question of whether TPO-negative women should be treated with SH remains controversial. The studies by Zhu et al. and Magri et al. have shown that women with SH and without thyroid autoimmunity have a higher prevalence of gestational diabetes, anemia, preeclampsia and fetuses small for gestational age [77,78]. LT4 treatment may be considered in TPOAb-positive pregnant women if TSH levels are above 2.5 mU/L and in TPOAb-negative pregnant women if TSH levels are above the pregnancy-specific reference range but do not exceed 10.0 mU/L (Figure 1) [58,68]. In addition, euthyroid women who test positive for TPOAb and/or TgAb are at risk of PPT within the first year after delivery due to an immune system rebound. Pregnant women with higher TPOAb levels have a higher risk of developing PPT [59]. The diagnosis of HT during pregnancy is difficult because the symptoms of hypothyroidism are like those commonly seen in pregnant women, and the timely determination of serum hormone concentration and TPO autoantibody titer is crucial. Pregnant women with subclinical hypothyroidism or borderline TSH levels early in pregnancy may not be able to meet the increased demand for thyroid hormones and may show signs of thyroid insufficiency during pregnancy [59].

It is important to emphasize that maternal and fetal thyroid functions are closely linked. The fetal thyroid gland concentrates and begins to fully synthesize thyroid hormones only after 18–20 weeks of gestation, but even after that, the fetus requires both maternal and its own thyroid hormones for normal development [74,79]. The adverse effects are thought to depend on the severity and timing of the maternal hormone deficiency. Therefore, overt hypothyroidism should be diagnosed early in pregnancy and treated promptly [74].

Given that AITD is the most common autoimmune disorder in young women, and considering its potential consequences—along with the fact that it can remain undiagnosed (and untreated) in its subclinical form—systematic screening for AITD during pregnancy has been recommended. Several studies have demonstrated the ineffectiveness of selective screening in identifying affected individuals. However, there is still no consensus in favor of the systematic screening of thyroid function in all pregnant women [80].

The complex pathophysiology of thyroid autoimmunity and the effects on thyroid dysfunction during pregnancy are still far from clear. Therefore, further studies are needed to help us uncover the underlying mechanisms and all factors involved.

4. Genetic Factors and Autoimmune Thyroid Diseases

Although HT and GD manifest with contrasting clinical presentations and represent opposite ends of the clinical spectrum of AITD, they share a common complex etiology involving the reciprocal interaction of the genetic basis with epigenetic and environmental factors [81]. AITD is considered a familial disease, as the familial clustering of AITD (risk ratio between siblings) is estimated to be 5.9 to >10, with a value of >5.0 considered significant. A high recurrence rate was found in first- and second-degree relatives of patients with AITD; among GD patients, 6.1% of first-degree relatives had GD, and among HT patients, 4.9% of first-degree relatives were affected [82]. Numerous recent studies have contributed significantly to a better understanding of the role of the genetic component in the development of mechanisms that promote thyroid autoimmunity [81–85]. This is certainly the basis for the earlier identification of individuals at increased risk of developing AITD and for earlier intervention, but also for the development of targeted therapeutic options.

4.1. Immune-Related Genes

HLA complex is a highly polymorphic genetic region that encodes several proteins that play a critical role in regulating the immune response and cellular self-recognition through antigen presentation and lymphocyte activation. More than 70 diseases have been linked to HLA polymorphisms, and many autoimmune diseases are associated with specific variations of the HLA class II gene [83]. Currently, the HLA-DR3 subtype is most consistently correlated with a higher risk of developing AITD. Evidence of this is the fact that 40–50% of GD patients have the HLA-DR3 gene, as opposed to 15–30% of the general population. Although the link between HLA-DR3 and HT was initially less conclusive, it has also been demonstrated [81,86].

The CTLA-4 gene is important for immune regulation as it plays a role as a down-regulator of the T-cell-mediated immune response, while CD152 is one of the expression products of the gene encoding the synthesis of CTLA-4 [82]. The mechanism by which CTLA-4 downregulates T-cell activation is by binding to the intracellular domain of CD152 during the early stage of activation and mediating the negative signaling that inhibits T-cell activation. The increased expression of CD152 on T cells in the late phase of immune activation leads to competition with CD28 for binding to B7 [85]. Consequently, even a subtle polymorphism in the CTLA-4 coding region can contribute to the development of decreased CTLA-4 expression, leading to a hyperactive and self-destructive immune response with increased production and secretion of thyroid autoantibodies and, eventually, AITD [82].

The CD40 is a transmembrane cell surface receptor that is classically expressed on B lymphocytes and other antigen-presenting cells and binds specifically to CD40 ligand (CD40L) on the surface of target cells [82]. Stimulation of the CD40 molecule controls the proliferation, expansion and activation of B cells. It also up-regulates major histocompatibility complex class II (MHC II) on B cells, drives plasma cell differentiation and promotes immunoglobulin isotype class switching and antibody secretion [81]. Some variants of the CD40 single nucleotide polymorphism (SNP) are associated with an increased risk of developing AITD. The variant rs1883832 was most clearly associated with a significant risk of GD, but no association with HT was found [82]. Studies, including immunohistochemistry and flow cytometry, confirmed the increased expression of CD40 in thyroid cells from individuals with GD (particularly in epithelial cells, follicular cells and fibroblasts). One possible mechanism that could explain the susceptibility to AITD is based on the hypothesis that autoantigens from GD patients are processed by the affected thyroid follicular epithelial cells and presented to infiltrating thyroid tissue T cells to induce their activation, while CD40/CD40L enhances the immune response during this process [81,87,88].

The PTPN22 gene plays a role in encoding lymphoid-specific tyrosine phosphatase (LYP), and polymorphism in this genetic region has been shown to have a strong and consistent association with the development of numerous autoimmune diseases. LYP is capable of suppressing kinases that mediate the activation and regulation of T lymphocytes but also plays an important role in B-lymphocyte signaling and is involved at multiple levels in the T-cell receptor signaling and activation cascade. Therefore, after HLA, the PTPN22 gene is the one most strongly associated with increased AITD risk, as it has regulatory effects on multiple cell types involved in the immune response and various signaling pathways [82].

The FOXP3 gene codes to produce the FOXP3 protein, which attaches to specific areas of DNA and helps to control the activities of genes involved in the regulation of the immune system. It is a crucial factor in the physiological development of T-regs. It has been shown that certain nucleotide polymorphism variants weaken the inhibitory function of T-regs and, thus, favor the development of an autoimmune reaction [89,90].

4.2. Thyroid-Specific Genes

The Tg gene is located on chromosome 8q24 and encodes a large glycoprotein homodimer molecule of Tg, which is the most quantitatively dominant autoantigen in the thyroid gland. Tg represents the matrix for thyroid hormone synthesis and the basic storage molecule for newly synthesized T3 and T4 [82]. TSH-R represents a major autoantigen of the thyroid gland, so many studies have been conducted to investigate the association between different TSH-R polymorphisms and the propensity to develop AITD, especially GD [82].

Intron 1 of the TSH-R gene was marked as a region of interest for GD and five GD-associated SNPs were mapped to TSH-R intron 1: rs179247, rs2284720, rs12101255, rs12101261 and rs2268458 [81]. In the current literature, two pathophysiological mechanisms have been proposed to explain the association between intron 1 variants and an increased risk of thyroid autoimmunity. The first mechanism is based on the disruption of peripheral tolerance and the development of an autoimmune reaction to TSH-R due to alterations in mRNA splicing of thyroid genes. The other theory is based on a lack of central immune tolerance due to a reduced expression of TSH-R in the thymus in individuals with the aforementioned SPNs [81,82].

The Tg gene contains more than 16,000 SNPs and certain Tg SNPs and allelic variations have been shown to correlate with AITD [82]. One of the possible underlying mechanisms is thought to be alternate endosomal Tg degradation leading to the release of immunogenic peptides [82]. Lee at al. note that in sequencing studies of the 5′UTR (untranslated region) of Tg, there is an A/G SNP at position 1623 (rs180195) that is strongly associated with AITD since it disrupts a regulatory element within the Tg promoter [81]. Furthermore, they mentioned three missense polymorphisms responsible for altering the amino acid sequence in the Tg molecule, possibly triggering the ER-to-lysosome-associated degradation (ERLAD) pathway of Tg and the generation of peptides that have an increasing binding affinity for HLA-DRb-Arg74 [81], thus resulting in significantly increased probability of GD occurrence [91].

The TPO gene is located on chromosome 2p25 and encodes TPO, a glycosylated hemoporotein located in the apical membrane of thyrocytes and consisting of a large extracellular, a short transmembrane domain and an intracellular C-terminal region. Its function is to catalyze the iodination of the tyrosine residues of Tg. Although TPO is considered one of the major thyroid antigens and AITD can result from several mechanisms (including total TPO dysfunction, heme cofactor binding disruption, inability to interact with the Tg substrate and disruption of localization with subcellular placement), the number of studies reporting the association of TPO gene polymorphisms with the development and prognosis of AITD is modest [82]. In their study, Tomari et al. genotyped eight single nucleotide polymorphisms in the TPO gene and demonstrated that TPO rs2071400 T carriers (CT + TT genotypes) and the TPO rs2071403 GG genotype were more common in individuals with AITD, including GD and HD patients [92]. However, no significant association was found between the SNPs and the prognosis of AITD. On the other hand, serum levels of TPOAb were significantly higher in AITD patients who were TPO rs2071400 T carriers (CT + TT genotypes) and TPO rs2048722 T carriers (CT + TT genotypes) than in those with the CC genotype [92].

4.3. Epigenetics Factors in Autoimmune Thyroid Disease

Since the AITD risk for some of the previously mentioned genes is rather low, it is thought that a synergy of environmental factors and genetic susceptibility may be necessary to trigger the development of AITD [82]. Epigenetics is considered a key factor in the integration of these genetic and environmental elements. Epigenetics provides insights into the mechanisms involved in the regulation of gene expression without changes in the underlying DNA sequence. The most important epigenetic mechanisms in AITD include DNA methylation, histone modifications, RNA interference by non-coding RNAs and inactivation of the X chromosome [93].

DNA methylation refers to the process of binding methyl groups to specific DNA regions, usually silencing gene expression [94]. In AITD, DNA methylation abnormalities affect the immune-related and thyroid-specific genes mentioned earlier. For example, in GD, the hypomethylation of genes related to immune activation contributes to the production of thyroid-stimulating antibodies. On the other hand, some genetic polymorphisms of DNA methylation-regulating genes can also lead to the dysfunction and maldevelopment of the DNA methylation process, further increasing the susceptibility to disease. Studies on DNA methylation are still limited and show high variability, but all agree with the conclusion that abnormal DNA methylation plays an important role in the pathogenesis of AITD [95].

Histone modifications play an important role in the control of chromatin compaction, nucleosome dynamics and DNA repair and can directly regulate transcription [96]. Like

DNA methylation, histone modifications are highly dynamic and can alter gene expression. Recent studies have provided evidence for their role in the modulation of immune tolerance and the development of autoimmune diseases [97]. Further research is needed to clarify the role of histone modifications in the pathogenesis of AITD, but also to elucidate their potential role as diagnostic biomarkers and predictors of treatment success in AITD patients [92].

Non-coding RNAs are small RNAs, especially microRNAs with a length of 18 to 25 nucleotides, which play an important role in the post-transcriptional regulation of gene expression [98]. Some miRNAs such as miR-223-3p and miR-155-5p also play an important role in regulating immune function and maintaining immune homeostasis. There-fore, it is not surprising that the abnormal expression of miRNAs involved in immune function may contribute to the development of autoimmune diseases [99–101]

Several recent studies have provided evidence of the abnormal expression of miR-155-5p and miR-146a-5p in AITD patients [102,103]. The abnormal expression of miR-155-5p and miR-146a-5p can certainly promote the development of AITD by disrupting immune homeostasis and immune tolerance [92]. Bernecker et al. found that patients with GD and HT had significantly lower levels of miR-146a-5p and miR-155-5p in thyroid tissue [104]. Currently, there are many studies investigating the differentially expressed miRNAs in AITD patients, but studies specifically exploring their clinical utility should be prioritized.

Inactivation of the X chromosome (XCI) is an important epigenetic trait that occurs randomly in females and involves the transcriptional silencing of an X chromosome. AITD has been shown to affect female patients more frequently, raising the question of a possible key role of XCI in the developmental process. An underlying mechanism could be distorted XCI, which may lead to a loss of balance of gene products and immune tolerance. Several previous studies have demonstrated an increased frequency of skewed XCI in AITD patients, while Ishido at al. found a non-significant difference in prevalence between GD patients and healthy individuals but demonstrated a correlation between skewed X chromosome and GD progression [105].

4.4. Environmental Factors

The key environmental factors involved in development of AITD are iodine excess, deficiency of selenium, iron and vitamin D, smoking, stress and infections [106,107] as shown on Figure 2.

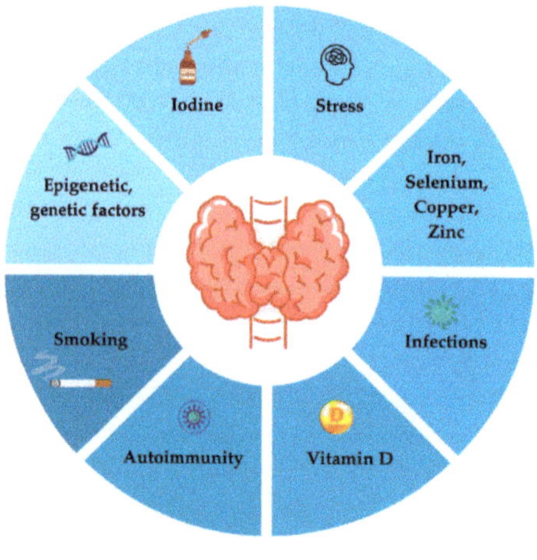

Figure 2. Key factors influencing thyroid function. Figure illustrates the most critical physiological, environmental, genetic and lifestyle factors that impact thyroid function.

4.4.1. Iodine Intake and Autoimmune Thyroid Disease

Of all the environmental factors that influence AITD, iodine is the most important because it is necessary for the synthesis of thyroid hormones [106,107]. Iodine is incorporated into the tyrosine residues of Tg, which ultimately leads to the production of the hormones T3 and T4. Iodine deficiency continues to be an important public issue and a common health problem worldwide. It is associated with decreased serum levels of thyroid hormones and leads to goiter, hypothyroidism, irreversible cognitive impairment, cretinism and even cancer [16,24]. On the other hand, it is also known that excess iodine can lead to thyroid dysfunction, resulting in either hypothyroidism or thyrotoxicosis through a transient destructive effect on thyroid cells or even hyperthyroidism if autonomously functioning thyroid tissue is present [108]. In addition, evidence has accumulated over the years that iodine prophylaxis is associated with an increased prevalence of thyroid autoimmunity, especially in areas previously deficient in iodine [109,110]. The exact cause of thyroid autoimmunity in relation to iodine is still not fully understood. The thyroid autoimmune process may be exacerbated or triggered by excessive or insufficient iodine intake [111]. The increasing prevalence and variety of thyroid disorders suggest possible negative effects of increased iodine intake. This trend is consistent with observations from studies conducted in both the United States and Europe [112,113]. There are data suggesting that iodine may be involved in triggering the process of lymphocytic intrathyroidal infiltration. One of the possible explanations is that iodine could increase the production of cytokines such as tumor necrosis factor (TNF)-alpha and chemokines and cause cell damage through oxidative stress [24,114,115]. In addition, a more-than-adequate iodine intake in the mouse model increases the expression of the intercellular adhesion molecule 1 on the thyroid cell, which leads to the increased infiltration of mononuclear cells and inflammation [116]. It has also been suggested that iodine may induce Th17 T cells in the thyroid gland and impair the development of T-reg cells and that, in excessive amounts, it could increase the antigenicity of thyroglobulin by altering its conformation [117]. In addition, increased TPOAb and TgAb titers have been found in regions with excessive iodine intake, also suggesting that excessive iodine consumption could lead to the development of AITD [110,118]. In Denmark, the iodized salt program in regions with moderate and mild iodine deficiency led to a steady increase in the incidence of hypothyroidism in young and middle-aged subjects [119]. On the other hand, there are studies that have found no change in thyroid autoimmunity over time following salt iodization [120,121]. A national cross-sectional survey in China in 2020 showed that after two decades of the salt iodization program, the prevalence of positive TPOAb was low and a more-than-adequate iodine intake was inversely related to TPOAb [122]. Studies have also shown that the iodine-induced early increase in thyroid antibody levels is usually transient but is also influenced by genetic and other environmental factors. It appears that adequate iodine intake, not exceeding a urinary iodine concentration of 300 μg, does not increase the risk of AITD according to the literature data, although further investigation is needed [24]. A controlled iodine prophylaxis program is recommended to avoid the adverse effects of iodine deficiency and iodine excess.

4.4.2. Iodine Disbalance During Pregnancy with Autoimmune Thyroid Disease

It is well known that increased maternal iodine intake during pregnancy is crucial and that the fetus is dependent on maternal thyroid hormones and maternal iodine reserves in all trimesters of pregnancy. The placenta stores iodine during pregnancy to provide the fetal thyroid gland with a sufficient concentration of iodine for adequate thyroid hormone synthesis and to prevent the negative consequences of iodine deficiency [123]. Adequate maternal iodine intake during pregnancy is required due to increased thyroid hormone production because of elevated levels of β-hCG, circulating estrogens and TBGs. In addition, renal iodine excretion is increased during pregnancy, as is the activity of placental deiodinases [124]. The hormones T4 and T3 are essential for the healthy neurological development of the fetus and are involved in highly sensitive processes such as neuronal migration, myelination, synaptic transmission and plasticity during the fetal and early postnatal period [125,126]. Therefore, it is known that severe iodine deficiency during pregnancy and the neonatal period can have serious adverse effects: an increased risk of pregnancy loss and infant death, neonatal hypothyroidism and neuropsychomotor developmental delay [127]. In addition, a prospective cohort study showed that pregnant women with adequate iodine supplementation had fewer maternal complications such as preeclampsia and placenta previa and a lower rate of fetal distress than pregnant women with severe iodine deficiency [128]. However, there are also studies that have found no association between iodine deficiency and adverse effects such as pregnancy loss, preeclampsia, gestational diabetes, anemia, postpartum hemorrhage, small for gestational age and preterm delivery, among several others [129,130]. Other factors besides iodine deficiency may play a role in pregnancy outcome and further investigation is needed. One of the most important factors to consider is maternal or fetal hypothyroxinemia, which may be exacerbated if iodine deficiency is combined with maternal thyroid autoimmunity during pregnancy. Since hypothyroidism in pregnant women with AITD may worsen during pregnancy, it would be very important to ensure adequate iodine intake to avoid the risk of an unfavorable pregnancy outcome (Figure 3).

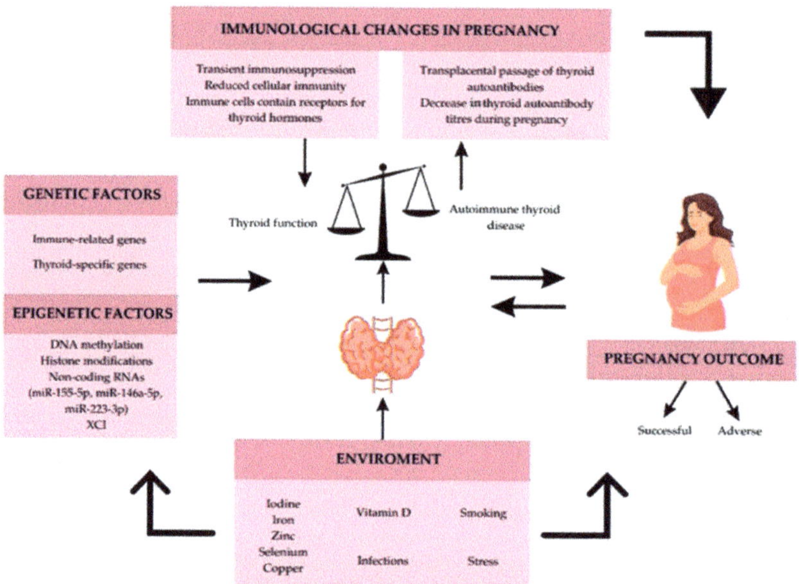

Figure 3. The complex network of factors that influence thyroid function and pregnancy outcome. Both thyroid function and a successful pregnancy are influenced by genetic and epigenetic predispositions as well as environmental factors that, when out of balance, can lead to AITD and an adverse pregnancy outcome. Immunomodulation during pregnancy, which is necessary for a successful pregnancy outcome, also affects thyroid function, especially in the presence of AITD. On the other hand, autoimmunity of the thyroid gland can affect the normal immunological changes and the outcome of pregnancy.

As iodine deficiency is preventable and can be avoided by adequate iodine supplementation during and before pregnancy, the importance of developing an effective strategy to avoid iodine imbalance becomes clear. Recent surveillance studies have shown that pregnant women have become moderately iodine deficient over the past decade [131,132]. Similar studies from various countries, including Australia [133], the United Kingdom [106], Spain [112], the Netherlands [113] and the United States [114], have also reported iodine deficiency in pregnant women. This global concern regarding maternal iodine supply has attracted much attention. Recent research in Shanghai also confirms that current iodine intake in pregnant women is inadequate [131].

Although the adverse maternal and fetal consequences of iodine deficiency have been extensively studied and are widely recognized, the effects of iodine excess have not received the same level of attention and warrant further investigation. Iodine is an essential micronutrient that must be obtained through diet, as the body cannot synthesize it on its own. However, excessive iodine intake can also lead to side effects and toxicity [134], especially during pregnancy. There is evidence that subclinical hypothyroidism can develop in pregnant women. An increased incidence of preterm birth has been described, and the neurological development of the fetus may also be impaired [135,136].

Given the significant prevalence of AITD in women of reproductive age and the knowledge that both iodine deficiency and iodine excess can lead to thyroid dysfunction, the careful monitoring of iodine prophylaxis is required to minimize the risk of adverse outcomes during pregnancy. These thyroid dysfunctions necessitate the careful management of iodine levels and monitoring of thyroid function in both the mother and fetus during pregnancy, especially in women with GD. Poor management can lead to notable neonatal morbidity, again emphasizing close monitoring and early intervention [58]. Further research is needed to clarify the impact of iodine status on thyroid autoimmunity, which will greatly contribute to the maintenance of normal pregnancy and the birth of a healthy child.

4.4.3. Selenium and Autoimmune Thyroid Disease: A Scientific Overview

In recent years, selenium, an essential trace element with significant antioxidant properties, has attracted attention for its potential role in AITD. Selenium has the highest concentration of all tissues, emphasizing its essential role in thyroid metabolism. Several selenoproteins have been documented to be expressed in thyroid cells, including the deiodinase isozymes DIO1 and DIO2, which convert T4 to the active hormone T3 [137,138]. These proteins also include glutathione peroxidases (GPX1, GPX3 and GPX4) and thioredoxin reductases (TXNRD1, TXNRD2 and TXNRD3), which regulate thyroid hormone levels and perform oxidoreductase activities. Although DIO3, which inactivates thyroid hormones, is not expressed in thyroid cells, it is expressed in the placenta and plays an important role in fetal development [139]. The thyroid gland is particularly vulnerable to oxidative stress during hormone production, and AITD exacerbates this damage. Selenium is an integral component of various selenoproteins that play a crucial role in redox regulation, thyroid hormone metabolism and immune function. In AITD, immune system attacks exacerbate oxidative damage. The role of selenium in reducing oxidative stress through the function of selenoproteins such as glutathione peroxidase (GPx) and thioredoxin reductase may mitigate tissue damage in the thyroid gland. Given the oxidative stress involved in thyroid inflammation, the antioxidant capacity of selenium, therefore, makes it a potential candidate for therapeutic intervention [140].

A recent large meta-analysis by Huwiler and coworkers [141] has shown that selenium was effective and safe in lowering TSH, TPOAb and malondialdehyde levels. Further studies have shown that selenium supplementation can enhance selenoenzyme activity and help lower inflammatory markers and oxidative stress in patients with HT, which may slow the progression of the autoimmune response and subsequent destruction of thyroid tissue [142]. Since this micronutrient is crucial for the conversion of the inactive hormone T4 to the active form T3 and the conversion is catalyzed by the selenium-dependent enzymes iodothyronine deiodinases, a selenium deficiency can impair this conversion process and contribute to the symptoms of hypothyroidism, even if the thyroid gland produces adequate amounts of T4. Ensuring adequate levels of selenium in the body may also help maintain efficient thyroid hormone metabolism [143].

The influence of selenium on immune function is particularly important in AITD. It can modulate the immune response by influencing both innate and adaptive immunity. Selenium has been shown to regulate the production of pro-inflammatory cytokines and shift the balance of T helper cells, which play a crucial role in autoimmune thyroid destruction. Selenium supplementation has been shown to reduce anti-TPOAbs, associated with the severity of thyroid inflammation and destruction [144,145]. However, mixed results were noted, and this variability in results could be due to differences in baseline selenium status, dosing, duration of supplementation and other patient-specific factors such as genetics and comorbidities. Indeed, long-term studies are needed to determine whether selenium supplementation can prevent the progression of AITD or improve clinical outcomes. In patients with AITD, selenium supplementation at a dose of 200 μg/day is considered safe. However, excessive selenium intake can lead to toxicity (selenosis). Therefore, supplementation should be carefully monitored, especially in regions where selenium levels in food and water are already high [146]. By reducing oxidative stress, modulating immune function and supporting thyroid hormone metabolism, selenium may help to alleviate some aspects of HT, particularly in selenium-deficient individuals. However, until definitive scientific and clinical conclusions are reached, selenium should be considered as an adjunct to conventional treatments under medical supervision [147].

4.4.4. Selenium and Autoimmune Thyroiditis in Pregnancy

Adequate selenium levels are crucial for maintaining appropriate thyroid hormone levels, especially during pregnancy when metabolic demands are increased. The appropriate management of thyroid function during pregnancy is crucial to avoid adverse outcomes. Selenium supplementation has been shown to be a possible adjunct therapy in women with AITD, although further studies are required to confirm its benefit [148]. A recent study showed that selenium levels were low in pregnant women with gestational diabetes compared to controls and selenium supplementation had a positive effect on blood glucose levels [149]. Pregnancy leads to significant changes in immune function, and PPT is a common complication in women with autoimmune thyroiditis. After childbirth, the immune system may be reactivated and attack the thyroid gland, leading to either transient hyperthyroidism or hypothyroidism. Selenium is generally considered safe to take during pregnancy, but dosing is crucial. A randomized controlled trial by Negro et al. examined the effect of selenium supplementation of 200 μg/day in euthyroid pregnant women with AITD and showed that selenium significantly lowered anti-TPO antibody levels during pregnancy and in the postpartum period while reducing the incidence of PPT [150]. These results suggest that selenium may contribute to the stabilization of thyroid function during pregnancy. Animal studies and observational studies have shown that selenium supplementation may support normal fetal development by ensuring adequate thyroid hormone levels [151]. Some studies suggest that selenium deficiency may be associated with neurodevelopmental delays in children. However, further research is needed to establish a direct link between maternal selenium intake and improved cognitive performance in offspring [152,153].

Although a positive role of selenium supplementation on thyroid function during pregnancy is suspected, especially in pregnant women with overt or subclinical hypothyroidism, most guidelines do not suggest routine selenium supplementation in pregnancy due to an overall lack of studies [59]. A 2017 review by Ventura et al. showed that selenium may contribute to thyroid health. However, they found that most studies measured thyroid antibodies but not selenium levels themselves. Since selenium has a narrow therapeutic index, supplementation could easily lead to toxicity [154]. Selenium supplementation may prevent complications such as preeclampsia, miscarriage and PPT, although this is not yet well established. Selenium plays an important role in the synthesis of thyroid hormones and antioxidant protection, but its supplementation regarding pregnancy complications is still under investigation [155].

In areas where selenium is deficient, selenium supplementation has also been considered to improve pregnancy outcomes, for example, by reducing preterm births, small-for-gestational-age babies and pregnancy-induced hypertension. Selenium supplementation, especially in the form of selenomethionine, has been shown to significantly lower levels of antithyroid anti-TPOAbs in euthyroid women with AITD throughout pregnancy. It may prevent the progression of hypothyroidism and reduce the inflammatory response during pregnancy, leading to better maternal and fetal outcomes. Selenium supplementation, while promising, is only recommended in some cases. Both the American and European Thyroid Associations urge further research to determine the optimal dosage and safety of routine selenium use during pregnancy. The benefits of selenium are more pronounced in selenium-deficient regions; therefore, geographic considerations are an important variable when making supplementation recommendations [69].

4.4.5. Autoimmune Thyroid Disease, Pregnancy and Iron—Causal Connections and Implications

Recent evidence emphasizes the role of iron in thyroid hormone synthesis and immune function, making iron status a very important factor in the management of AITD in pregnancy [156]. Iron plays a crucial role in both thyroid function and immune system regulation, making it particularly important for pregnant women with AITD. Iron is a co-factor for TPO, which is essential to produce thyroid hormones. If the iron supply is insufficient, the activity of TPO is impaired, which leads to the reduced synthesis of thyroid hormones [157]. Iron deficiency can impair the production of thyroid hormones and, thereby, exacerbate hypothyroidism, especially in women with AITD, which can lead to complications such as fatigue, anemia or the worsening of thyroid dysfunction [158]. Iron plays an important role in regulating the immune system and helps to maintain the balance between pro-inflammatory and anti-inflammatory responses. Iron deficiency can impair immune function and make the body more susceptible to exaggerated inflammatory responses, potentially exacerbating thyroid autoimmunity, which can lead to increased thyroid damage [159].

Low iron and ferritin levels during pregnancy can lead to anemia, which, in combination with thyroid dysfunction, can increase the risk of miscarriage, preeclampsia and premature birth. Women with AITD already have a higher risk of these complications, so iron deficiency further increases the risks [160]. Adequate thyroid function is critical for fetal neurologic development, especially in the first trimester, and iron deficiency predicts poor maternal thyroid status during pregnancy [161]. Since the fetus is dependent on maternal thyroid hormones, iron deficiency leading to hypothyroidism may impair fetal brain development and increase the risk of cognitive impairment and developmental delay [162]. For pregnant women with AITD, the monitoring and treatment of iron levels is crucial. Therefore, the appropriate management of iron levels is critical for optimizing maternal and fetal health. Iron supplementation may be necessary to prevent the exacerbation of thyroid dysfunction as it helps to stabilize TPO activity, improve thyroid hormone production and reduce the risk of complications [159].

4.4.6. Vitamin D and Thyroid Dysfunction

A growing body of research suggests that vitamin D, which is also a secosteroid hormone, may play a role in thyroid health and the development of thyroid disease [163]. Vitamin D receptors (VDR) are found in many tissues, including immune cells, suggesting that they play a critical role in regulating the immune response. The active form of vitamin D, 1,25-dihydroxyvitamin D (calcitriol), exerts immunoregulatory effects, particularly in autoimmune diseases. Scientific evidence confirms that insufficient vitamin D levels can lead to immune dysregulation, possibly contributing to autoimmune thyroid diseases, although conflicting results have been found [164]. Nevertheless, numerous studies have shown that patients with HT tend to have lower vitamin D levels compared to healthy controls. The presence of TPOAb and lower vitamin D levels are often associated with higher antibody titers, indicating a more active autoimmune process [165]. Similarly, hyperthyroidism due to GD has been associated with lower vitamin D levels. Studies suggest that vitamin D deficiency may exacerbate disease severity, although the scientific evidence is less consistent compared to hypothyroidism [166,167].

Several biological mechanisms have been proposed that could explain the link between vitamin D deficiency and thyroid dysfunction, of which the immuno-modulatory effect of vitamin D seems to be the most important [168]. Vitamin D is known to regulate both innate and adaptive immune responses and can modulate the proliferation of T cells and the differentiation of T-regs, which are crucial for the maintenance of immune tolerance [169]. Vitamin D deficiency may impair these mechanisms and, thus, contribute to the development and/or progression of AITD and other autoimmune diseases [170,171]. In addition, VDRs are expressed in thyroid cells, suggesting that vitamin D may influence thyroid function. Recent findings show an association between VDR gene polymorphism, vitamin D status and AITD [172]. Vitamin D is also known for its anti-inflammatory properties, and its deficiency may lead to increased inflammation and oxidative stress in thyroid tissues. Chronic inflammation is a key component of AITD, and vitamin D supplementation has been suggested as a potential means of reducing this inflammation, although clinical trials examining the effects of vitamin D supplementation on thyroid function are still limited [173].

Numerous epidemiological studies have shown a link between low vitamin D levels and thyroid disease [174]. However, the question of whether vitamin D deficiency is a cause or a consequence of thyroid dysfunction remains a topic of ongoing research, as the results are not yet conclusive. Indeed, further research is needed to determine whether vitamin D supplementation can serve as a therapeutic or preventive measure for thyroid dysfunction.

4.4.7. Smoking and Autoimmune Thyroid Disease

Cigarette smoking is considered one of the environmental factors affecting thyroid function and appears to have different effects on the development of autoimmune thyroid disease. Data on the effects of cigarette smoking on thyroid function and the triggering of thyroid autoimmunity are varied and conflicting. It has been suggested that the chemical components of tobacco may affect hormone production, hormone transport and secretion [175]. Smoking has been reported to increase the size of the thyroid gland and the development of non-toxic goiter [176]. There are studies showing that smokers have higher thyroid hormone levels and lower TPOAb levels than non-smokers [177], but other studies have not confirmed these results [178,179]. The results of most studies relied on questionnaires to assess smoking status, which is associated with limitations such as information bias and subjectivity [175]. Several studies investigated serum cotinine as a measure of nicotine exposure to more objectively determine smoking status [180,181]. Soldin et al. reported decreased TSH and T4 levels in active smokers [182], while Kim et al. found that cigarette smoking was associated with decreased TSH levels in men and women and increased TPOAb levels in male subjects [175]. In addition, they reported that urinary cotinine levels were negatively associated with TSH levels after controlling for age, height, weight, health behaviors and urinary iodine levels. The authors suggest that smoking may have a stimulating effect on the thyroid gland by increasing serum TBG and T3 concentrations and lowering serum TSH levels [175]. Cigarette smoking may impair iodide transport and iodide organization. One hypothetical explanation is that thiocyanate, a metabolite of cigarette smoke, inhibits the sodium iodide symporter and, thus, impairs iodine uptake and thyroid function, especially in iodine-deficient women. This could lead to the development of autoimmune thyroid dysfunction and increased production of thyroid hormones, which, in turn, lowers TSH levels [183,184]. This was supported by the research conducted by Shields et al., which showed that smoking lowers thyroid antibody levels, possibly due to the inhibitory effect of thiocyanate, on the sodium iodide symporter, which affects iodine uptake in the thyroid gland. It was also found that smokers were less likely to test positive for TPOAbs, again supporting the hypothesis of immune modulation by smoking that suppresses the autoimmune responses of the immune system, thus explaining the lower risk of hypothyroidism in active smokers. The study also found that this protective effect wears off after quitting smoking and that people return to their baseline risk of hypothyroidism a few years after quitting [185].

To date, cigarette smoking has been shown to be associated with a twofold increased risk of GD and a higher likelihood of relapse in GD or GO [16,186]. The mechanism is not yet fully understood, but smoking is thought to increase the risk by increasing the formation of reactive oxygen species and decreasing the production of antioxidants [16]. However, the effects of smoking in HT are not so clear and mixed results have been reported. There is evidence that cigarette smoking is associated with a lower prevalence of TPOAb [176,187,188]. On the other hand, there are studies that find no significant correlation between smoking and TPOAbs [189]. Although the data are contradictory, smoking appears to lower the overall risk of TPOAb, TgAbs and autoimmune hypothyroidism by a factor of about 40%. It has been suggested that nicotine alters immune responses by activating nicotinic receptors on immune cells, shifting the autoimmune profile away from the Th1 and Th17 pathways [190]. Smoking can impair cell-mediated immunity and inhibit the activity of natural killer cells and reduce the number of cytotoxic CD8+ T cells [191] which could reduce the risk of the thyroid autoimmunity [176]. In addition to autoimmunity and iodine status, the effect of smoking on thyroid function might depend on several factors, such as age, the duration and intensity of smoking, physical health and comorbidities and other environmental factors [192].

4.4.8. Smoking and Thyroid Function During Pregnancy

Smoking during pregnancy can have harmful effects on the development of the fetus. It is associated with an increased risk of miscarriage, growth failure and malformations, e.g., orofacial cleft, congenital heart defects or neural tube defects [193–196]. Quelhas et al. reported that active tobacco use during pregnancy was associated with significantly higher rates of small for gestational age, shorter length and smaller head circumference at birth [193]. One of the suggested mechanisms is oxidative stress in the placenta caused by tobacco, which can impair the transport of oxygen and nutrients to the growing fetus [197]. Yuan et al. showed, in a Mendelian randomization investigation, a positive association between smoking initiation and increased risk of pregnancy loss [198]. A long-term consequence was also found to be impaired intellectual development [199]. However, data on the effects of smoking on thyroid function during pregnancy are limited and contradictory. Smoking during pregnancy has been shown to increase the risk of subsequent hyperthyroidism, while paradoxically, it also has a protective effect against hypothyroidism [59]. Andersen et al. showed lower TSH, higher T3 and lower or unchanged T4 in pregnant women who smoked [200]. One of the possible explanations is that smoking affects the activity of deiodinase, especially D2, during pregnancy and the delicate balance of the sympathetic nervous system [124]. Andersen et al. also reported that women who quit smoking during pregnancy had higher TSH, lower T4 and higher T3 [200]. Previous research suggests that smoking lowers the risk of positive thyroid autoantibody concentrations, which may be one reason for the protective effects of smoking on hypothyroidism in this population. Shields et al. investigated thyroid function in a cross-sectional study of two independent cohorts of pregnant women without a history of thyroid disease or with overt biochemical thyroid dysfunction [185]. They reported that pregnant women who smoked had lower TSH and higher FT3 levels than non-smoking pregnant women, while FT4 levels were similar in both groups, as was the prevalence of TPOAbs. TSH levels were also lower in the cord blood of babies born to mothers who had smoked during pregnancy [185]. A meta-analysis showed that smoking was associated with an increased risk of both HT and GD. In the population at risk for AITD, an inverse association was found between smoking and the presence of TPOAb, a finding that was later confirmed in other population-based studies [16]. Curiously, smoking during pregnancy was associated with a lower risk of developing thyroiditis, but increased the incidence of PPT [185].

Despite this protection against hypothyroidism, smoking during pregnancy carries many other risks, including an increased risk of low birth weight, preterm birth and infant mortality. Healthcare providers should, therefore, watch for symptoms of hyperthyroidism in women who smoke, especially in the first two years after giving birth. Although smoking during pregnancy has decreased, a large proportion of pregnant women still smoke, which means that public health efforts need to continue.

Clearly, further research is needed to investigate the effects of maternal thyroid autoimmunity and smoking on fetal development and adverse pregnancy outcomes and to identify the complex underlying mechanisms.

4.4.9. Infections and Autoimmune Thyroid Disease

The immunological basis of AITD has both an innate and an adaptive component. The innate mechanisms of immune responses are primarily cell-mediated and represent a rapid defense against pathogens, whereas the adaptive mechanisms are antigen-specific and elicit antibodies against specific targets. Autoimmune thyrocyte destruction in HT is a cell-mediated phenomenon represented by lymphocytic infiltration into thyroid follicles. Recent evidence suggests that stromal cells in the thyroid gland of HT patients may drive the recruitment of inflammatory cells into organized lymphoid structures called tertiary lymphoid organs. The resulting tissue destruction leads to exposure to thyroid antigens, triggering the production of autoantibodies. In contrast, GD shows less aggressive lymphocytic infiltration and a predominant humoral immune response, although these processes are interdependent [83].

While adaptive immunity in AITD is well documented, recent attention has focused on the innate immune cells involved, such as neutrophils, NK cells, NKT cells, monocytes, macrophages and dendritic cells [83,201]. The activation of innate immune pathways usually leads to the release of cytokines, infiltration of lymphocytes and tissue destruction. Although innate immunity is classically considered to be non-specific, some degree of specificity has been established [202].

NK cells are components of innate immunity and work together with T lymphocytes as major effectors of cell-mediated immunity. NK cells make up 10–15% of lymphocytes in peripheral blood and have been categorized into two subsets based on the cell surface density of the neuronal cell adhesion molecule (N-CAM), also known as CD56: one subset comprises cells often referred to as $CD56^{dim}$ cells, which are highly cytotoxic and account for 90% of NK cells, and the remaining fraction consists of $CD56^{bright}$ cells, which are immunoregulatory cells and produce cytokines [203,204]. Due to their cytotoxic nature, they can destroy virus-infected and malignant cells without prior sensitization, a unique property compared to T lymphocytes. NK cells are activated by the proinflammatory cytokines IL-2, IFN-γ, IFN-β and IL-12 and may take on regulatory functions via their interactions with T cells and dendritic cells, thereby modulating both innate and acquired immunity [203].

In viral infections, NK cells play the most important role due to their ability to rapidly eliminate virus-infected cells. The activity of NK cells is controlled by a delicate balance of activating and inhibitory receptors on their surface that control cytotoxic responses [205]. NK cells kill target cells via two main pathways: a direct cytotoxic release of granules and binding to "death receptors" such as Fas/FasL on the target cells. The activated NK cells produce cytokines such as IFN-γ, TNF-α and TNF-β, which help in immune regulation and apoptosis. NK cells are also involved in autoimmune diseases such as multiple sclerosis and Crohn's disease, where viral antigens interfere with NK cell function. Chronic viral infection has been shown to downregulate NK cytotoxicity, promote viral persistence and contribute to autoimmunity through its effects on B- and T-cell responses.

During pregnancy, there is a functional change in NK cells. In a normal pregnancy, the number and activity of NK cells increase in the first trimester and then decrease in the later stages. However, high NK cell activity has been associated with miscarriage and recurrent pregnancy loss, suggesting a role in immune regulation at the feto-maternal interface [83]. The exacerbation of autoimmune thyroid disorders of AITD, such as HT and GD after delivery, has also been associated with increased NK cell activity [205]. These findings emphasize that NK cells play a Janus-like role both in the protection against viral infections and the development of autoimmune diseases and pregnancy complications. In summary, NK cells play a crucial role in viral immunity and the control of autoimmunity, and functional changes in diseases such as AITD, viral infections and pregnancy suggest that they are involved in the immune response [206].

4.4.10. Stress and Autoimmune Thyroid Disease

There is growing evidence that stressful life events are among the environmental factors that may contribute to the development of autoimmunity in genetically predisposed individuals [207]. Stress is known to lead to the excessive secretion of glucocorticoids and catechol-amines through activation of the hypothalamic–pituitary–adrenal axis and sympathoadrenal system, which can disrupt immune homeostasis and cause the Th1/Th2 imbalance associated with autoimmunity and the pathogenesis of AITD [208]. Elevated glucocorticoid levels affect the cytokine network by inhibiting the synthesis of IL-1, IL-2, TNF and IFN and stimulating the production of IL-4, IL-10 and IL-13, thereby shifting the immune profile towards a humoral response, which is mainly involved in the etiopathogenesis of GD [209]. There is also evidence that elevated glucocorticoid levels can downregulate antioxidant enzymes [210]. There are studies that establish a link between stress and the development of GD [115]. However, the results are not yet clear. Stressful life events have been reported to favor the onset and recurrence of GD in patients who have been observed for at least 5 years after the exclusion of thyrostatic therapy [211]. On the other hand, there was a prospective 5-year follow-up study that showed no causal relationship between stress and GD [208,212].

The influence of stress on the development of HT is also far from clear, although there are accumulating data suggesting that the pathogenesis of HT is more complex and involves both cellular and humoral immune mechanisms [213]. The authors also suggested that acute stress could lead to the progression of HT, while chronic stress induces a Th2 immune response and increased levels of TPOAb and Tg autoantibodies [209]. Interestingly, Vaivode et al. investigated the relationship between the number and impact of stressful life events in AITD patients and the Th1/Th2/Th17 immune response and found no significant differences in the number of stressful life events between patients with HT, patients with GD and controls. There was a positive correlation between the number of major life events and life events with negative effects on TPO and Tg antibody levels [208]. The exact role of TPOAbs in the pathogenesis of HT is not clear, but they appear to be associated with oxidative stress, as higher oxidative parameters have been found in euthyroid, untreated HT patients [214]. Markomanolaki et al. reported that after an 8-week stress management intervention, patients showed a statistically significant decrease in TgAb titers and stress, depression and anxiety scores compared to the control group [213]. The study by Corso et al. provides the first evidence that stressful events such as emotional neglect and abuse are potential risk factors for the development of AITD [215]. In a pilot study investigating the relationship between thyroid function and perceived stress in newly diagnosed hypothyroid women of reproductive age, a significant difference was found between clinical and subclinical hypothyroid women in terms of the mean score of the Perceived Stress Scale (PSS), which measures the individual perception of people exposed to stressful situations. A significant positive correlation was found between PSS scores and TSH levels [207]. A recent cross-sectional study also showed a positive but non-significant correlation between PSS and TSH in women of reproductive age with normal thyroid function and with SH [216].

4.4.11. Stress and Thyroid Function During Pregnancy

Data from the literature suggest that stress during pregnancy increases the risk of pregnancy complications and unfavorable outcomes such as low birth weight, preterm birth [217] and impaired fetal neurodevelopment [218]. Maternal stress has also been associated with an increased risk of pregnancy loss [219], gestational diabetes [220], birth complications [221,222], hypertension and pre-eclampsia [223]. Stressful events during pregnancy can cause changes in glucocorticoid levels through activation of the hypothalamic–pituitary–adrenal axis. It has been found that both decreased and increased concentrations of glucocorticoids can affect fetal neurodevelopment [224]. Glucocorticoids are involved in structural and neurochemical processes that are important for brain maturation [225].

The literature data on the effects of stress on pregnancy with AITD are insufficient, but it has been shown that activation of the hypothalamic–pituitary–adrenal axis and increased glucocorticoids affect thyroid hormone metabolism during pregnancy by lowering TSH levels and inhibiting the peripheral conversion of T4 to the active T3 form [226]. It has also been described that glucocorticoids can alter iodine metabolism, thyrocyte secretory activity and the differentiation of deiodinase activity. Thyroid hormones are essential for normal fetal development, especially for brain maturation and neurophysiological processes such as neuron and glial cell differentiation and synaptogenesis [227]. T3 plays the main role in fetal neurodevelopment, and T3 receptors are already present in the brain in early pregnancy. Most of the fetal T3 in the central nervous system is locally converted from maternal T4, which is actively transported into the fetal central nervous system [227]. In pregnant women with HT and reduced thyroid reserve due to an autoimmune process, stress-related events could further jeopardize transplacental delivery and the supply of T4 to the growing fetus. Therefore, stress-related abnormalities in thyroid hormone and glucocorticoid levels during pregnancy, especially in autoimmune hypothyroidism, could have short- and long-term consequences for the offspring. We cannot rule out stressful events during pregnancy, but maintaining maternal TSH and thyroid hormone levels within a strict normal range contributes to a successful pregnancy and birth, as well as safe and normal fetal development.

5. Conclusions

During pregnancy, maintaining normal thyroid function is crucial for both the mother and the developing fetus. Since maternal and fetal thyroid function are closely interconnected, any changes in the mother's thyroid health can influence the course and outcome of the pregnancy, as well as the condition of the fetus. AITD is relatively common in pregnant women, and pregnancy itself can exacerbate AITD due to various hormonal changes. Often, AITD remains undiagnosed and untreated, particularly in its subclinical form. Therefore, both preventing the onset of AITD and managing existing cases during pregnancy are of utmost importance. To effectively address AITD in pregnancy, it is essential to understand the factors that contribute to its development and take steps to mitigate them. Current knowledge suggests that AITD develops in genetically predisposed individuals, influenced by environmental factors and mediated by epigenetic mechanisms. The genetic background plays a role in immune regulation and may predispose the thyroid gland to autoimmune responses triggered by environmental factors. While modifiable environmental factors present a promising target for the prevention and treatment of AITD, there is still a lack of established protocols on how to intervene effectively. At present, ensuring adequate iodine intake remains a key focus, with iodized salt being the primary method of implementation. Research has also linked insufficient selenium and vitamin D levels to thyroid autoimmunity during pregnancy, but routine supplementation with these nutrients is not yet recommended. Additionally, avoiding smoking and managing stress have been shown to have beneficial effects on thyroid health. One promising approach is systematic screening for AITD during pregnancy, which could significantly help in preventing adverse pregnancy outcomes and developmental disorders in the child. However, due to the substantial financial resources and health system involvement required, this approach has not yet been widely implemented.

Author Contributions: Conceptualization, T.B.C., B.Ć.-C., V.S. and L.B.; writing—original draft preparation, T.B.C., B.Ć.-C., V.S., N.G., M.I.T., A.K., I.K., T.Š., I.P., L.B. and S.K.; writing—review and editing, T.B.C., B.Ć.-C., V.S. and L.B.; visualization, A.K.; supervision, T.B.C., B.Ć.-C., V.S. and L.B.; project administration, T.B.C. All authors have read and agreed to the published version of the manuscript.

Funding: This research was funded by the grant of the University of Rijeka (grant no. uniri-iskusni-biomed-23-61, main researcher: T.B.C.).

Institutional Review Board Statement: Not applicable.

Informed Consent Statement: Not applicable.

Data Availability Statement: No new data were generated with this research.

Conflicts of Interest: The authors declare no conflicts of interest.

References

1. Bogusławska, J.; Godlewska, M.; Gajda, E.; Piekiełko-Witkowska, A. Cellular and molecular basis of thyroid autoimmunity. *Eur. Thyroid J.* **2022**, *11*, e210024. [CrossRef]
2. Martínez-Hernández, R.; Sánchez de la Blanca, N.; Sacristán-Gómez, P.; Serrano-Somavilla, A.; Muñoz De Nova, J.L.; Sánchez Cabo, F.; Heyn, H.; Sampedro-Núñez, M.; Marazuela, M. Unraveling the molecular architecture of autoimmune thyroid diseases at spatial resolution. *Nat. Commun.* **2024**, *15*, 5895. [CrossRef]
3. Anaya, J.M.; Shoenfeld, Y.; Rojas-Villarraga, A.; Levy, R.A.; Cervera, R. (Eds.) *Autoimmunity: From Bench to Bedside*; El Rosario University Press: Bogota, Colombia, 2013.
4. Caturegli, P.; De Remigis, A.; Rose, N.R. Hashimoto thyroiditis: Clinical and diagnostic criteria. *Autoimmun. Rev.* **2014**, *13*, 391–397. [CrossRef]
5. Csaba, G. Hormones in the immune system and their possible role. A critical review. *Acta. Microbiol. Immunol. Hung.* **2014**, *61*, 241–260. [CrossRef] [PubMed]
6. Tomer, Y. Mechanisms of autoimmune thyroid diseases: From genetics to epigenetics. *Annu. Rev. Pathol.* **2014**, *9*, 147–156. [CrossRef] [PubMed]
7. Rostami, R.; Nourooz-Zadeh, S.; Mohammadi, A.; Khalkhali, H.R.; Ferns, G.; Nourooz-Zadeh, J. Serum Selenium Status and Its Interrelationship with Serum Biomarkers of Thyroid Function and Antioxidant Defense in Hashimoto's Thyroiditis. *Antioxidants* **2020**, *9*, 1070. [CrossRef]
8. Chao, G.; Zhu, Y.; Fang, L. Correlation Between Hashimoto's Thyroiditis-Related Thyroid Hormone Levels and 25-Hydroxyvitamin D. *Front. Endocrinol* **2020**, *11*, 4. [CrossRef] [PubMed]
9. Cyna, W.; Wojciechowska, A.; Szybiak-Skora, W.; Lacka, K. The Impact of Environmental Factors on the Development of Autoimmune Thyroiditis—Review. *Biomedicines* **2024**, *12*, 1788. [CrossRef]
10. Yang, C.; Xiao, J.; Xu, Z.; Wang, Z. Gut Microbiota Changes and Its Potential Relations with Thyroid Disorders: From Composition to Therapeutic Targets. *Int. J. Gen. Med.* **2024**, *17*, 3719–3731. [CrossRef]
11. Shen, S.; Wong, C.H. Bugging inflammation: Role of the gut microbiota. *Clin. Transl. Immunol.* **2016**, *5*, e72. [CrossRef]
12. Chou, S.M.; Yeh, H.J.; Lin, T.M.; Chang, Y.S.; Hsu, H.C.; Shen, Y.C.; Kuo, T.T.; Chen, J.H.; Chen, S.H.; Chang, C.C. Association of interferon-based therapy with risk of autoimmune diseases in patients with chronic hepatitis C virus infection: A population-based Taiwanese cohort study. *Front. Immunol.* **2022**, *13*, 992819. [CrossRef]
13. Luo, W.; Wu, S.; Chen, H.; Wu, Y.; Peng, J. Thyroid dysfunction is associated with the loss of hepatitis B surface antigen in patients with chronic hepatitis B undergoing treatment with a-interferon. *J. Int. Med. Res.* **2021**, *49*, 3000605211025139. [CrossRef] [PubMed]
14. Ajjan, R.A.; Weetman, A.P. The Pathogenesis of Hashimoto's Thyroiditis: Further Developments in our Understanding. *Horm. Metab. Res.* **2015**, *47*, 702–710. [CrossRef]
15. Wiersinga, W.M. Clinical relevance of environmental factors in the pathogenesis of autoimmune thyroid disease. *Endocrinol. Metab.* **2016**, *31*, 213. [CrossRef]
16. Ferrari, S.M.; Fallahi, P.; Antonelli, A.; Benvenga, S. Environmental Issues in Thyroid Diseases. *Front. Endocrinol.* **2017**, *8*, 50. [CrossRef] [PubMed]
17. Stathatos, N.; Daniels, G.H. Autoimmune thyroid disease. *Curr. Opin. Rheumatol.* **2012**, *24*, 70–75. [CrossRef]
18. Dayan, C.M.; Daniels, G.H. Chronic autoimmune thyroiditis. *N. Engl. J Med.* **1996**, *335*, 99–107. [CrossRef]
19. Menconi, F.; Oppenheim, Y.L.; Tomer, Y. Graves disease. In *Diagnostic Criteria in Autoimmune Diseases*; Humana Press: Totowa, NJ, USA, 2008; pp. 231–235.
20. Brent, G.A. Clinical practice. Graves' disease. *N. Engl. J. Med.* **2008**, *358*, 2594–2605. [CrossRef]
21. Pokhrel, B.; Bhusal, K. *Graves Disease*; StatPearls: Treasure Island, FL, USA, 2023.
22. Hussain, Y.S.; Hookham, J.C.; Allahabadia, A.; Balasubramanian, S.P. Epidemiology, management and outcomes of Graves' disease-real life data. *Endocrine* **2017**, *56*, 568–578. [CrossRef]
23. Cooper, D.S. Hyperthyroidism. *Lancet* **2003**, *362*, 459–468. [CrossRef] [PubMed]
24. Kravchenko, V.; Zakharchenko, T. Thyroid hormones and minerals in immunocorrection of disorders in autoimmune thyroid diseases. *Front. Endocrinol.* **2023**, *14*, 1225494. [CrossRef] [PubMed]
25. Hashimoto, H. Zur Kenntniss der lymphoatosen Veranderung der Schilddrüse (Struma lymphomatoa). *Langenbecks. Arch. Klin. Chirurg.* **1912**, *97*, 219–248.
26. Zhang, Q.Y.; Ye, X.P.; Zhou, Z.; Zhu, C.F.; Li, R.; Fang, Y.; Zhang, R.J.; Li, L.; Liu, W.; Wang, Z.; et al. Lymphocyte infiltration and thyrocyte destruction are driven by stromal and immune cell components in Hashimoto's thyroiditis. *Nat. Commun.* **2022**, *13*, 775. [CrossRef] [PubMed]

27. Witebsky, E.; Rose, N.R.; Terplan, K.; Paine, J.R.; Egan, R.W. Chronic thyroiditis and autoimmunization. *J. Am. Med. Assoc.* **1957**, *164*, 1439–1447. [CrossRef] [PubMed]
28. Ralli, M.; Angeletti, D.; Fiore, M.; D'Aguanno, V.; Lambiase, A.; Artico, M.; de Vincentiis, M.; Greco, A. Hashimoto's thyroiditis: An update on pathogenic mechanisms, diagnostic protocols, therapeutic strategies, and potential malignant transformation. *Autoimmun. Rev.* **2020**, *19*, 102649. [CrossRef] [PubMed]
29. Franco, J.S.; Amaya-Amaya, J.; Anaya, J.M. Thyroid disease and autoimmune diseases. In *Autoimmunity: From Bench to Bedside*; Anaya, J.M., Shoenfeld, Y., Rojas-Villarraga, A., Eds.; El Rosario University Press: Bogota, Colombia, 2013; Chapter 30. Available online: https://www.ncbi.nlm.nih.gov/books/NBK459466/ (accessed on 3 October 2024).
30. Ragusa, F.; Fallahi, P.; Elia, G.; Gonnella, D.; Paparo, S.R.; Giusti, C.; Churilov, L.P.; Ferrari, S.M.; Antonelli, A. Hashimotos' thyroiditis: Epidemiology, pathogenesis, clinic and therapy. *Best. Pract. Res. Clin. Endocrinol. Metab.* **2019**, *33*, 101367. [CrossRef]
31. Wu, G.; Zou, D.; Cai, H.; Liu, Y. Ultrasonography in the diagnosis of Hashimoto's thyroiditis. *Front. Biosci.* **2016**, *21*, 1006–1012. [CrossRef]
32. Aljarad, M.; Alhalabi, N.; Hamad, A.; Nmr, N.; Abbas, F.; Alkhatib, A.; Alhalabi, M.; Al-Hammami, H.; Ibrahim, N. Prevalence of Thyroid Autoimmune Antibodies in Women Seeking Fertility Care in Damascus, Syria. *Cureus* **2019**, *11*, e5315. [CrossRef] [PubMed]
33. Biondi, B.; Cappola, A.R.; Cooper, D.S. Subclinical hypothyroidism: A review. *JAMA* **2019**, *322*, 153–160. [CrossRef] [PubMed]
34. Selmer, C.; Olesen, J.B.; Hansen, M.L.; von Kappelgaard, L.M.; Madsen, J.C.; Hansen, P.R.; Pedersen, O.D.; Faber, J.; Torp-Pedersen, C.; Gislason, G.H. Subclinical and overt thyroid dysfunction and risk of all-cause mortality and cardiovascular events: A large population study. *J. Clin. Endocrinol. Metab.* **2014**, *99*, 2372–2382. [CrossRef] [PubMed]
35. Klubo-Gwiezdzinska, J.; Wartofsky, L. Hashimoto thyroiditis: An evidence-based guide to etiology, diagnosis and treatment. *Pol. Arch. Intern. Med.* **2022**, *132*, 16222. [CrossRef]
36. Martinez Quintero, B.; Yazbeck, C.; Sweeney, L.B. Thyroiditis: Evaluation and Treatment. *Am. Fam. Physician* **2021**, *104*, 609–617. [PubMed]
37. Botta, A.; Rizzo, F.; Antonielli, T.; Ciliberti, A.; Garufi, E.; Lanzone, A.; Garufi, C.; De Carolis, S. The Detrimental Effect of Thyroiditis on Pregnancy Outcome of Patients Affected by Autoimmune Diseases: An Open Question. *Front. Pharmacol.* **2022**, *13*, 827735. [CrossRef]
38. Weng, J.; Couture, C.; Girard, S. Innate and Adaptive Immune Systems in Physiological and Pathological Pregnancy. *Biology* **2023**, *12*, 402. [CrossRef]
39. Kareva, I. Immune Suppression in Pregnancy and Cancer: Parallels and Insights. *Transl. Oncol.* **2020**, *13*, 100759. [CrossRef] [PubMed]
40. Croce, L.; Di Dalmazi, G.; Orsolini, F.; Virili, C.; Brigante, G.; Gianetti, E.; Moleti, M.; Napolitano, G.; Tonacchera, M.; Rotondi, M. Graves' Disease and the Post-partum Period: An Intriguing Relationship. *Front. Endocrin.* **2019**, *10*, 853. [CrossRef] [PubMed]
41. Moleti, M.; Di Mauro, M.; Sturniolo, G.; Russo, M.; Vermiglio, F. Hyperthyroidism in the pregnant woman: Maternal and fetal aspects. *J. Clin. Transl. Endocrinol.* **2019**, *16*, 100190. [CrossRef] [PubMed]
42. Marx, H.; Amin, P.; Lazarus, J.H. Hyperthyroidism and pregnancy. *BMJ* **2008**, *336*, 663–667. [CrossRef] [PubMed]
43. Cooper, D.S.; Laurberg, P. Hyperthyroidism in pregnancy. *Lancet Diabetes Endocrinol.* **2013**, *1*, 238–249. [CrossRef]
44. Kung, A.W.; Lau, K.S.; Kohn, L.D. Epitope mapping of tsh receptor-blocking antibodies in Graves' disease that appear during pregnancy. *J. Clin. Endocrinol. Metab.* **2001**, *86*, 3647–8653. [PubMed]
45. Kung, A.W.; Jones, B.M. A change from stimulatory to blocking antibody activity in Graves' disease during pregnancy. *J. Clin. Endocrinol. Metab.* **1998**, *83*, 514–518. [CrossRef]
46. Ueta, Y.; Fukui, H.; Murakami, H.; Yamanouchi, Y.; Yamamoto, R.; Murao, A.; Santou, Y.; Taniguchi, S.; Mitani, Y.; Shigemasa, C. Development of primary hypothyroidism with the appearance of blocking-type antibody to thyrotropin receptor in Graves' disease in late pregnancy. *Thyroid* **1999**, *9*, 179–182. [CrossRef]
47. Gargallo Fernández, M. Hyperthyroidism and pregnancy. *Endocrinol. Nutr.* **2013**, *60*, 535–543. [CrossRef] [PubMed]
48. Negro, R.; Stagnaro-Green, A. Clinical aspects of hyperthyroidism, hypothyroidism, and thyroid screening in pregnancy. *Endocr. Pract.* **2014**, *20*, 597–607. [CrossRef] [PubMed]
49. Nguyen, C.T.; Mestman, J.H. Graves' hyperthyroidism in pregnancy. *Curr. Opin. Endocrinol. Diabetes Obes.* **2019**, *26*, 232–240. [CrossRef] [PubMed]
50. Sorah, K.; Alderson, T.L. *Hyperthyroidism in Pregnancy*; StatPearls Publishing: Treasure Island, FL, USA, 2024; p. 32644629.
51. Illouz, F.; Luton, D.; Polak, M.; Besançon, A.; Bournaud, C. Graves' disease and pregnancy. *Ann. Endocrinol.* **2018**, *79*, 636–646. [CrossRef]
52. Laurberg, P.; Andersen, S.L. Endocrinology in pregnancy: Pregnancy and the incidence, diagnosing and therapy of Graves' disease. *Eur. J. Endocrinol.* **2016**, *175*, 219–230. [CrossRef] [PubMed]

53. De Groot, L.; Abalovich, M.; Alexander, E.K.; Amino, N.; Barbour, L.; Cobin, R.H.; Eastman, C.J.; Lazarus, J.H.; Luton, D.; Mandel, S.J.; et al. Management of thyroid dysfunction during pregnancy and postpartum: An Endocrine Society clinical practice guideline. *J. Clin. Endocrinol. Metab.* **2012**, *97*, 2543–2565. [CrossRef]
54. King, J.R.; Lachica, R.; Lee, R.H.; Montoro, M.; Mestman, J. Diagnosis and Management of Hyperthyroidism in Pregnancy: A Review. *Obstet. Gynecol. Surv.* **2016**, *71*, 675–685. [CrossRef]
55. Kobaly, K.; Mandel, S.J. Hyperthyroidism and Pregnancy. *Endocrinol. Metab. Clin. N. Am.* **2019**, *48*, 533–545. [CrossRef]
56. Sarkar, S.; Bischoff, L.A. Management of Hyperthyroidism during the Preconception Phase, Pregnancy, and the Postpartum Period. *Semin. Reprod. Med.* **2016**, *34*, 317–322. [CrossRef]
57. Luz, I.R.; Martins, J.R.; Jerónimo, M.; Caetano, J.S.; Cardoso, R.; Dinis, I.; Mirante, A. Neonates Born to Mothers with Graves' Disease: 15 Year Experience of a Pediatric Endocrinology Department. *Acta Med. Port.* **2020**, *33*, 483–490. [CrossRef] [PubMed]
58. Pyrżak, B.; Rumińska, M.; Witkowska-Sędek, E.; Kucharska, A. Follow-Up of Thyroid Function in Children with Neonatal Hyperthyroidism. *Front. Endocrinol.* **2022**, *13*, 877119. [CrossRef] [PubMed]
59. Alexander, E.K.; Pearce, E.N.; Brent, G.A.; Brown, R.S.; Chen, H.; Dosiou, C.; Grobman, W.A.; Laurberg, P.; Lazarus, J.H.; Mandel, S.J.; et al. Guidelines of the American Thyroid Association for the Diagnosis and Management of Thyroid Disease During Pregnancy and the Postpartum. *Thyroid* **2017**, *27*, 315–389. [CrossRef]
60. Kahaly, G.J.; Bartalena, L.; Hegedüs, L.; Leenhardt, L.; Poppe, K.; Pearce, S.H. European Thyroid Association Guideline for the Management of Graves' Hyperthyroidism. *Eur. Thyroid J.* **2018**, *7*, 167–186. [CrossRef]
61. Sheffield, J.S.; Cunningham, F.G. Thyrotoxicosis and heart failure that complicate pregnancy. *Am. J. Obstet. Gynecol.* **2004**, *190*, 211–217. [CrossRef] [PubMed]
62. Lee, S.Y.; Pearce, E.N. Hyperthyroidism: A Review. *JAMA* **2023**, *17*, 1472–1483. [CrossRef]
63. Moleti, M.; Sturniolo, G.; Di Mauro, M.; Russo, M.; Vermiglio, F. Autoimmune thyroid diseases and pregnancy. *Ann. Thyroid* **2018**, *3*, 18. [CrossRef]
64. Earl, R.; Crowther, C.A.; Middleton, P. Interventions for hyperthyroidism pre-pregnancy and during pregnancy. *Cochrane Database Syst. Rev.* **2013**, *19*, CD008633. [CrossRef] [PubMed]
65. Sarantaki, A.; Tsiorou, K.; Gourount, K. The impact of Hashimoto's disease on female fertility: A systematic review. *Int. J. Reprod. Contracept. Obstet. Gynecol.* **2022**, *11*, 583–589. [CrossRef]
66. Li, C.; Zhou, J.; Huang, Z.; Pan, X.; Leung, W.; Chen, L.; Zhang, Y.; Wang, L.; Sima, Y.; Gober, H.J.; et al. The Clinical Value and Variation of Antithyroid Antibodies during Pregnancy. *Dis. Markers* **2020**, *2020*, 8871951. [CrossRef]
67. Karkoszka, N.; Gibula-Tarlowska, E.; Kotlinska, J.; Bielenica, A.; Gawel, K.; Kedzierska, E. Selenium Intake and Postnatal Depression—A brief overview. *Nutrients* **2024**, *18*, 1926. [CrossRef] [PubMed]
68. Oken, E.; Rifas-Shiman, S.L.; Amarasiriwardena, C.; Jayawardene, I.; Bellinger, D.C.; Hibbeln, J.R.; Wright, R.O.; Gillman, M.W. Maternal prenatal fish consumption and cognition in mid childhood: Mercury, fatty acids, and selenium. *Neurotoxicol. Teratol.* **2016**, *57*, 71–78. [CrossRef] [PubMed]
69. Filipowicz, D.; Majewska, K.; Kalantarova, A.; Szczepanek-Parulska, E.; Ruchała, M. The rationale for selenium supplementation in patients with autoimmune thyroiditis, according to the current state of knowledge. *Endokrynol. Pol.* **2021**, *72*, 153–162. [CrossRef] [PubMed]
70. Gać, P.; Czerwińska, K.; Macek, P.; Jaremkow, A.; Mazur, G.; Pawlas, K.; Poreba, R. The importance of selenium and zinc deficiency in cardiovascular disorders. *Environ. Toxicol. Pharmacol.* **2021**, *82*, 103553. [CrossRef]
71. Kuria, A.; Tian, H.; Li, M.; Wang, Y.; Aaseth, J.O.; Zang, J.; Cao, Y. Selenium status in the body and cardiovascular disease: A systematic review and meta-analysis. *Crit. Rev. Food. Sci. Nutr.* **2020**, *61*, 3616–3625. [CrossRef] [PubMed]
72. Bastola, M.M.; Locatis, C.; Maisiak, R.; Fontelo, P. Selenium, copper, zinc and hypertension: An analysis of the National Health and Nutrition Examination Survey (2011–2016). *BMC Cardiovasc. Disord.* **2020**, *20*, 45. [CrossRef] [PubMed]
73. Vinceti, M.; Chawla, R.; Filippini, T.; Dutt, C.; Cilloni, S.; Loomba, R.; Bargellini, A.; Orsini, N.; Dhillon, K.S.; Whelton, P. Blood pressure levels and hypertension prevalence in a high selenium environment: Results from a cross-sectional study. *Nutr. Metab. Cardiovasc. Dis.* **2019**, *29*, 398–408. [CrossRef] [PubMed]
74. Korevaar, T.I.M.; Medici, M.; Visser, T.J.; Peeters, R.P. Thyroid disease in pregnancy: New insights in diagnosis and clinical management. *Nat. Rev. Endocrinol.* **2017**, *13*, 610–622. [CrossRef] [PubMed]
75. Lazarus, J.; Brown, R.S.; Daumerie, C.; Hubalewska-Dydejczyk, A.; Negro, R.; Vaidya, B. European thyroid association guidelines for the management of subclinical hypothyroidism in pregnancy and in children. *Eur. Thyroids J.* **2014**, *3*, 76–94. [CrossRef]
76. Korevaar, T.I.M.; Derakhshan, A.; Taylor, P.N.; Meima, M.; Chen, L.; Bliddal, S.; Carty, D.M.; Meems, M.; Vaidya, B.; Shields, B.; et al. Association of thyroid function test abnormalities and thyroid autoimmunity with preterm birth: A systematic review and meta-analysis. *JAMA* **2019**, *322*, 632–641. [CrossRef]

77. Zhu, P.; Chu, R.; Pan, S.; Lai, X.; Ran, J.; Li, X. Impact of subclinical TPOAb-negative maternal hypothyroidism in early pregnancy on adverse pregnancy outcomes. *Ther. Adv. Endocrinol. Metab.* **2021**, *12*, 20420188211054690. [CrossRef] [PubMed]
78. Magri, F.; Bellingeri, C.; De Maggio, I.; Croce, L.; Coperchini, F.; Rotondi, M.; Chiovato, L.; Spinillo, A.; Beneventi, F. First trimester serum TSH in the range of 4–10 mIU/L is associated with obstetric complications in thyroid peroxidase antibody-negative women. *J. Endocrinol. Investig.* **2023**, *46*, 1407–1414. [CrossRef]
79. Poppe, K.G. Levothyroxine in Pregnancy. In *70 Years of Levothyroxine*; Kahaly, G.J., Ed.; Springer: Cham, Switzerland, 2021; pp. 47–60.
80. Solha, S.T.G.; Mattar, R.; Teixeira, P.F.D.S.; Chiamolera, M.I.; Maganha, C.A.; Zaconeta, A.C.M.; Souza, R.T. Screening, diagnosis and management of hypothyroidism in pregnancy. *Rev. Bras. Ginecol. Obstet.* **2022**, *44*, 999–1010. [CrossRef] [PubMed]
81. Lee, H.J.; Stefan-Lifshitz, M.; Li, C.W.; Tomer, Y. Genetics and epigenetics of autoimmune thyroid diseases: Translational implications. *Best Pract. Res. Clin. Endocrinol. Metab.* **2023**, *37*, 101661. [CrossRef]
82. Vargas Uricoechea, H. Molecular Mechanisms in Autoimmune Thyroid Disease. *Cells* **2023**, *12*, 918. [CrossRef] [PubMed]
83. Jacobson, E.M.; Tomer, Y. The CD40, CTLA-4, thyroglobulin, TSH receptor, and PTPN22 gene quintet and its contribution to thyroid autoimmunity: Back to the future. *J. Autoimmun.* **2007**, *28*, 85–98. [CrossRef] [PubMed]
84. Bogović Crnčić, T.; Girotto, N.; Ilić Tomaš, M.; Krištović, I.; Klobučar, S.; Batičić, L.; Ćurko-Cofek, B.; Sotošek, V. Innate Immunity in Autoimmune Thyroid Disease during Pregnancy. *Int. J. Mol. Sci.* **2023**, *24*, 15442. [CrossRef]
85. Chen, X.; Mei, Y.; He, B.; Li, H.; Wang, X.; Hu, R.; Li, L.; Ding, Z. General and Specific Genetic Polymorphism of Cytokines-Related Gene in AITD. *Mediators. Inflamm.* **2017**, *2017*, 3916395.
86. Jacobson, E.M.; Huber, A.; Tomer, Y. The HLA gene complex in thyroid autoimmunity: From epidemiology to etiology. *J. Autoimmun.* **2008**, *30*, 58–62. [CrossRef]
87. Metcalfe, R.A.; McIntosh, R.S.; Marelli-Berg, F.; Lombardi, G.; Lechler, R.; Weetman, A.P. Detection of CD40 on human thyroid follicular cells: Analysis of expression and function. *J. Clin. Endocrinol. Metab.* **1998**, *83*, 1268–1274. [CrossRef]
88. Mysliwiec, J.; Oklota, M.; Nikolajuk, A.; Waligorski, D.; Gorska, M. Serum CD40/CD40L system in Graves' disease and Hashimoto's thyroiditis related to soluble Fas, FasL and humoral markers of autoimmune response. *Immunol. Investig.* **2007**, *36*, 247–257. [CrossRef] [PubMed]
89. Mazzieri, A.; Montanucci, P.; Basta, G.; Calafiore, R. The role behind the scenes of Tregs and Th17s in Hashimoto's thyroiditis: Toward a pivotal role of FOXP3 and BACH2. *Front. Immunol.* **2022**, *13*, 1098243. [CrossRef] [PubMed]
90. Ramirez, R.N.; Chowdhary, K.; Leon, J.; Mathis, D.; Benoist, C. FoxP3 associates with enhancer-promoter loops to regulate Treg-specific gene expression. *Sci. Immunol.* **2022**, *7*, eabj9836. [PubMed]
91. Mizuma, T.; Watanabe, M.; Inoue, N.; Arakawa, Y.; Tomari, S.; Hidaka, Y.; Iwatani, Y. Association of the polymorphisms in the gene encoding thyroglobulin with the development and prognosis of autoimmune thyroid disease. *Autoimmunity* **2017**, *50*, 386–392. [CrossRef] [PubMed]
92. Tomari, S.; Watanabe, M.; Inoue, N.; Mizuma, T.; Yamanaka, C.; Hidaka, Y.; Iwatani, Y. The polymorphisms in the thyroid peroxidase gene were associated with the development of autoimmune thyroid disease and the serum levels of anti-thyroid peroxidase antibody. *Endocr. J.* **2017**, *64*, 1025–1032. [CrossRef]
93. Wang, B.; Shao, X.; Song, R.; Xu, D.; Zhang, J.A. The Emerging Role of Epigenetics in Autoimmune Thyroid Diseases. *Front. Immunol.* **2017**, *8*, 396. [CrossRef] [PubMed]
94. Moore, L.D.; Le, T.; Fan, G. DNA methylation and its basic function. *Neuropsychopharmacology* **2013**, *38*, 23–38. [CrossRef]
95. Lafontaine, N.; Wilson, S.G.; Walsh, J.P. DNA Methylation in Autoimmune Thyroid Disease. *J. Clin. Endocrinol. Metab.* **2023**, *108*, 604–613. [CrossRef] [PubMed]
96. Zhang, Y.; Sun, Z.; Jia, J.; Du, T.; Zhang, N.; Tang, Y.; Fang, Y.; Fang, D. Overview of Histone Modification. *Adv. Exp. Med. Biol.* **2021**, *1283*, 1–16.
97. Haga, E.; Inoue, N.; Iwatani, Y.; Arakawa, Y.; Morita, E.; Hashimoto, H.; Noguchi, Y.; Hidaka, Y.; Watanabe, M. Intraindividual variation in histone acetylation and its impact on autoimmune thyroid diseases. *Endocr. J.* **2023**, *70*, 1169–1174. [CrossRef] [PubMed]
98. Mehta, A.; Baltimore, D. MicroRNAs as regulatory elements in immune system logic. *Nat. Rev. Immunol.* **2016**, *16*, 279–294. [CrossRef]
99. Vicente, R.; Noel, D.; Pers, Y.M.; Apparailly, F.; Jorgensen, C. Deregulation and therapeutic potential of microRNAs in arthritic diseases. *Nat. Rev. Rheumatol.* **2016**, *12*, 211–220. [CrossRef] [PubMed]
100. Seddiki, N.; Brezar, V.; Ruffin, N.; Levy, Y.; Swaminathan, S. Role of miR-155 in the regulation of lymphocyte im-mune function and disease. *Immunology* **2014**, *142*, 32–38. [CrossRef] [PubMed]
101. Chen, J.Q.; Papp, G.; Szodoray, P.; Zeher, M. The role of microRNAs in the pathogenesis of autoimmune diseases. *Autoimmun. Rev.* **2016**, *15*, 1171–1180. [CrossRef] [PubMed]

102. Rodriguez-Munoz, A.; Martinez-Hernandez, R.; Ramos-Levi, A.M.; Serrano-Somavilla, A.; Gonzalez-Amaro, R.; Sanchez-Madrid, F.; de la Fuente, H.; Marazuela, M. Circulating microvesicles regulate Treg and Th17 differentiation in human autoimmune thyroid disorders. *J. Clin. Endocrinol. Metab.* **2015**, *100*, e1531–e1539. [CrossRef] [PubMed]
103. Wang, Z.; Fan, X.; Zhang, R.; Lin, Z.; Lu, T.; Bai, X.; Li, W.; Zhao, J.; Zhang, Q. Integrative analysis of mRNA and miRNA array data reveals the suppression of retinoic acid pathway in regulatory T cells of Graves' disease. *J. Clin. Endocrinol. Metab.* **2014**, *99*, e2620–e2627. [CrossRef] [PubMed]
104. Bernecker, C.; Lenz, L.; Ostapczuk, M.S.; Schinner, S.; Willenberg, H.; Ehlers, M.; Vordenbäumen, S.; Feldkamp, J.; Schott, M. MicroRNAs miR-146a1, miR-155_2, and miR-200a1 are regulated in autoimmune thyroid diseases. *Thyroid* **2012**, *22*, 1294–1295. [CrossRef]
105. Ishido, N.; Inoue, N.; Watanabe, M.; Hidaka, Y.; Iwatani, Y. The relationship between skewed X chromosome inactivation and the prognosis of Graves' and Hashimoto's diseases. *Thyroid* **2015**, *25*, 256–261. [CrossRef] [PubMed]
106. Chen, X.; Wu, C.; Wang, Z.; Wu, C.; Guo, Y.; Zhu, X.; Hu, Y.P.; Shi, Z.; Song, Q.; Cui, X.; et al. Iodine nutrition status and thyroid autoimmunity during pregnancy: A cross-sectional study of 4635 pregnant women. *Nutr. J.* **2022**, *21*, 7. [CrossRef]
107. Zhang, L.; Shang, F.; Liu, C.; Zhai, X. The correlation between iodine and metabolism: A review. *Front. Nutr.* **2024**, *19*, 1346452. [CrossRef]
108. Farebrother, J.; Zimmermann, M.B.; Andersson, M. Excess iodine intake: Sources, assessment, and effects on thyroid function. *Ann. N. Y. Acad Sci.* **2019**, *1446*, 44–65. [CrossRef]
109. Luo, Y.; Kawashima, A.; Ishido, Y.; Yoshihara, A.; Oda, K.; Hiroi, N.; Ito, T.; Ishii, N.; Suzuki, K. Iodine excess as an environmental risk factor for autoimmune thyroid disease. *Int. J. Mol. Sci.* **2014**, *15*, 12895–12912. [CrossRef] [PubMed]
110. Teti, C.; Panciroli, M.; Nazzari, E.; Pesce, G.; Mariotti, S.; Olivieri, A.; Bagnasco, M. Iodoprophylaxis and thyroid autoimmunity: An update. *Immunol. Res.* **2021**, *69*, 129–138. [CrossRef]
111. Chen, X.; Chen, L.; Lian, X.; Liu, C.; Shan, Z.; Shi, B.; Shi, L.; Tong, N.; Weng, J.; Zhao, J.; et al. Urinary iodine concentration is inversely associated with thyroglobulin antibodies. *Endocr. Pract.* **2019**, *25*, 454–460. [CrossRef] [PubMed]
112. Herrick, K.A.; Perrine, C.G.; Aoki, Y.; Caldwell, K.L. Iodine status and consumption of key iodine sources in the U.S. population with special attention to reproductive age women. *Nutrients* **2018**, *10*, 874. [CrossRef] [PubMed]
113. Dineva, M.; Rayman, M.P.; Levie, D.; Guxens, M.; Peeters, R.P.; Vioque, J.; González, L.; Espada, M.; Ibarluzea, J.; Sunyer, J.; et al. Similarities and differences of dietary and other determinants of iodine status in pregnant women from three European birth cohorts. *Eur. J. Nutr.* **2020**, *59*, 371–387. [CrossRef] [PubMed]
114. Tsatsoulis, A. The role of iodine versus selenium in the rising trend of autoimmune thyroiditis in iodine-sufficient countries. *Endocrinol. Metab. Int.* **2018**, *6*, 412–414.
115. Wémeau, J.L.; Klein, M.; Sadoul, J.L.; Briet, C.; Vélayoudom-Céphise, F.L. Graves' disease: Introduction, epidemiology, endogenous and environmental pathogenic factors. *Ann. Endocrinol.* **2018**, *79*, 599–607. [CrossRef] [PubMed]
116. Burek, C.L.; Talor, M.V. Environmental triggers of autoimmune thyroiditis. *J. Autoimmun.* **2009**, *33*, 183–189. [CrossRef]
117. Carayanniotis, G. Molecular parameters linking thymoglobulin iodination with autoimmune thyroiditis. *Hormones* **2011**, *10*, 27–35. [CrossRef] [PubMed]
118. Duntas, L.H. The catalytic role of iodine excess in loss of homeostasis in autoimmune thyroiditis. *Curr. Opin. Endocrinol. Diabetes Obes.* **2018**, *25*, 347–352. [CrossRef] [PubMed]
119. Petersen, M.; Knudsen, N.; Carlé, A.; Andersen, S.; Jørgensen, T.; Perrild, H.; Ovesen, L.; Rasmussen, L.B.; Thuesen, B.H.; Pedersen, I.B. Increased incidence rate of hypothyroidism after iodine fortification in Denmark: A 20-year prospective population-based study. *J. Clin. Endocrinol. Metab.* **2019**, *104*, 1833–1840. [CrossRef] [PubMed]
120. Hong, A.; Stokes, B.; Otaha, L.P.; Owens, D.; Burgess, J.R. Temporal trends in thyroid- stimulating hormone (TSH) and thyroid peroxidase antibody (ATPO) testing across two phases of iodine fortification in Tasmania (1995–2013). *Clin. Endocrinol.* **2017**, *87*, 386–393. [CrossRef] [PubMed]
121. Khattak, R.M.; Ittermann, T.; Nauck, M.; Below, H.; Völzke, H. Monitoring the prevalence of thyroid disorders in the adult population of Northeast Germany. *Popul. Health Metr.* **2016**, *14*, 1–11. [CrossRef] [PubMed]
122. Teng, D.; Yang, W.; Shi, X.; Li, Y.; Ba, J.; Chen, B.; Du, J.; He, L.; Lai, X.; Li, Y.; et al. An inverse relationship between iodine intake and thyroid antibodies: A national cross-sectional survey in mainland China. *Thyroid* **2020**, *30*, 1656–1665. [CrossRef] [PubMed]
123. De la Vieja, A.; Santisteban, P. Role of iodide metabolism in physiology and cancer. *Endocr. Relat. Cancer* **2018**, *25*, 225–245. [CrossRef] [PubMed]
124. Moleti, M.; Trimarchi, F.; Vermiglio, F. Thyroid physiology in pregnancy. *Endocr. Pract.* **2014**, *20*, 589–596. [CrossRef] [PubMed]
125. Zimmermann, M.B. Iodine deficiency in pregnancy and the effects of maternaliodine supplementation on the offspring: A review. *Am. J. Clin. Nutr.* **2009**, *89*, 668–672. [CrossRef]
126. Toloza, F.J.K.; Motahari, H.; Maraka, S. Consequences of Severe Iodine Deficiency in Pregnancy: Evidence in Humans. *Front. Endocrinol.* **2020**, *11*, 409. [CrossRef]

127. Pearce, E.N.; Lazarus, J.H.; Moreno-Reyes, R.; Zimmermann, M.B. Consequences of iodine deficiency and excess in pregnant women: An overview of current knowns and unknowns. *Am. J. Clin. Nutr.* **2016**, *104*, 918–923. [CrossRef] [PubMed]
128. Yang, J.; Liu, Y.; Liu, H.; Zheng, H.; Li, X.; Zhu, L.; Wang, Z. Associations of maternal iodine status and thyroid function with adverse pregnancy outcomesin Henan Province of China. *J. Trace Elem. Med. Biol.* **2018**, *47*, 104–110. [CrossRef] [PubMed]
129. Mills, J.L.; Ali, M.; Buck Louis, G.M.; Kannan, K.; Weck, J.; Wan, Y.; Maisog, J.; Giannakou, A.; Sundaram, R. Pregnancy loss and iodine status: The LIFE prospective cohort study. *Nutrients* **2019**, *11*, 534. [CrossRef]
130. Leung, A.M.; Braverman, L.E. Consequences of excess iodine. *Nat. Rev. Endocrinol.* **2014**, *10*, 136–142. [CrossRef] [PubMed]
131. Wang, Z.; Liu, P.; Su, X.; Zou, S.; Song, J.; Liu, S. A comparison of iodine status in children and pregnant women after a policy change in the iodized salt standard in Shanghai, China. *Biol. Trac Elem. Res.* **2018**, *185*, 275–281. [CrossRef] [PubMed]
132. Wang, Z.; Liu, P.; Su, X.; Zou, S.; Song, J.; Liu, S. A Comparative Study of Iodized Salt Programs: Shanghai and Switzerland. *Biol. Trace Elem. Res.* **2019**, *187*, 59–64. [CrossRef] [PubMed]
133. Hurley, S.; Eastman, C.J.; Gallego, G. The impact of mandatory iodine fortification and supplementation on pregnant and lactating women in Australia. *Asia Pac. J. Clin. Nutr.* **2019**, *28*, 15–22.
134. Southern, A.P.; Anastasopoulou, C.; Jwayyed, S. *Iodine Toxicity*; StatPearls Publishing: Treasure Island, FL, USA, 2024; p. 32644629.
135. Rebagliato, M.; Murcia, M.; Alvarez-Pedrerol, M.; Espada, M.; Fernández-Somoano, A.; Lertxundi, N.; Navarrete-Muñoz, E.M.; Forns, J.; Aranbarri, A.; Llop, S.; et al. Iodine supplementation during pregnancy and infant neuropsychological development. INMA Mother and Child Cohort Study. *Am. J. Epidemiol.* **2013**, *177*, 944–953. [CrossRef]
136. Purdue-Smithe, A.C.; Männistö, T.; Bell, G.A.; Mumford, S.L.; Liu, A.; Kannan, K.; Kim, U.J.; Suvanto, E.; Surcel, H.M.; Gissler, M.; et al. The Joint Role of Thyroid Function and Iodine Status on Risk of Preterm Birth and Small for Gestational Age: A Population-Based, Nested Case-Control Study of Finnish Women. *Nutrients* **2019**, *11*, 2573. [CrossRef] [PubMed]
137. Winther, K.H.; Rayman, M.P.; Bonnema, S.J.; Hegedus, L. Selenium in thyroid disorders—Essential knowledge for clinicians. *Nat. Rev. Endocrinol.* **2020**, *16*, 165–176. [CrossRef]
138. Schomburg, L. Selenium Deficiency Due to Diet, Pregnancy, Severe Illness, or COVID-19-A Preventable Trigger for Autoimmune Disease. *Int. J. Mol. Sci.* **2021**, *22*, 8532. [CrossRef] [PubMed]
139. Minnetti, M.; Sada, V.; Feola, T.; Giannetta, E.; Pozza, C.; Gianfrilli, D.; Isidori, A.M.; Cozzolino, A. Selenium Supplementation in Pregnant Women with Autoimmune Thyroiditis: A Practical Approach. *Nutrients* **2022**, *14*, 2234. [CrossRef]
140. Huang, S.; Ziros, P.G.; Chartoumpekis, D.V.; Psarias, G.; Duntas, L.; Zuo, X.; Li, X.; Ding, Z.; Sykiotis, G.P. Traditional Chinese Medicine for Hashimoto's Thyroiditis: Focus on Selenium and Antioxidant Phytochemicals. *Antioxidants* **2024**, *13*, 868. [CrossRef]
141. Huwiler, V.V.; Maissen-Abgottspon, S.; Stanga, Z.; Mühlebach, S.; Trepp, R.; Bally, L.; Bano, A. Selenium Supplementation in Patients with Hashimoto Thyroiditis: A Systematic Review and Meta-Analysis of Randomized Clinical Trials. *Thyroid* **2024**, *34*, 295–313. [CrossRef]
142. Wang, Y.S.; Liang, S.S.; Ren, J.J.; Wang, Z.Y.; Deng, X.X.; Liu, W.D.; Yan, Y.L.; Song, G.H.; Li, X.X. The Effects of Selenium Supplementation in the Treatment of Autoimmune Thyroiditis: An Overview of Systematic Reviews. *Nutrients* **2023**, *15*, 3194. [CrossRef] [PubMed]
143. Shulhai, A.M.; Rotondo, R.; Petraroli, M.; Patianna, V.; Predieri, B.; Iughetti, L.; Esposito, S.; Street, M.E. The Role of Nutrition on Thyroid Function. *Nutrients* **2024**, *16*, 2496. [CrossRef]
144. Wang, W.; Jiang, Q.L.; Xu, Q.; Zeng, Y.; Jiang, R.; Jiang, J. Selenium regulates T cell differentiation in experimental autoimmune thyroiditis in mice. *Int. Immunopharmacol.* **2023**, *124*, 110993. [CrossRef] [PubMed]
145. Hu, Y.; Feng, W.; Chen, H.; Shi, H.; Jiang, L.; Zheng, X.; Liu, X.; Zhang, W.; Ge, Y.; Liu, Y.; et al. Effect of selenium on thyroid autoimmunity and regulatory T cells in patients with Hashimoto's thyroiditis: A prospective randomized- controlled trial. *Clin. Tansl. Sci.* **2021**, *14*, 1390–1402. [CrossRef] [PubMed]
146. Kong, X.Q.; Qiu, G.Y.; Yang, Z.B.; Tan, Z.X.; Quan, X.Q. Clinical efficacy of selenium supplementation in patients with Hashimoto thyroiditis: A systematic review and meta-analysis. *Medicin* **2023**, *102*, e33791. [CrossRef]
147. Köhrle, J. Selenium and the thyroid. *Curr. Opin. Endocrinol. Diabetes Obes.* **2015**, *22*, 392–401. [CrossRef]
148. McDougall, A.R.; Dore, G.; Aboud, L.; Makama, M.; Nguyen, P.Y.; Mills, K.; Sanderson, B.; Hastie, R.; Ammerdorffer, A.; Vogel, J.P. The effect of selenium supplementation in pregnant women on maternal, fetal, and newborn outcomes: A systematic review and meta-analysis. *Am. J. Obstet. Gynecol. MFM* **2023**, *5*, 101160. [CrossRef] [PubMed]
149. Yigit, E.; Sayar, I. Selenium Supplementation and Gestational Diabetes: A Randomised Controlled Trial. Journal of the College of Physicians and Surgeons—Pakistan. *JCPSP* **2024**, *34*, 561–567. [PubMed]
150. Negro, R.; Greco, G.; Mangieri, T.; Pezzarossa, A.; Dazzi, D.; Hassan, H. The influence of selenium supplementation on postpartum thyroid status in pregnant women with thyroid peroxidase autoantibodies. *J. Clin. Endocrinol. Metabol.* **2007**, *92*, 1263–1268. [CrossRef] [PubMed]
151. Pitts, M.W.; Byrns, C.N.; Ogawa-Wong, A.N.; Kremer, P.; Berry, M.J. Selenoproteins in nervous system development and function. *Biol. Trace Elem. Res.* **2014**, *161*, 231–245. [CrossRef]

152. Demircan, K.; Chillon, T.S.; Jensen, R.C.; Jensen, T.K.; Sun, Q.; Bonnema, S.J.; Glintborg, D.; Bilenberg, N.; Andersen, M.S.; Schomburg, L. Maternal selenium deficiency during pregnancy in association with autism and ADHD traits in children: The Odense Child Cohort. *Free Radic. Biol. Med.* **2024**, *1*, 324–332. [CrossRef]
153. Lee, A.S.E.; Ji, Y.; Raghavan, R.; Wang, G.; Hong, X.; Pearson, C.; Mirolli, G.; Bind, E.; Steffens, A.; Mukherjee, J.; et al. Maternal prenatal selenium levels and child risk of neurodevelopmental disorders: A prospective birth cohort study. *Autism. Res.* **2021**, *14*, 2533–2543. [CrossRef] [PubMed]
154. Ventura, M.; Melo, M.; Carrilho, F. Selenium and thyroid disease: From pathophysiology to treatment. *Int. J. Endocrinol.* **2017**, *31*, 1–9. [CrossRef] [PubMed]
155. Hubalewska-Dydejczyk, A.; Duntas, L.; Gilis-Januszewska, A. Pregnancy, thyroid, and the potential use of selenium. *Hormones* **2020**, *19*, 47–53. [CrossRef] [PubMed]
156. Garofalo, V.; Condorelli, R.A.; Cannarella, R.; Aversa, A.; Calogero, A.E.; La Vignera, S. Relationship between Iron Deficiency and Thyroid Function: A Systematic Review and Meta-Analysis. *Nutrients* **2023**, *15*, 4790. [CrossRef] [PubMed]
157. Luo, J.; Wang, X.; Yuan, L.; Guo, L. Iron Deficiency, a Risk Factor of Thyroid Disorders in Reproductive-Age and Pregnant Women: A Systematic Review and Meta-Analysis. *Front. Endocrinol.* **2021**, *25*, 629831. [CrossRef] [PubMed]
158. Abbas, W.; Elmugabil, A.; Hamdan, H.Z.; Rayis, D.A.; Adam, I. Iron deficiency and thyroid dysfunction among sudanese women in first trimester of pregnancy: A cross-sectional study. *BMC Endocr. Disord.* **2023**, *13*, 223. [CrossRef]
159. Huang, X.; Mao, M.; Guo, T.; Wu, Y.; Xu, Q.; Dai, J.; Huang, Y. Iron Status, Thyroid Dysfunction, and Iron Deficiency Anemia: A Two-Sample Mendelian Randomization Study. *Ann. Nutr. Metab.* **2024**, *10*, 1–12. [CrossRef] [PubMed]
160. Li, X.; Zhang, Z.; Cai, W.; Zhou, X.; Zhang, Y.; Wu, C.; Xu, X.; Wu, H. Association Between Serum Ferritin Levels in Early Pregnancy and Thyroid Function and Pregnancy Outcomes in Chinese Population. *Int. J. Womens Health* **2023**, *11*, 1951–1957. [CrossRef]
161. Zimmermann, M.B.; Burgi, H.; Hurrell, R.F. Iron deficiency predicts poor maternal thyroid status during pregnancy. *J. Clin. Endocrinol. Metab.* **2007**, *92*, 3436–3440. [CrossRef] [PubMed]
162. Veltri, F.; Decaillet, S.; Kleynen, P.; Grabczan, L.; Belhomme, J.; Rozenberg, S.; Pepersack, T.; Poppe, K. Prevalence of thyroid autoimmunity and dysfunction in women with iron deficiency during early pregnancy: Is it altered? *Eur. J. Endocrinol.* **2016**, *175*, 191–199. [CrossRef]
163. Pleić, N.; Babić Leko, M.; Gunjača, I.; Zemunik, T. Vitamin D and thyroid function: A mendelian randomization study. *PLoS ONE* **2024**, *19*, e0304253. [CrossRef] [PubMed]
164. Khozam, S.A.; Sumaili, A.M.; Alflan, M.A.; Shawabkeh, R.A.S. Association Between Vitamin D Deficiency and Autoimmune Thyroid Disorder: A Systematic Review. *Cureus* **2022**, *12*, e25869. [CrossRef]
165. Durá-Travé, T.; Gallinas-Victoriano, F. Autoimmune Thyroiditis and Vitamin, D. *Int. J. Mol. Sci.* **2024**, *9*, 3154. [CrossRef] [PubMed]
166. Pang, B.; Li, L.; Liu, X.; Cao, Z.; Pang, T.; Wang, Q.; Wei, J. Association between serum vitamin D level and Graves' disease: A systematic review and meta-analysis. *Nutr. J.* **2024**, *7*, 60. [CrossRef]
167. Waterhouse, M.; Pham, H.; Rahman, S.T.; Baxter, C.; Duarte Romero, B.; Armstrong, B.K.; Ebeling, P.R.; English, D.R.; Hartel, G.; van der Pols, J.C.; et al. The Effect of Vitamin D Supplementation on Hypothyroidism in the Randomized Controlled D-Health Trial. *Thyroid* **2023**, *33*, 1302–1310. [CrossRef] [PubMed]
168. Bellastella, G.; Maiorino, M.I.; Petrizzo, M.; De Bellis, A.; Capuano, A.; Esposito, K.; Giugliano, D. Vitamin D and autoimmunity: What happens in autoimmune polyendocrine syndromes? *J. Endocrinol. Investig.* **2015**, *38*, 629–633. [CrossRef] [PubMed]
169. Gallo, D.; Baci, D.; Kustrimovic, N.; Lanzo, N.; Patera, B.; Tanda, M.L.; Piantanida, E.; Mortara, L. How Does Vitamin D Affect Immune Cells Crosstalk in Autoimmune Diseases? *Int. J. Mol. Sci.* **2023**, *28*, 4689. [CrossRef]
170. Altieri, B.; Muscogiuri, G.; Barrea, L.; Mathieu, C.; Vallone, C.V.; Mascitelli, L.; Bizzaro, G.; Altieri, V.M.; Tirabassi, G.; Balercia, G.; et al. Does vitamin D play a role in autoimmune endocrine disorders? A proof of concept. *Rev. Endocr. Metab. Disord.* **2017**, *18*, 335–346. [CrossRef]
171. Houen, G. Auto-immuno- deficiency syndromes. *Autoimmun. Rev.* **2024**, *23*, 103610. [CrossRef]
172. Sinharay, M.; Dasgupta, A.; Karmakar, A. Association between Vitamin D Receptor Gene Polymorphism (Fok 1), Vitamin D Status and Autoimmune Thyroiditis. *Mymensingh Med. J.* **2024**, *33*, 914–922. [PubMed]
173. Soda, M.; Priante, C.; Pesce, C.; De Maio, G.; Lombardo, M. The Impact of Vitamin D on Immune Function and Its Role in Hashimoto's Thyroiditis: A Narrative Review. *Life* **2024**, *17*, 771. [CrossRef]
174. Wu, J.; Li, J.; Yan, Z.; Yu, X.; Huang, H. Higher prevalence of thyroid-specific autoibodies (TPOAb and TgAb) is related to a higher prevalence of fractures in females: Results from NHANES 2007-2010. *Osteoporos. Int.* **2024**, *35*, 1213–1221. [CrossRef] [PubMed]
175. Kim, S.J.; Kim, M.J.; Yoon, S.G.; Myong, J.P.; Yu, H.W.; Chai, Y.J.; Choi, J.Y.; Lee, K.E. Impact of smoking on thyroid gland: Dose-related effect of urinary cotinine levels on thyroid function and thyroid autoimmunity. *Sci. Rep.* **2019**, *12*, 4213. [CrossRef]

176. Zhang, Y.; Shi, L.; Zhang, Q.; Peng, N.; Chen, L.; Lian, X.; Liu, C.; Shan, Z.; Shi, B.; Tong, N.; et al. The association between cigarette smoking and serum thyroid stimulating hormone, thyroid peroxidase antibodies and thyroglobulin antibodies levels in Chinese residents: A cross-sectional study in 10 cities. *PLoS ONE* **2019**, *25*, e0225435. [CrossRef] [PubMed]
177. Kadkhodazadeh, H.; Amouzegar, A.; Mehran, L.; Gharibzadeh, S.; Azizi, F.; Tohidi, M. Smoking status and changes in thyroid-stimulating hormone and free thyroxine levels during a decade of follow-up: The Tehran thyroid study. Caspian. *J. Intern. Med.* **2020**, *11*, 47–52.
178. Vestergaard, P.; Rejnmark, L.; Weeke, J.; Hoeck, H.C.; Nielsen, H.K.; Rungby, J.; Laurberg, P.; Mosekilde, L. Smoking as a risk factor for Graves' disease, toxic nodular goiter, and autoimmune hypothyroidism. *Thyroid* **2002**, *12*, 69–75. [CrossRef] [PubMed]
179. Tohidi, M.; Derakhshan, A.; Akbarpour, S.; Amouzegar, A.; Mehran, L.; Baghbani-Oskouei, A.; Azizi, F.; Hadaegh, F. Thyroid Dysfunction States and Incident Cardiovascular Events: The Tehran Thyroid Study. *Horm. Metab. Res.* **2018**, *50*, e1. [PubMed]
180. Kunutsor, S.K.; Dey, R.S.; Touw, D.J.; Bakker, S.J.L.; Dullaart, R.P.F. Urine cotinine versus self-reported smoking and the risk of chronic kidney disease. *Nephrol. Dial. Transplant.* **2024**, *39*, 1683–1691. [CrossRef] [PubMed]
181. Gruppen, E.G.; Kootstra-Ros, J.; Kobold, A.M.; Connelly, M.A.; Touw, D.; Bos, J.H.J.; Hak, E.; Links, T.P.; Bakker, S.J.L.; Dullaart, R.P.F. Cigarette smoking is associated with higher thyroid hormone and lower TSH levels: The PREVEND study. *Endocrine* **2020**, *67*, 613–622. [CrossRef] [PubMed]
182. Soldin, O.P.; Goughenour, B.E.; Gilbert, S.Z.; Landy, H.J.; Soldin, S.J. Thyroid hormone levels associated with active and passive cigarette smoking. *Thyroid* **2009**, *19*, 817–823. [CrossRef] [PubMed]
183. Karbownik-Lewińska, M.; Stępniak, J.; Iwan, P.; Lewiński, A. Iodine as a potential endocrine disruptor—A role of oxidative stress. *Endocrine* **2022**, *78*, 219–240. [CrossRef] [PubMed]
184. Andersen, S.L.; Olsen, J.; Wu, C.S.; Laurberg, P. Smoking reduces the risk of hypothyroidism and increases the risk of hyperthyroidism: Evidence from 450,842 mothers giving birth in Denmark. *Clin. Endocrinol.* **2014**, *80*, 307–314. [CrossRef] [PubMed]
185. Shields, B.; Hill, A.; Bilous, M.; Knight, B.; Hattersley, A.T.; Bilous, R.W.; Bijay, V. Cigarette Smoking during Pregnancy Is Associated with Alterations in Maternal and Fetal Thyroid Function. *J. Clin. Endocrinol. Metab.* **2009**, *94*, 570–574. [CrossRef]
186. Rashad, R.; Pinto, R.; Li, E.; Sohrab, M.; Distefano, A.G. Thyroid Eye Disease. *Life* **2022**, *12*, 2084. [CrossRef]
187. Kang, J.; Kong, E.; Choi, J. Associations of urinary cotinineverified active and passive smoking with thyroid function: Analysis of population-based nationally representative data. *Thyroid* **2018**, *28*, 583–592. [CrossRef]
188. Mehran, L.; Amouzgar, A.; Delshad, H.; Azizi, F. The association of cigarette smoking with serum TSH concentration and thyroperoxidase antibody. *Exp. Clin. Endocrinol. Diabetes* **2012**, *120*, 80–83. [CrossRef] [PubMed]
189. Cho, N.H.; Choi, H.S.; Kim, K.W.; Kim, H.L.; Lee, S.Y.; Choi, S.H.; Lim, S.; Park, Y.J.; Park, D.J.; Jang, H.C.; et al. Interaction between cigarette smoking and iodine intake and their impact on thyroid function. *Clin. Endocrinol.* **2010**, *73*, 264–270. [CrossRef]
190. Mahmoudzadeh, L.; Abtahi Froushani, S.M.; Ajami, M.; Mahmoudzadeh, M. Effect of Nicotine on Immune System Function. *Adv. Pharm. Bull.* **2023**, *13*, 69–78. [CrossRef] [PubMed]
191. Qiu, F.; Liang, C.L.; Liu, H.; Zeng, Y.Q.; Hou, S.; Huang, S.; Lai, X.; Dai, Z. Impacts of cigarette smoking on immune responsiveness: Up and down or upside down? *Oncotarget* **2017**, *8*, 268–284. [CrossRef] [PubMed]
192. Brown, S.J.; Bremner, A.P.; Hadlow, N.C.; Feddema, P.; Leedman, P.J.; O'Leary, P.C.; Walsh, J.P. The log TSH-free T4 relationship in a community-based cohort is nonlinear and is influenced by age, smoking and thyroid peroxidase antibody status. *Clin. Endocrinol.* **2016**, *85*, 789–796. [CrossRef]
193. Quelhas, D.; Kompala, C.; Wittenbrink, B.; Han, Z.; Parker, M.; Shapiro, M.; Downs, S.; Kraemer, K.; Fanzo, J.; Morris, S.; et al. The association between active tobacco use during pregnancy and growth outcomes of children under five years of age: A systematic review and metaanalysis. *BMC Public Health* **2018**, *13*, 1372. [CrossRef] [PubMed]
194. Gunnerbeck, A.; Edstedt Bonamy, A.K.; Wikström, A.K.; Granath, F.; Wickström, R.; Cnattingius, S. Maternal snuff use and smoking and the risk of oral cleft malformations: A population- based cohort study. *PLoS ONE* **2014**, *15*, e84715. [CrossRef] [PubMed]
195. Leite, M.; Albieri, V.; Kjaer, S.K.; Jensen, A. Maternal smoking in pregnancy and risk for congenital malformations: Results of a Danish register-based cohort study. *Acta Obstet. Gynecol. Scand.* **2014**, *93*, 825–834. [CrossRef] [PubMed]
196. Sabbagh, H.J.; Hassan, M.H.A.; Innes, N.P.T.; Elkodary, H.M.; Little, J.; Mossey, P.A. Passive smoking in the etiology of non-syndromic orofacial clefts: A systematic review and meta-analysis. *PLoS ONE* **2015**, *10*, e0116963. [CrossRef] [PubMed]
197. Suter, M.A.; Aagaard, K.M. The impact of tobacco chemicals and nicotine on placental development. *Prenat. Diagn.* **2020**, *40*, 1193–1200. [CrossRef]
198. Yuan, S.; Liu, J.; Larsson, S.C. Smoking, alcohol and coffee consumption and pregnancy loss: A Mendelian randomization investigation. *Fertil. Steril.* **2021**, *116*, 1061–1067. [CrossRef]
199. Lange, S.; Probst, C.; Rehm, J.; Popova, S. National, regional, and global prevalence of smoking during pregnancy in the general population: A systematic review and meta-analysis. *Lancet Glob. Health* **2018**, *6*, e769–e776. [CrossRef] [PubMed]

200. Andersen, S.L.; Knøsgaard, L.; Handberg, A.; Vestergaard, P.; Andersen, S. Maternal adiposity, smoking, and thyroid function in early pregnancy. *Endocr. Connect.* **2021**, *10*, 1125–1133. [CrossRef] [PubMed]
201. Ebbo, M.; Crinier, A.; Vely, F.; Vivier, E. Innate lymphoid cells: Major players in inflammatory diseases. *Nat. Rev. Immunol.* **2017**, *17*, 665–678. [CrossRef] [PubMed]
202. Domínguez-Andrés, J.; Novakovic, B.; Li, Y.; Scicluna, B.P.; Gresnigt, M.S.; Arts, R.J.W.; Oosting, M.; Moorlag, S.J.C.F.M.; Groh, L.A.; Zwaag, J.; et al. The Itaconate Pathway Is a Central Regulatory Node Linking Innate Immune Tolerance and Trained Immunity. *Cell. Metab.* **2019**, *29*, 211–220. [CrossRef] [PubMed]
203. Bjorkstrom, N.K.; Ljunggren, H.G.; Michaelsson, J. Emerging insights into natural killer cells in human peripheral tissues. *Nat. Rev. Immunol.* **2016**, *16*, 310–320. [CrossRef]
204. Cooper, M.A.; Fehniger, T.A.; Caligiuri, M.A. The biology of human natural killer-cell subsets. *Trends Immunol.* **2001**, *22*, 633–640. [CrossRef] [PubMed]
205. Lee, E.K.; Sunwoo, J.B. Natural Killer Cells and Thyroid Diseases. *Endocrinol. Metab.* **2019**, *34*, 132–137. [CrossRef] [PubMed]
206. Wisgalla, A.; Ramien, C.; Streitz, M.; Schlickeiser, S.; Lupu, A.R.; Diemert, A.; Tolosa, E.; Arck, P.C.; Bellmann-Strobl, J.; Siebert, N.; et al. Alterations of NK Cell Phenotype during Pregnancy in Multiple Sclerosis. *Front. Immunol.* **2022**, *13*, 907994. [CrossRef]
207. Harinarayan, C.V.; Akhila, H.; Shanthisree, E. Modern India and Dietary Calcium Deficiency-Half a Century Nutrition Data-Retrospect-Introspect and the Road Ahead. *Front. Endocrinol.* **2021**, *12*, 583654. [CrossRef] [PubMed]
208. Vaivode, I.; Zake, T.; Strele, I.; Upmale-Engela, S.; Gogins, D.; Gersone, G.; Skesters, A.; Dambrova, M.; Konrade, I. Stress-Related Immune Response and Selenium Status in Autoimmune Thyroid Disease Patients. *Int. J. Mol. Sci.* **2023**, *24*, 2440. [CrossRef]
209. Dhabhar, F.S. Effects of stress on immune function: The good, the bad, and the beautiful. *Immunol. Res.* **2014**, *58*, 193–210. [CrossRef]
210. Torres, D.J.; Alfulaij, N.; Berry, M.J. Stress and the Brain: An Emerging Role for Selenium. *Front. Neurosci* **2021**, *15*, 666601. [CrossRef] [PubMed]
211. Vita, R.; Lapa, D.; Trimarchi, F.; Benvenga, S. Stress triggers the onset and the recurrences of hyperthyroidism in patients with Graves' disease. *Endocrine* **2015**, *48*, 254–263. [CrossRef] [PubMed]
212. Effraimidis, G.; Strieder, T.G.; Tijssen, J.G.; Wiersinga, W.M. Natural history of the transition from euthyroidism to overt autoimmune hypo- or hyperthyroidism: A prospective study. *Eur. J. Endocrinol.* **2011**, *164*, 107–113. [CrossRef] [PubMed]
213. Markomanolaki, Z.S.; Tigani, X.; Siamatras, T.; Bacopoulou, F.; Tsartsalis, A.; Artemiadis, A.; Megalooikonomou, V.; Vlachakis, D.; Chrousos, G.P.; Darviri, C. Stress Management in Women with Hashimoto's thyroiditis: A Randomized Controlled Trial. *J. Mol. Biochem.* **2019**, *8*, 3–12. [PubMed]
214. Ruggeri, R.M.; Vicchio, T.M.; Cristani, M.; Certo, R.; Caccamo, D.; Alibrandi, A.; Giovinazzo, S.; Saija, A.; Campennì, A.; Trimarchi, F.; et al. Oxidative Stress and Advanced Glycation End Products in Hashimoto's Thyroiditis. *Thyroid* **2016**, *26*, 504–511. [CrossRef] [PubMed]
215. Corso, A.; Engel, H.; Müller, F.; Fiacco, S.; Mernone, L.; Gardini, E.; Ehlert, U.; Fischer, S. Early life stress in women with autoimmune thyroid disorders. *Sci. Rep.* **2023**, *13*, 22341. [CrossRef] [PubMed]
216. Puttaswamy, S.H.; Nandibewur, N.P.; Kumar, P.; Venkataiah, V.; Pinjar, M.J. A Cross-Sectional Study of the Relationship Between Perceived Stress and Thyroid Function Among Apparently Normal Women in the Reproductive Age. *Cureus* **2024**, *16*, 55567. [CrossRef] [PubMed]
217. Staneva, A.; Bogossian, F.; Pritchard, M.; Wittkowski, A. The effects of maternal depression, anxiety, and perceived stress during pregnancy on preterm birth: A systematic review. *Women Birth* **2015**, *28*, 179–193. [CrossRef]
218. Van den Bergh, B.R.; Dahnke, R.; Mennes, M. Prenatal stress and the developing brain: Risks for neurodevelopmental disorders. *Dev. Psychopathol.* **2018**, *30*, 743–762. [CrossRef]
219. Qu, F.; Wu, Y.; Zhu, Y.H.; Barry, J.; Ding, T.; Baio, G.; Muscat, R.; Todd, B.K.; Wang, F.F.; Hardiman, P.J. The association between psychological stress and miscarriage: A systematic review and meta-analysis. *Sci. Rep.* **2017**, *7*, 1731. [CrossRef] [PubMed]
220. Cai, S.; Tan, S.; Gluckman, P.D.; Godfrey, K.M.; Saw, S.M.; Teoh, O.H.; Chong, Y.S.; Meaney, M.J.; Kramer, M.S.; Gooley, J.J.; et al. Sleep quality and nocturnal sleep duration in pregnancy and risk of gestational diabetes mellitus. *Sleep* **2017**, *40*, 5–12. [CrossRef] [PubMed]
221. Slade, P.; Sheen, K.; Weeks, A.; Wray, S.; De Pascalis, L.; Lunt, K.; Bedwell, C.; Thompson, B.; Hill, J.; Sharp, H. Do stress and anxiety in early pregnancy affect the progress of labor: Evidence from theWirral Child Health and Development Study. *Acta Obstet. Gynecol. Scand.* **2021**, *100*, 1288–1296. [CrossRef]
222. Sanni, K.R.; Eeva, E.; Noora, S.M.; Laura, K.S.; Linnea, K.; Hasse, K. The influence of maternal psychological distress on the mode of birth and duration of labor: Findings from the FinnBrain Birth Cohort Study. *Arch. Womens Ment. Health* **2022**, *25*, 463–472. [CrossRef]
223. Tang, Y.; Zhang, J.; Dai, F.; Razali, N.S.; Tagore, S.; Chern, B.S.; Tan, K.H. Poor sleep is associated with higher blood pressure and uterine artery pulsatility index in pregnancy: A prospective cohort study. *BJOG Int. J. Obstet. Gynaecol.* **2021**, *128*, 1192–1199. [CrossRef] [PubMed]

224. Anifantaki, F.; Pervanidou, P.; Lambrinoudaki, I.; Panoulis, K.; Vlahos, N.; Eleftheriades, M. Maternal Prenatal Stress, Thyroid Function and Neurodevelopment of the Offspring: A Mini Review of the Literature. *Front. Neurosci.* **2021**, *15*, 692446. [CrossRef]
225. Heim, C.M.; Entringer, S.; Buss, C. Translating basic research knowledge on the biological embedding of early-life stress into novel approaches for the developmental programming of lifelong health. *Psychoneuroendocrinology* **2019**, *105*, 123–137. [CrossRef] [PubMed]
226. Benker, G.; Raida, M.; Olbricht, T.; Wagner, R.; Reinhardt, W.; Reinwein, D. TSH secretion in Cushing's syndrome: Relation to glucocorticoid excess, diabetes, goitre, and the 'sick euthyroid syndrome. *Clin. Endocrinol.* **1990**, *33*, 777–786. [CrossRef] [PubMed]
227. Miranda, A.; Sousa, N. Maternal hormonal milieu influence on fetal brain development. *Brain Behav.* **2018**, *8*, e00920. [CrossRef] [PubMed]

Journal of
Clinical Medicine

MDPI

Case Report

Resistance to Thyroid Hormone in a Boy with a Severe, Complex, Congenital Heart Defect (CHD) Requiring Multiple Cardiac Surgeries—Whether and How to Prepare Child for the Surgery

Anna Fedorczak [1], Beata Kruk [2], Anna Mazurek-Kula [2], Łukasz Kępczyński [3] and Renata Stawerska [1,4,*]

[1] Department of Endocrinology and Metabolic Diseases, Polish Mother's Memorial Hospital–Research Institute, 93-338 Lodz, Poland; anna.fedorczak@outlook.com
[2] Department of Cardiology, Polish Mother's Memorial Hospital–Research Institute, 93-338 Lodz, Poland; b.slap@interia.pl (B.K.); qla@op.pl (A.M.-K.)
[3] Department of Genetics, Polish Mother's Memorial Hospital–Research Institute, 93-338 Lodz, Poland; lukasz.kepczynski@iczmp.edu.pl
[4] Department of Pediatric Endocrinology, Medical University of Lodz, 93-339 Lodz, Poland
* Correspondence: renata.stawerska@icloud.com

Abstract: Background: Resistance to thyroid hormones (RTH) is a rare, genetically determined disease characterised by reduced tissue sensitivity to thyroid hormones (THs). It is caused by mutations in genes encoding the receptors for thyroid hormones, α (THRα) or β (THRβ), the distribution of which varies between tissues. Therefore, patients present with elevated TH levels with unsuppressed TSH levels, and symptoms of both hypothyroidism and hyperthyroidism may be present. **Methods**: Hence, we report the case of a boy with a complex, cyanotic, congenital heart defect who was also diagnosed with TH resistance syndrome. **Results**: Because of the clinical features of hyperthyroidism in preparation for cardiac surgery, thiamazole was administered, resulting in the normalisation of TH effects on the α-receptor for HTs. Due to the effectiveness of the proposed treatment, it was further introduced before the further stages of cardiac surgeries. **Conclusions**: The management of RTH is a constant challenge for clinicians and must be individualised.

Keywords: resistance to thyroid hormones; thyroid hormone receptor β; cardiac defect; child; surgery

1. Introduction

Thyroid hormone (TH) resistance syndrome (RTH) is a rare, genetically determined disease characterised by reduced tissue sensitivity to THs [1]. The condition results from mutations that impair the function of thyroid hormone receptors (THR), leading to dysregulated hormone action in various tissues. The estimated incidence of the disease is one in 40,000 live births [2,3]. The most commonly identified cause of RTH is point mutations in the *THRB* gene, which encodes the thyroid hormone receptor beta (THRβ), while mutations in the *THRA* gene, encoding thyroid hormone receptor alpha (THRα), are much less frequent [4]. Clinically, RTH presents with a biochemical profile characterised by elevated levels of circulating thyroid hormones (fT3 and fT4) with unsuppressed thyroid-stimulating hormone (TSH) levels. Due to the differential distribution and function of TH receptors in various tissues, affected individuals may exhibit symptoms of both hypothyroidism (e.g., short stature) and/or hyperthyroidism (e.g., tachycardia—heart rate depends on the effect of THs on the non-defective THRα) [5,6]. In most cases, symptoms are sparse, and patients do not need treatment, whereas patients exhibiting symptoms may require treatment with β-blockers, antithyroid medications, or synthetic thyroid hormones.

However, to our knowledge, no case has yet been described of a patient with resistance to thyroid hormones and a serious congenital heart defect. Furthermore, the optimal perioperative management of patients with RTH undergoing surgical interventions remains undefined. Thus, the aim of this study was to present a currently 5-year-old boy with a complex, congenital heart defect requiring multistage cardiac surgery, who was also diagnosed with RTH due to mutations in the gene encoding THRβ.

2. Materials and Methods

The data were collected from a retrospective analysis of the medical, laboratory, and genetic records of a patient who was under the care of the Department of Cardiology, the Department of Cardiac Surgery, and the Department of Endocrinology and Metabolic Diseases Clinics at the Polish Mother's Memorial Hospital–Research Institute in Lodz. The study was carried out with prior informed parental consent. As this was a retrospective study, the Bioethical Committee of the Medical University of Lodz declared that special ethical approval was not required.

Serum TSH, FT4, and FT3 concentrations were measured by the electroimmunochemiluminescent method (ECLIA), Roche, Elecsys ® Systems 1010/2010/modular analytics E170. For TSH, the analytical sensitivity was 0.005 μIU/mL, ranging up to 100 μIU/mL, with an intra-assay coefficient of variance (CV) of 1.5–8.6% and accuracy of 1.1–3.0%. The analytical range for FT4 was 0.023–7.77 ng/mL, the intra-assay CV was 1.4–2.9%, and the accuracy was 2.7–6.6%. For FT3, the analytical range was 0.26–32.55 pg, the intra-assay CV was 3.7–9.5%, and the accuracy was 3.8–11.2%.

Sanger sequencing of THRB exons 3, 4, 5, 6, and 8 was performed on patients' genomic DNA isolated from the whole blood sample. The primers were designed via Primer3 input software (version 0.4.0). PCR amplification was conducted via PCR Master Mix (Promega Corporation, Cat. No. M7423, Madison, WI, USA). Following the amplification step, the resulting products were purified before sequencing. The BigDye Terminator v3.1 Cycle Sequencing Kit (Thermo Fisher Scientific, No. 4337455, Waltham, MA, USA) was used for sequencing, which was conducted on a 3500 Genetic Analyzer instrument (Thermo Fisher Scientific, Waltham, MA, USA). The heterozygous, pathogenic variant NM_000461.5(THRB):c.947G>A p.(Arg316His) was detected. Variant classification was performed using ACMG-AMP guidelines with ClinGen modifications.

3. Detailed Case Description

A 12-month-old boy with a complex, cyanotic, congenital heart defect was admitted to the Department of Cardiology at PMMH-RI in order to prepare for the subsequent stage of surgical treatment—Glen bidirectional surgery. The boy's complex heart defect was characterised by a double outlet right ventricle (DORV) with a ventricular septal defect (VSD), pulmonary stenosis (PS), and hypoplasia of the left ventricle (LV).

Birth history: The baby was born from a first pregnancy and first birth at 38 gestational weeks by caesarean section, with a weight of 3240 g. He was prenatally diagnosed with a heart defect (DORV + VSD + PS). At birth, the baby presented features of circulatory insufficiency and an infusion of prostaglandins was administered; then, captopril and spironolactone were introduced to the treatment with clinical improvement. In the neonatal period, the child had poor weight gain and temporarily required feeding by gastric tube. At 4 months of age, the surgical removal of an atrial septal defect (ASD) and right ventricular outflow tract (RVOT) dilatation was performed.

Upon admission, the patient was in good general condition. His height was 75 cm (25th–50th percentile) and his weight was 8.5 kg (10th–25th percentile). Arterial blood pressure was 95/60 mmHg and blood saturation was 85–88%. Physical examination revealed tachycardia, with a heart rate of 125 bpm; no other abnormalities were noted. The following tests were performed before qualifying him for the surgery:

Electrocardiographic examination (ECG): Sinus rhythm, regular, 130/min. PQ = 160 ms, QRS = 60 ms, QTc = 413 ms. Features of right ventricular hypertrophy with overload.

Chest radiograph: Bilateral small interstitial thickening dependent on congestive changes. Otherwise, lung areas were without focal changes. Diaphragm and diaphragmatic–rib angles were free. The cardiac silhouette was enlarged in the transverse dimension with a cardiothoracic ratio (CRT) of 0.69. The left mediastinal outline was convex—most probably a thymus outline.

Echocardiography: Mitral valve with a narrow mitral annulus with a limited opening to approx. 5 mm with a flow of up to 1.7 m/s; tricuspid valve with normal flow and moderate central regurgitation and at the base of the STL; in IAS, a cavity with a diameter of approx. 12 mm with a left-to-right leak without restriction was found. In IVS, a cavity with a diameter of approx. 9 mm for the restoration of septo-aortic continuity of approx. 14 mm was found. We observed an aortic valve with laminar flow; a hypoplastic pulmonary trunk with predominant subvalvular stenosis up to 4.8 mm and significant flow acceleration up to 5.3 m/s; and pulmonary branches at the level of bifurcation of about 5 mm each. The thymus was visible in the subcostal view. IVC—8 mm; SVC—7 mm; Ao asc—11 mm; Ao thoracic—6.6 m; Ao abdominal—6 mm; aortic arch left; Ao desc without features of stenosis. Heart cavities: right ventricle above normal, left ventricle at the lower limit of normal; in 2D RVDd—28 mm, LVDd—16 mm RV/LV—1.75; contractility was good; E = 73%. Conclusions: double outlet right ventricle (DORV) + ventricular septal defect (VSD) + pulmonary artery (PA) hypoplasia + pulmonary stenosis (PS) + mitral valve (MV) hypoplasia + left ventricle (LV) hypoplasia; status post-surgical removal of an atrial septal defect (ASD) and the right ventricular outflow tract (RVOT) dilatation.

Blood test results revealed elevated levels of free thyroid hormones FT3 (6.39 pg/mL; N: 2.41–5.5) and FT4 (2.3 ng/mL; N: 0.96–1.77) with the absence of thyrotropin suppression (TSH = 2.93 mIU/L; N: 0.7–5.97) (Table 1).

Table 1. Results of the patient's hormonal panel.

Hormone	Range	Diagnosis	Surgery Preparation (Thiamazole 0.5 mg/kg)	Surgery Preparation (Thiamazole 2 mg/kg)	Between the Surgeries
TSH [mIU/L]	0.7–5.97	2.56	4.87	12.12	2.55
FT3 [pg/mL]	2.41–5.5	7.16	6.41	4.71	6.72
FT4 [ng/mL]	0.96–1.77	2.4	2.3	1.65	2.55

TSH—Thyroid-stimulating hormone; FT3—Free Triiodothyronine; FT4—Free Thyroxine.

Therefore, an endocrinology consultation was requested and the diagnostics were expanded to antithyroid antibodies and thyroid ultrasonography. Anti-peroxidase (anti-TPO, 20.87; N: <34 IU/mL), anti-thyroglobulin (anti-TG, 11.74, N: <115 IU/mL), and anti-TSH receptor (anti-TSHR, <0.3; N: <1.75 IU/L) antibodies were negative.

Thyroid ultrasound: The thyroid gland is typically located on the neck; the lower poles of both lobes do not descend below the sternal notch. The left lobe measured 23 × 8 × 8 mm and the right lobe measured 19 × 9 × 6 mm. The thickness of the isthmus was 2 mm. The echogenicity of both lobes was slightly hypoechoic and homogeneous. No focal changes were visualised. The organ showed a normal vascularisation pattern.

Thyroid hormone resistance (RTH) was suspected and genetic testing was ordered. Sanger sequencing of exons 3, 4, 5, 6, 8 of the *THRB* gene revealed heterogenous NH_000461.4: c.947G>A, p.(Arg316His), a variant classified as pathogenic, which confirmed the diagnosis of RTH. As a mutation indicating RTH was diagnosed and a pituitary RMI would have required general anaesthesia; we waived the pituitary RMI until the boy is older.

To reduce the potential risk of cardiac arrhythmias during surgery in a boy with a low cardiac ejection fraction and tachycardia, in preparation for cardiac surgery (BG Glenn type), we decided to use thiamazole to decrease FT4 and FT3 levels and the effect of their excessive concentration on THRα receptors. We initially administered the drug at typically used doses (0.5 mg/kg body mass) for 7 days, without achieving the normalisation of FT3 and FT4. Therefore, a dose of 2 mg/kg body mass thiamazole was applied for a period of 7 days, achieving the normalisation of FT3 (4.71 pg/mL) and FT4 (1.65 ng/mL) as well as normal heart function. At the same time, excessive TSH secretion was observed (12.12 mIU/L) (Table 1). Elevated TSH levels did not constitute an endocrinological contraindication to the procedure (the dysregulation between TSH and FT3 and FT4 was determined by disease). Thus, the patient was qualified for Glenn surgery; the course of the procedure was successful and no arrhythmias or other cardiac complications were observed. In the postoperative period, the treatment (thiamazole) was gradually reduced and the test results returned to baseline.

Given the clinical efficacy of the proposed management, the same treatment (thiamazole in dose 2 mg/kg body weight for 10–14 days) was implemented prior to subsequent stages of cardiac surgeries (Table 2). In the periods between surgeries, the patient did not receive any endocrine treatment. We did not consider therapy with propranolol, because propranolol reduces the cardiac ejection fraction and is not recommended in patients with a univentricular heart. At 5 years of age, the staged treatment was completed.

Table 2. Stages of treatment for a complex, congenital heart defect.

No.	Name of Performed Surgery	Age
1.	Surgical removal of an atrial septal defect (ASD) and right ventricular outflow tract (RVOT) dilatation	4 months
2.	Glenn bidirectional surgery	13 months
3.	Cardiac catheterisation with the implantation of a Valeo stent into proximal segments of pulmonary arteries	20 months
4.	Cardiac catheterisation with closure of the pulmonary artery trunk using an Amlatzer Vascular Plug	2 years
5.	Fontan operation without fenestration—anastomosis of the inferior vena cava with the right branch of the pulmonary artery using a vascular prosthesis under extracorporeal circulation	4 years
6.	Cardiac catheterisation with closure of a veno-venous fistula in the left venous angle with an Amlatzer Vascular Plug	5 years

Currently, the boy remains under cardiological and endocrinological care. He displays features of hyperactivity, with normal intellectual development. His growth rate and height are within the normal range with respect to age and sex (107 cm, 50th–75th percentile). In the patient's family, the same point mutation was detected in the boy's father, with no known impact on the cardiovascular system or other aspects of health.

4. Discussion

Thyroid hormones (THs) act through α (THRα) and β (THRβ) receptors. Their distribution is variable and depends on the type of tissue: the α type predominates in the brain, the β type in the liver, and both types are present in the myocardium [1,7]. The metabolic effects of TH mainly depend on TRβ1, whereas the cardiac effects of TH are mediated by TRα [8]. TH resistance (RTH) may be caused by a mutation in *THRβ*, or, far less frequently, in *THRα* [8]. Patients with this syndrome usually have elevated FT4 and FT3 concentrations with normal or increased TSH levels [9,10]. The described clinical features of RTH include goitre, tachycardia, emotional disturbances, attention deficit hyperactivity disorder, hyperkinetic behaviour, hearing loss, low body mass index, short stature, and delayed bone age, among others [9]. Tachycardia occurs in 75–94% of patients with RTH and is often the finding that prompts diagnosis [11]. A few cases of the coexistence of TH and atrial fibrillation have also been reported [12,13]. Sometimes the aetiology of hyperthyroidism may be difficult to establish—like in a newborn with RTH, born to a mother with Graves' disease [14]. Distinguishing between RTH and TSH-producing pituitary tumours may be challenging, as there are no significant differences in TSH and TH concentrations in both conditions. Therefore, pituitary imaging as well as the results of TRH testing and genetic testing would be helpful [15].

There is no therapy that corrects a defect in thyroid hormone receptor function. Patients with adequate compensation by enhanced TH production without thyrotoxic symptoms do not require treatment [16], whereas patients with hyperthyroid and/or hypothyroid symptoms may require ß-blockers, antithyroid drugs, or synthetic forms of thyroid hormones. The rationale for the antithyroid drugs treatment in patients with RTH remains controversial. The administration of antithyroid drugs further raises TSH and may consequently induce goitre and or pituitary thyrotrophic hyperplasia [17]. On the other hand, several cases of successful thiamazole therapy in children diagnosed with RTH and hyperthyroidism symptoms were also reported. One of them described that therapy with antithyroid drugs in a 2-year-old patient diagnosed with RTHβ improved behaviour, sleep, and body weight and reduced tachycardia [16]. Another case report presented a girl treated with thiamazole followed by levothyroxine replacement therapy, achieving notable improvement in intelligence, verbal skills, and behaviour [18]. The introduction of thiamazole and propranolol in a 15-year-old girl with hyperactivity, behaviour disorders, and tachycardia improved clinical symptoms but also increased TSH levels [19]. In conclusion, indications for treatment in RTH patients should be discussed individually.

Ultimately, we did not find any publications on how to prepare a patient with RTH for surgery. As our patient was diagnosed with the c.947G>A, p.(Arg316His) variant in one allele of the *THRβ* gene, the symptoms presented by the boy were attributed to an excessive effect of THs on the THRα, which was not affected by the mutation. Given the fact that the boy presented selective symptoms of hyperthyroidism (tachycardia), we decided to introduce cardiac surgery preparation with thiamazole. This approach aimed to reduce the impact of THs on the THRα, which mainly mediates the cardiac effects of THs [8].

It is well known that thyroid dysfunction is associated with elevated cardiovascular risk [20]. The cardiovascular effects of TH excess include an increase in heart rate, stroke volume, and cardiac output [21]. Hyperthyroidism enhances the risk of atrial fibrillation, cardiovascular disease, and heart failure [22]. Therefore, the aim of preparing patients with thyroid dysfunction for surgery is to normalise TH levels before surgical intervention whenever possible [23,24]. Being concerned about the impact of THs on THRα in the heart, we decided to proceed with this case similarly to patients with hyperthyroidism, where antithyroid drugs are recommended as a fundamental treatment and preoperative approach [24]. Antithyroid drugs act to suppress the synthesis of thyroid hormones by inhibiting the enzyme thyroperoxidase, which adds iodine to tyrosine residues on the hormone precursor—thyroglobulin. Thiamazole, as well as propylthiouracil, are absorbed immediately and accumulate in the thyroid gland, inhibiting the synthesis process of THs [25]. Recently, only thiamazole has been recommended as an antithyroid drug due to the elevated risk of hepatitis induced by propylthiouracil [25].

To date, no similar case report has been reported in the literature. We conclude that this description is important to provide some clues for the management of patients with RTH requiring complex surgical interventions.

5. Conclusions

The majority of patients with RTH do not require treatment and the observed abnormalities in hormonal test results do not constitute a contraindication to surgery. However, the simultaneous occurrence of a severe complex heart defect and RTH in a child presenting with selective clinical symptoms of hyperthyroidism prompted us to apply atypical preoperative treatment (antithyroid drugs), which resulted in the normalisation of TH effects on the THRα. The management of RTH is an ongoing challenge for clinicians and must be individualised.

Author Contributions: Conceptualisation—R.S.; software—A.F.; formal analysis—R.S.; investigation—R.S., B.K., Ł.K., and A.M.-K.; data curation—A.F.; writing—original draft preparation—A.F.; writing—review and editing—A.M.-K., B.K., A.F., Ł.K., and R.S.; visualisation—A.F.; supervision—R.S. All authors have read and agreed to the published version of the manuscript.

Funding: The costs of publishing this article were funded by Polish Mother's Memorial Hospital–Research Institute in Lodz, Poland.

Institutional Review Board Statement: The study was conducted in accordance with the Declaration of Helsinki, and the Bioethical Committee of the Medical University of Lodz was requested for approval. The committee declared that this retrospective case report did not require special ethical approval.

Informed Consent Statement: Written informed consent has been obtained from the patient to publish this paper.

Data Availability Statement: Data are contained within the article.

Conflicts of Interest: The authors declare no conflicts of interest.

References

1. Ortiga-Carvalho, T.M.; Sidhaye, A.R.; Wondisford, F.E. Thyroid Hormone Receptors and Resistance to Thyroid Hormone Disorders. *Nat. Rev. Endocrinol.* **2014**, *10*, 582–591. [CrossRef] [PubMed]
2. Prakash, K.; Hamid, P. Thyroid Hormone Resistance Syndrome: From Molecular Mechanisms to Its Potential Contribution to Hypertension. *Cureus* **2023**, *15*, e49913. [CrossRef] [PubMed]
3. Sun, H.; Cao, L.; Zheng, R.; Xie, S.; Liu, C. Update on Resistance to Thyroid Hormone Syndromeβ. *Ital. J. Pediatr.* **2020**, *46*, 168. [CrossRef]
4. Pappa, T.; Refetoff, S. Resistance to Thyroid Hormone Beta: A Focused Review. *Front. Endocrinol.* **2021**, *12*, 656551. [CrossRef] [PubMed]
5. Cannarella, R.; Musmeci, M.; Garofalo, V.; Timpanaro, T.A.; Leone, G.; Caruso, M.; Maltese, P.E.; Condorelli, R.A.; La Vignera, S.; Calogero, A.E. Resistance to Thyroid Hormones: A Case-Series Study. *Int. J. Mol. Sci.* **2022**, *23*, 11268. [CrossRef]
6. Chiesa, A.; Olcese, M.; Papendieck, P.; Martínez, A.; Vieites, A.; Bengolea, S.; Targovnik, H.; Rivolta, C.; Rivolta, C.; Gruñeiro-Papendieck, L. Variable Clinical Presentation and Outcome in Pediatric Patients with Resistance to Thyroid Hormone (RTH). *Endocrine* **2011**, *41*, 130–137. [CrossRef] [PubMed]
7. Refetoff, S.; Weiss, R.E.; Usala, S.J. The Syndromes of Resistance to Thyroid Hormone. *Endocr. Rev.* **1993**, *14*, 348–399. [CrossRef]
8. Zucchi, R. Thyroid Hormone Analogues: An Update. *Thyroid* **2020**, *30*, 1099–1105. [CrossRef] [PubMed]

9. Metwalley, K.; Farghaly, H. Hormone Resistance in Children: What Primary Care Physicians Need to Know. *Acta Biomed.* **2021**, *92*, e2021255. [CrossRef]
10. Foryś-Dworniczak, E.A.; Moran, C.; Kalina-Faska, B.; Małecka-Tendera, E.; Zachurzok, A. Resistance to Thyroid Hormone with a Mutation of the Thyroid β Receptor Gene in an Eight-Month-Old Infant—A Case Report. *Endokrynol. Pol.* **2019**, *70*, 124–130. [CrossRef] [PubMed]
11. Beck-Peccoz, P.; Chatterjee, V.K. The Variable Clinical Phenotype in Thyroid Hormone Resistance Syndrome. *Thyroid* **1994**, *4*, 225–232. [CrossRef]
12. Zimering, M.B. Thyroid Hormone Resistance in Identical Twin Sisters with Atrial Fibrillation: Case Report and Review of the Literature. *J. Endocrinol. Diabetes* **2018**, *5*. [CrossRef]
13. Sato, H.; Tomita, Y. Resistance to Thyroid Hormone Accompanied by Atrial Fibrillation. *Endocrinol. Diabetes Metab. Case Rep.* **2018**, *2018*, EDM180100. [CrossRef]
14. Seetharaman, S.; Quintos, J.B.; Salas-Lucia, F. Resistance to Thyroid Hormone Beta in a Patient Born to a Mother With Undiagnosed Graves' Disease. *AACE Clin. Case Rep.* **2023**, *9*, 63–66. [CrossRef] [PubMed]
15. Deng, F.; Yang, Z.; Zhang, Y.; Wang, Y.; Hu, J.; Zhang, F. TSH Adenoma and Syndrome of Resistance to Thyroid Hormones—Two Cases Report of Syndrome of Inappropriate Secretion of Thyrotropin. *Brain Behav.* **2021**, *11*, e02081. [CrossRef] [PubMed]
16. Tsai, S.L.; Ahmet, A. Treatment with Methimazole in a 3-Year-Old Male with Thyroid Hormone Resistance. *Horm. Res. Paediatr.* **2012**, *77*, 402–406. [CrossRef] [PubMed]
17. Glymph, K.; Gosmanov, A.R. Methimazole-Induced Goitrogenesis in an Adult Patient With the Syndrome of Resistance to Thyroid Hormone. *J. Investig. Med. High. Impact Case Rep.* **2014**, *2*, 2324709614555768. [CrossRef] [PubMed]
18. Kim, T.J.; Travers, S. Case Report: Thyroid Hormone Resistance and Its Therapeutic Challenges. *Curr. Opin. Pediatr.* **2008**, *20*, 490–493. [CrossRef]
19. Rezgani, I.; Chihaoui, M.; Oueslati, I.; Chaker, F.; Nagi, S.; Yazidi, M. Thyroid Hormone Resistance Syndrome Caused by a Novel Mutation in the Thyroid Hormone Receptor-Beta Gene (THRB, GLU457LYS) Treated with Methimazole. *Clin. Case Rep.* **2022**, *10*, e6543. [CrossRef] [PubMed]
20. Collet, T.-H.; Gussekloo, J.; Bauer, D.C.; den Elzen, W.P.J.; Cappola, A.R.; Balmer, P.; Iervasi, G.; Åsvold, B.O.; Sgarbi, J.A.; Völzke, H.; et al. Subclinical Hyperthyroidism and the Risk of Coronary Heart Disease and Mortality. *Arch. Intern. Med.* **2012**, *172*, 799–809. [CrossRef]
21. Kohl, B.A.; Schwartz, S. Surgery in the Patient with Endocrine Dysfunction. *Med. Clin. N. Am.* **2009**, *93*, 1031–1047. [CrossRef]
22. Biondi, B. Mechanisms in Endocrinology: Heart Failure and Thyroid Dysfunction. *Eur. J. Endocrinol.* **2012**, *167*, 609–618. [CrossRef] [PubMed]
23. Palace, M.R. Perioperative Management of Thyroid Dysfunction. *Health Serv. Insights* **2017**, *10*, 1178632916689677. [CrossRef] [PubMed]
24. Xu, T.; Zheng, X.; Wei, T. Preoperative Preparation for Graves' Disease. *Front. Endocrinol.* **2023**, *14*, 1234056. [CrossRef] [PubMed]
25. Yamakawa, H.; Kato, T.S.; Noh, J.Y.; Yuasa, S.; Kawamura, A.; Fukuda, K.; Aizawa, Y. Thyroid Hormone Plays an Important Role in Cardiac Function: From Bench to Bedside. *Front. Physiol.* **2021**, *12*, 606931. [CrossRef]

Journal of
Clinical Medicine

MDPI

Article

Evaluation of Changes in Clinicopathological Features and Prognosis in Patients with Thyroid Cancer

Özlem Doğan [1], Melin Aydan Ahmed [2], Ömer Burak Ekinci [3], Anıl Yıldız [4] and Izzet Dogan [5,*]

1 Department of Endocrinology, Health Sciences University, Haseki Training and Research Hospital, Istanbul 34265, Turkey
2 Department of Medical Oncology, Institute of Oncology, Istanbul University, Istanbul 34193, Turkey
3 Department of Medical Oncology, Health Sciences University, Prof. Dr. Cemil Tascioglu City Hospital, Istanbul 34284, Turkey
4 Department of Medical Oncology, Health Sciences University, Basaksehir Cam and Sakura City Hospital, Istanbul 34480, Turkey
5 Department of Medical Oncology, Acıbadem Healthcare Group, Istanbul 34140, Turkey
* Correspondence: izzet.dogan@istanbul.edu.tr

Abstract: Background: In this study, we evaluated the changes in clinicopathological features and prognosis in patients with thyroid cancer in the last two decades using the Surveillance, Epidemiology, and End Results Database (SEER) data. **Methods:** Data from the SEER-12 registry (1992–2021) were analyzed, focusing on patients diagnosed with malignant thyroid cancer between 2001 and 2020. The study population was divided into Cohort 1 (2001–2010) and Cohort 2 (2011–2020). Cohorts 1 and 2 were compared regarding clinicopathological features and prognosis. **Results:** The study included 94,892 patients diagnosed with thyroid cancer between 2001 and 2020, with 39,265 patients in Cohort 1 and 55,627 in Cohort 2. Compared to Cohort 1, in Cohort 2 showed a statistically significant increase in the proportion of patients aged 60+ (+4.2%), male patients (+2.1%), and cases of papillary cancer (+5.3%) and regional disease (+3.7%) (all $p < 0.001$). Although Cohort 2 demonstrated an 8% improvement in survival compared to Cohort 1, this result was not statistically significant ($p = 0.057$). Prognostic factors were identified, such as disease stage at diagnosis, age, gender, and origin. Among pathological subtypes, the patients with papillary + FV had the best prognosis (HR: 0.78), compared to patients in the other group, mainly comprising anaplastic tumors and sarcomas, which had the worst prognosis (HR: 9.61). **Conclusions:** In this large-scale study of thyroid cancer patients, we found significant differences between the two cohorts. In Cohort 2, the proportion of patients aged $\geq$60 years, male, and with papillary thyroid cancer was increased. We found that age, sex, origin, histopathological subtype, and stage at diagnosis were prognostic factors in patients with thyroid cancer. Also, we observed a trend toward improved survival in Cohort 2.

Keywords: thyroid cancer; SEER database; prognosis; clinicopathological features

1. Introduction

Thyroid cancer is the most commonly diagnosed malignancy of the endocrine system, with an increasing global incidence over the past few decades [1]. It accounts for approximately 2% of all cancers and is predominantly diagnosed in women, with a notable age-related distribution, often affecting individuals between the ages of 20 and 55 [2]. The majority of thyroid cancers are differentiated, including papillary and follicular subtypes, which typically have a favorable prognosis. However, more aggressive forms, such as anaplastic and medullary thyroid cancers, are less common and are associated with poorer outcomes. Advances in early detection, imaging techniques, and improved surgical treatments contribute to an overall improvement in survival rates, yet regional and metastatic disease remains a significant concern [3].

Studies have identified various clinical and pathological factors that affect the prognosis of thyroid cancer patients. The main prognostic factors include age at diagnosis, gender, tumor size, lymph node involvement, extrathyroidal spread, and distant metastasis [4]. However, the most important prognostic factor is the tumor's histological subtype. Papillary thyroid carcinoma (PTC) is generally associated with a better prognosis, while follicular, medullary, and anaplastic thyroid cancers (ATC) tend to have worse prognosis [5]. Studies in thyroid cancer also highlight the role of genetic mutations, such as those in the BRAF and RAS genes, which are linked to more aggressive disease and poorer survival outcomes [6]. Understanding prognostic factors is critical for tailoring individualized treatment plans and improving patient outcomes.

Today, the incidence of thyroid cancer has increased significantly, especially in small and localized PTCs, probably due to the increased use of neck ultrasonography and fine needle aspiration (FNA) [7]. This increased detection rate has led to earlier diagnosis, but it has also raised concerns about overtreatment. Economic, social, and demographic changes occurring in societies may lead to lifestyle changes in areas such as nutrition, smoking, alcohol use, and sports [8]. These changes necessitate a re-evaluation of prognostic factors and survival outcomes using large population-based databases. In this study, we evaluated the changes in clinicopathological and survival characteristics of thyroid cancer patients in the SEER database between 2001–2010 and 2011–2020.

2. Materials and Methods

2.1. Patients and Data Selection

This study was designed as a retrospective cohort study. The patients included in the study were obtained from the SEER Program of the National Cancer Institute (NCI), and the patient data were anonymized. The study was conducted in accordance with the declaration of Helsinki and good clinical practice guidelines. We obtained data for this study from the US NCI's SEER-12 registry [November 2023 (1992–2021)]. SEER*Stat program version 8.4.4 was used to extract data. The patient population to be included in the study was determined by selecting Site recode ICD-O-3/WHO 2008 = ''thyroid'' and Behavior code ICD-O-3 = ''malignant'' from the SEER*Stat program. Patients to be included in the study were restricted as Age recode with < 1-year olds = "20–24, 25–29, . . ., 80–84 and 85 years +" and Year of diagnosis= "2001, 2002, 2003, . . ., 2019, and 2020". From the SEER*Stat program, patients' Sex, Race recode, Origin recode, AYA site recode 2020 Revision, Histologic Type ICD-O-3, Combined Summary Stage (2004+), Summary stage 2000 (1998–2017), RX Summ--Scope Reg LN Sur (2003+), Radiation recode, Chemotherapy recode (yes, no/unk), and SEER cause-specific death classification data was saved.

The patient group was divided into two cohorts. Patients registered between 2001–2010 were considered Cohort 1, and patients registered between 2011–2020 were assigned to Cohort 2. Patients' ages were divided into 20–39, 40–59, and 60+. Patients registered according to AYA site recode 2020 revision were recorded as "Other" except for papillary, papillary with follicular variant (FV), follicular, hurthle cell, and medullary. Surgery status, according to RX Summ-Surg Prim Site (1998+), and lymph node sampling status, according to RX Summ-Scope Reg LN Sur (2003+), were divided into three groups as "Yes, No and Unknown". Radiation recode is divided into four groups as: "Radioisotopes, Radiotherapy (Implant and/or external), Radioisotopes+Radiotherapy, and None/Unknown". While calculating the overall survival (OS) of the patients, "Survival months" were taken as the duration, and analysis was performed with patients coded "Dead (attributable to this cancer dx)" according to SEER cause-specific death classification. In addition, univariate and multivariate analyses were performed to determine the factors affecting OS.

2.2. Statistical Analysis

The SPSS 25.0 software (IBM, Armonk, NY, USA) and MedCalc statistical software version 23.0.9 (Ostend, Belgium) were used to perform the study statistics. The characteristics of patients in Cohorts 1 and 2 were compared using the Chi-square test. We used the Kaplan–Meier technique to analyze survival. Cox regression test was performed for univariate and multivariate analysis to evaluate the factors affecting survival in patients with thyroid cancer. Hazard ratios (HRs) and their 95% confidence intervals (CI) were estimated. Statistically significant variables from the univariate model have been included in the multivariate model. Chemotherapy, radiotherapy, radioisotope therapy, and surgical treatments were not included in multivariate analysis because they were correlated with tumor stage at diagnosis in patients with thyroid cancer. Statistical significance was accepted as a p-value < 0.05.

3. Results

3.1. Patient Characteristics and Treatment Modalities

A total of 94,892 patients were included in the study. The number of patients in Cohort 1 was 39,265, while the number in Cohort 2 was 55,627. The female/male ratio of patients included in the study was 3.01. The proportion of patients over the age of 60 in the study was determined to be 28.7%. The most common pathological subtypes were papillary, papillary with FV, and follicular types, respectively. Only 3.7% of patients were metastatic at the time of diagnosis, while the majority of patients presented with localized disease (58.4%). General characteristics and treatment characteristics of the patients are presented in Table 1.

Table 1. General characteristics of thyroid cancer patients in the SEER database included between 2001 and 2020.

		Number N: 94,892	**%**
Age	*20–39 years*	25,609	27.0
	40–59 years	41,993	44.3
	60 years+	27,290	28.7
Sex	*Female*	71,235	75.1
	Male	23,657	24.9
Cohort	*Cohort 1 (2001–2010 years)*	39,265	41.4
	Cohort 2 (2011–2020 years)	55,627	58.6
Race Recode	*White*	73,448	77.5
	Asian or Pacific Islander	14,181	14.9
	Black	5120	5.4
	American Indian/Alaska Native	981	1.0
	Unknown	1162	1.2
Origin Recode	*Spanish-Hispanic-Latino*	16,958	17.9
	Non-Spanish-Hispanic-Latino	77,934	82.1
Histologic Subtypes	*Papillary*	62,057	65.4
	Papillary with FV	21,775	22.9
	Follicular	4723	5.0
	Hurthle cell carcinoma	1979	2.1
	Medullary	1573	1.7
	Other	2785	2.9

Table 1. *Cont.*

		Number N: 94,892	%
Stage at Diagnosis	*Localized*	55,420	58.4
	Regional	25,303	26.7
	Distant	3504	3.7
	Unknown	10,665	11.2
Surgery	*Yes*	89,605	94.4
	No	5030	5.3
	Unknown	257	0.3
Lymph Node Sampling	*Yes*	46,400	48.9
	No	42,163	44.4
	Unknown	6329	6.7
Radiotherapy and/or RAI	*RAI*	38,615	40.7
	RAI + Radiotherapy	308	0.3
	Radiotherapy	2558	2.7
	None/Unknown	53,411	56.3
Chemotherapy	*None/Unknown*	93,867	98.9
	Yes	1025	1.1
Thyroid Cancer-Related Death	*Alive or Other Causes Dead*	90,906	95.8
	Yes	3986	4.2

3.2. Differences Between Cohort Groups

Cohort 1 and Cohort 2 were compared in terms of several parameters. In Cohort 2, the proportion of patients aged 60+ (+4.2%) and male patients (+2.1% increase) was detected to be increased (both $p < 0.001$). The origin rates were statistically significantly different between the two groups. When evaluated in terms of pathological subtype, there was a statistically significant increase of 5.3% in the proportion of patients with PTC ($p < 0.001$). There was also a 3.7% increase in the proportion of regional disease ($p < 0.001$). General and treatment-related differences in Cohort 2 compared to Cohort 1 are shown in Table 2.

Table 2. Comparison of General Characteristics of Patient Groups in Cohorts 1 and 2.

		Cohort 1		Cohort 2		*p*-Value
		N	%	N	%	
Age	*20–39 years*	10,905	27.8	14,704	26.4	$p < 0.001$
	40–59 years	18,041	45.9	23,952	43.1	
	60 years+	10,319	26.3	16,971	30.5	
		39,265	100.0	55,627	100.0	
Sex	*Female*	29,946	76.3	41,289	74.2	$p < 0.001$
	Male	9319	23.7	14,338	25.8	
		39,265	100.0	55,627	100.0	
Race Recode	*White*	31,244	80.2	42,204	77.1	$p < 0.001$
	Asian or Pacific Islander	5368	13.7	8813	16.1	
	Black	2019	5.2	3101	5.6	
	American Indian/Alaska Native	348	0.9	633	1.2	
		38,979	100.0	54,751	100.0	
Origin Recode	*Spanish-Hispanic-Latino*	6132	15.6	10,826	19.5	$p < 0.001$
	Non-Spanish-Hispanic-Latino	33,133	84.4	44,801	80.5	
		39,265	100.0	55,627	100.0	
Histologic Subtypes	*Papillary*	24,452	62.3	37,605	67.6	$p < 0.001$
	Papillary with FV	9583	24.3	12,192	21.9	
	Follicular	2272	5.8	2451	4.4	
	Hurthle cell	1050	2.7	929	1.7	
	Medullary	691	1.8	882	1.6	
	Other	1217	3.1	1568	2.8	
		39,265	100.0	55,627	100.0	

Table 2. *Cont.*

		Cohort 1 N	Cohort 1 %	Cohort 2 N	Cohort 2 %	p-Value
Stage at Diagnosis	*Localized*	20,077	67.7	35,343	64.8	$p < 0.001$
	Regional	8200	27.6	17,103	31.3	
	Distant	1391	4.7	2113	3.9	
		29,668	100.0	54,559	100.0	
Surgery	*Yes*	37,293	95.1	52,312	94.4	$p < 0.001$
	No	1906	4.9	3124	5.6	
		39,199	100.0	55,436	100.0	
Lymph Node Samplin	*Yes*	15,742	47.4	30,658	55.4	$p < 0.001$
	No	17,497	52.6	24,666	44.6	
		33,239	100.0	55,324	100.0	
Radiotherapy and/or RAI	*RAI*	18,443	92.5	20,172	93.6	$p < 0.001$
	RAI + Radiotherapy	178	0.9	130	0.6	
	Radiotherapy	1311	6.6	1247	5.8	
		19,932	100.0	21,549	100.0	
Chemotherapy	*None/Unknown*	38,872	99.0	54,995	98.9	$p = 0.047$
	Yes	393	1.0	632	1.1	
		39,265	100.0	55,627	100.0	
Thyroid Cancer-Related Death	*Alive or Other Causes*	37,082	94.4	53,824	96.8	$p < 0.001$
	Yes	2183	5.6	1803	3.2	
		39,265	100.0	55,627	100.0	

3.3. Survival Outcomes and Prognosis

Of the patients included in the study, 3986 (4.2%) had died due to thyroid cancer. Univariate and multivariate analyses were performed to evaluate the factors affecting survival, and significant differences were observed between the Cohorts (Table 3). Although an 8% increase in survival was found in Cohort 2 compared to Cohort 1, this result remained below the statistical significance limit ($p = 0.057$) (Figure 1A). As expected, the disease stage at diagnosis was a prognostic factor (Figure 1B).

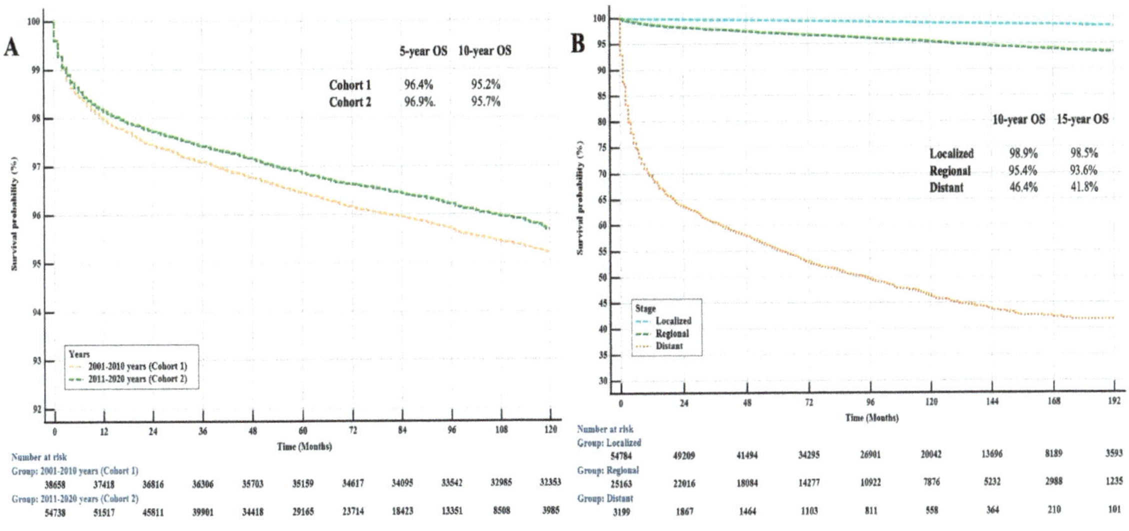

Figure 1. Kaplan–Meier Curves for OS by Cohorts (**A**) and Stages at Diagnosis (**B**) in Patients with Thyroid Cancer.

Table 3. Univariate and multivariate analysis for factors affecting OS in thyroid cancer patients included in the SEER database between 2001 and 2020.

	Univariate Analysis		Multivariate Analysis	
	Hazard Ratio (CI 95%)	p-Value	Hazard Ratio (CI 95%)	p-Value
Age				
20–39 years	Reference		Reference	
40–59 years	4.54 (3.76–5.48)	**<0.001**	4.84 (3.85–6.08)	**<0.001**
60 years+	26.62 (22.22–31.89)	**<0.001**	16.12 (12.91–20.15)	**<0.001**
Sex				
Female	Reference		Reference	
Male	2.50 (2.35–2.67)	**<0.001**	1.42 (1.32–1.53)	**<0.001**
Cohorts				
Cohort 1	Reference		Reference	
Cohort 2	0.88 (0.82–0.94)	**<0.001**	0.92 (0.86–1.00)	0.057
Race				
White	Reference		Reference	
Asian or Pacific Islander	1.18 (1.08–1.28)	**<0.001**	1.04 (0.94–1.14)	0.41
Black	1.25 (1.10–1.42)	**0.001**	1.09 (0.94–1.26)	0.22
American Indian/Alaska Native	1.08 (0.79–1.48)	0.595	1.22 (0.86–1.73)	0.26
Origin				
Spanish-Hispanic-Latino	Reference		Reference	
Non-Spanish-Hispanic-Latino	0.88 (0.81–0.96)	**0.004**	0.79 (0.71–0.86)	**<0.001**
Histopathological subtype				
Papillary	Reference		Reference	
Papillary with FV	0.64 (0.57–0.72)	**<0.001**	0.78 (0.69–0.89)	**<0.001**
Follicular	2.41 (2.13–2.74)	**<0.001**	1.76 (1.52–2.05)	**<0.001**
Hurthle Cell	2.83 (2.39–3.36)	**<0.001**	2.43 (2.01–2.95)	**<0.001**
Medullary	5.58 (4.83–6.46)	**<0.001**	2.71 (2.30–3.20)	**<0.001**
Other	34.54 (32.08–37.18)	**<0.001**	9.61 (8.74–10.57)	**<0.001**
Stage at diagnosis				
Localized	Reference		Reference	
Regional	4.61 (4.13–5.14)	**<0.001**	4.89 (4.38–5.46)	**<0.001**
Distant	81.49 (73.62–90.21)	**<0.001**	29.54 (26.42–33.02)	**<0.001**

Multivariate analysis model p-value < 0.001.

Age (95% CI, HR: 4.84) (Figure 2A) and gender (95% CI, HR: 1.42) (Figure 2B) were shown to be significant prognostic factors in patients with thyroid cancer. In addition, we showed that origin had a prognostic factor in patients with thyroid cancer (95% CI, HR: 0.79) in the multivariate analysis.

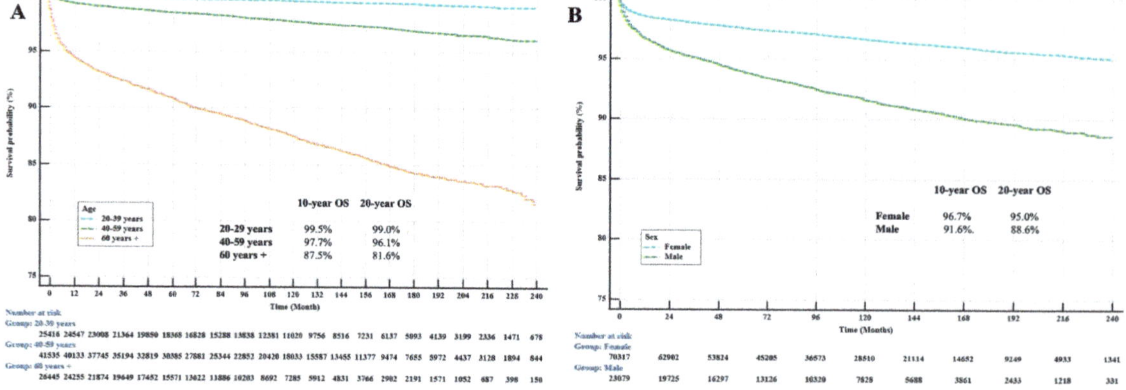

Figure 2. Kaplan–Meier Curves for OS by Age (**A**) and Sex (**B**) in Patients with Thyroid Cancer.

When evaluated in terms of pathological subtypes, the type with the best prognosis compared to the papillary type was papillary + FV (95% CI, HR: 0.78), and the type with the worst prognosis was the other group (95% CI, HR: 9.61) (Figure 3). The other group mainly included ATC and sarcomas.

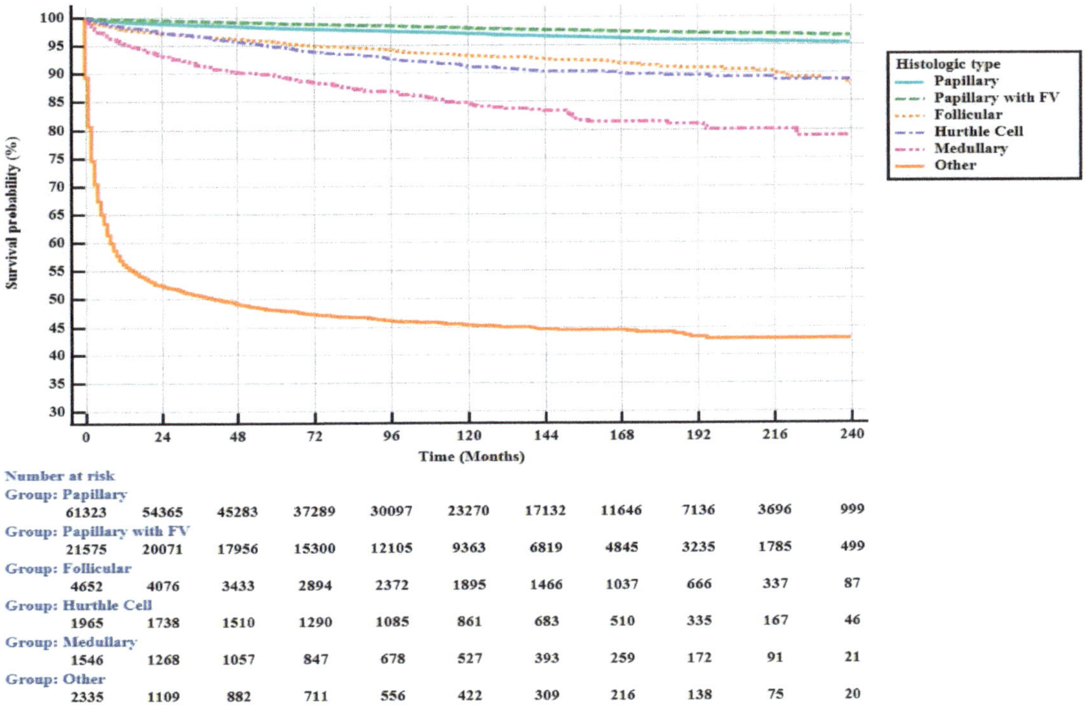

Figure 3. Kaplan–Meier Curves for OS by Pathologic Subgroups in Patients with Thyroid Cancer.

4. Discussion

In this study, we compared the clinical features and prognoses of patients with thyroid cancer registered between 2001–2010 and 2011–2020 in the SEER database. Over the past several decades, advancements in early detection, treatment strategies, and molecular profiling have significantly influenced various cancers' clinical presentation and prognosis. In particular, improvements in screening methods (such as mammography for breast cancer and colonoscopy for colorectal cancer) have contributed to earlier detection and, consequently, improved survival rates. In our study, comparing Cohort 1 and Cohort 2, we found that the proportion of patients aged 60+ and male patients tended to increase in recent years. Few studies in the literature have examined trends in thyroid cancer demographics with different findings regarding age and gender distributions. A study analyzing US data from 1976 to 2005 also observed that PTC incidence rates increased faster in women than in men, with the gender gap widening over time [9]. In particular, the female-to-male incidence ratio decreases with age, from over five in individuals aged 20–24 to approximately one in individuals aged 80 and over, showing a convergence in incidence rates between the sexes in older age groups. Consistent with our findings, a study conducted in the Balearic Islands between 2000 and 2020 reported that the mean age at diagnosis increased from 47.3 years in the previous decade to 52.1 years in the following decade [10]. These changes may reflect aging populations and improved diagnostic practices that detect thyroid cancer in older adults. However, gender trends remained consistent in this study, with proportionally similar thyroid cancer incidence in women compared to men throughout the study period.

One of the significant results we found in our study was the changes in the disease stages at diagnosis in the patients. Although diagnostic possibilities have increased over the years, we have shown that, contrary to expectations, there has been an increase in the proportion of patients in the regional stage and a decrease in the proportion of patients diagnosed with localized disease. A study conducted in Switzerland between 1998 and 2012 noted a significant increase in early-stage thyroid cancer diagnoses without an increase in advanced-stage cases, reinforcing the idea that less aggressive cancers are being overdiagnosed due to improved detection technologies and diagnostic practices [11]. This pattern contrasts with the decrease in rates of early-stage disease observed in our study and likely reflects differences in health systems or population characteristics. Another analysis noted that shifts in staging criteria, such as the adoption of the eighth edition of the TNM staging system, led to systematic downstaging of many cases of differentiated thyroid cancer [12]. This can be useful for interpreting trends over time, as changes in staging systems can affect the proportion of cases categorized as localized or regional. Direct comparisons of stage distributions are further complicated by the focus of modern staging systems on predicting mortality rather than recurrence.

We found a 5.3% increase in the frequency of PTC in the histopathological subgroup assessment in Cohort 2. Similarly, many studies have reported an increase in the frequency of PTC due to advances in diagnostic techniques such as high-resolution ultrasound and FNA biopsy. Similarly, this increase has been observed in various populations. For example, studies have shown that the incidence of PTC has more than doubled in certain regions, including South Korea, in recent decades, and this has been attributed primarily to increased screening efforts [13]. This trend has also been confirmed in other countries, with studies highlighting a significant rise in PTC diagnoses due to the more widespread use of imaging and pathological examinations [14]. Additionally, molecular alterations, such as those in the TERT promoter, have been shown to correlate with more aggressive PTC subtypes, further complicating the prognosis and treatment strategies [15].

In the survival analysis of patients with thyroid cancer, we determined that age, gender, origin, stage at diagnosis, and histopathological subtypes significantly affected survival statistically. The best prognostic group in histopathology was papillary + FV, while the worst was the other group, which mainly included ATC and sarcomas. Few studies in the literature have also examined prognostic factors affecting survival in thyroid cancer patients. A population-based study found that tumor differentiation status, age, and stage at diagnosis were strong predictors of survival, with increasing age being associated with lower relative survival for each histological type [16]. Similarly, another study reported that age greater than 60 years is associated with a worse prognosis in patients with PTC [17]. However, while race is a significant determinant in some studies, it appears to interact with other factors like age and stage rather than acting as an independent prognostic factor [18]. In the literature, there are studies on factors affecting overall survival in patients with thyroid cancer, as well as different studies examining factors affecting recurrence. In a recently published study evaluating factors predicting recurrence in patients with early-stage thyroid cancer, the presence of extrathyroid tumor extension and neck lymph node metastasis in patients with PTC were found to be statistically significant prognostic factors [19].

When comparing the cohorts in terms of prognosis, we found that, although the frequency of patients with regional-stage disease was increased in our study, there was a trend towards improved prognosis in patients with thyroid cancer in Cohort 2. There was an 8% survival improvement in patients in Cohort 2 compared with Cohort 1. This situation is thought to be possible due to the new drugs that have been used in cancer treatment in recent years. Several studies have examined the impact of new therapies on the prognosis of thyroid cancer, finding similar trends of survival improvement linked to novel therapies. In a recent study, it was found that combining targeted therapies and immunotherapy significantly improved overall survival in patients with ATC [20]. Additionally, studies on ATC, which is known to be aggressive, demonstrate significant survival improvements over the past two decades with personalized treatment regimens that include targeted therapies such as BRAF mutation inhibitors [21]. Similarly, in a study focused on differentiated thyroid cancer with lung metastases, it was indicated that radioiodine therapy (RAI) had a positive effect on survival, particularly in younger patients and those with fewer metastases [22].

This study has some limitations as it is a retrospective cohort study. It is difficult to demonstrate causal relationships in retrospective studies as they cannot account for all possible confounding variables since the results have already been reported. In addition, different studies or institutions may have different standards for the quality and consistency of data collection, which may have led to a heterogeneous collection of information. Retrospective studies using historical data may lead to a sample that is less representative of the current population, which may limit the generalizability of the results. In addition, The NCI SEER Dataset is a very comprehensive database containing data on cancer patients. This database was created with data from many different cancer centers [23]. The differences in diagnosis, treatment, and imaging methods among cancer centers are a limitation in obtaining standardized data. Also, there are deficiencies regarding patient treatment data in the NCI SEER Dataset [24]. This situation makes it difficult to perform more in-depth statistical analyses.

5. Conclusions

In this large-scale study of twenty years of data from patients with thyroid cancer, we investigated the main factors affecting survival outcomes and prognosis. In the study, we revealed significant differences between the two cohorts; we found an increase in the proportion of older patients, males, and PTC in Cohort 2. Though an increasing trend in survival rates was observed in Cohort 2, the results were not statistically significant. We found that age, sex, gender, origin, stage at diagnosis, and pathological subtype, including papillary + FV subtype, were critical prognostic indicators. The strengths of this study were its large sample size and the comprehensive examination of survival data across multiple variables, which increased the reliability and generalizability of the study. Identifying age, gender, and cancer subtype as essential factors for prognosis may facilitate clinical decision-making and guide more personalized treatment strategies for thyroid cancer patients. In addition, by demonstrating changes in patient characteristics and survival over time, this study sets a valuable precedent for future studies to improve patient outcomes and understand the evolving nature of thyroid cancer.

Author Contributions: Conception and design: All authors; Development of methodology, analysis, and interpretation of data: All authors; Data acquisition: All authors; Manuscript writing: All authors; Final approval of manuscript: All authors. All authors have read and agreed to the published version of the manuscript.

Funding: This research received no external funding.

Institutional Review Board Statement: All data is openly accessible, and ethical approval is not needed.

Informed Consent Statement: Since the article was taken from the SEER database, which contains deidentified patient data from the National Cancer Institute (NCI) in the United States, patient consent was waived.

Data Availability Statement: The datasets generated and/or analyzed during the current study are available in the Surveillance, Epidemiology, and End Results (SEER) Program repository, https://seer.cancer.gov/data-software/ (accessed on 15 December 2024)

Conflicts of Interest: The authors declared that there are no potential conflicts of interest.

References

1. Sung, H.; Ferlay, J.; Siegel, R.L.; Laversanne, M.; Soerjomataram, I.; Jemal, A.; Bray, F. Global Cancer Statistics 2020: GLOBOCAN Estimates of Incidence and Mortality Worldwide for 36 Cancers in 185 Countries. *CA Cancer J. Clin.* **2021**, *71*, 209–249. [CrossRef]
2. Kitahara, C.M.; Sosa, J.A. The changing incidence of thyroid cancer. *Nat. Rev. Endocrinol.* **2016**, *12*, 646–653. [CrossRef] [PubMed]
3. Haugen, B.R.; Alexander, E.K.; Bible, K.C.; Doherty, G.M.; Mandel, S.J.; Nikiforov, Y.E.; Pacini, F.; Randolph, G.W.; Sawka, A.M.; Schlumberger, M.; et al. 2015 American Thyroid Association Management Guidelines for Adult Patients with Thyroid Nodules and Differentiated Thyroid Cancer: The American Thyroid Association Guidelines Task Force on Thyroid Nodules and Differentiated Thyroid Cancer. *Thyroid* **2016**, *26*, 1–133. [CrossRef] [PubMed]
4. Glikson, E.; Alon, E.; Bedrin, L.; Talmi, Y.P. Prognostic Factors in Differentiated Thyroid Cancer Revisited. *Isr. Med. Assoc. J.* **2017**, *19*, 114–118. [PubMed]
5. Ulisse, S.; Baldini, E.; Lauro, A.; Pironi, D.; Tripodi, D.; Lori, E.; Ferent, I.C.; Amabile, M.I.; Catania, A.; Di Matteo, F.M.; et al. Papillary Thyroid Cancer Prognosis: An Evolving Field. *Cancers* **2021**, *13*, 5567. [CrossRef] [PubMed]
6. Ahmadi, S.; Landa, I. The prognostic power of gene mutations in thyroid cancer. *Endocr. Connect.* **2024**, *13*, e230297. [CrossRef]
7. Davies, L.; Welch, H.G. Increasing incidence of thyroid cancer in the United States, 1973–2002. *JAMA* **2006**, *295*, 2164–2167. [CrossRef] [PubMed]
8. Rahelić, V.; Perković, T.; Romić, L.; Perković, P.; Klobučar, S.; Pavić, E.; Rahelić, D. The Role of Behavioral Factors on Chronic Diseases—Practice and Knowledge Gaps. *Healthcare* **2024**, *12*, 2520. [CrossRef] [PubMed]
9. Kilfoy, B.A.; Devesa, S.S.; Ward, M.H.; Zhang, Y.; Rosenberg, P.S.; Holford, T.R.; Anderson, W.F. Gender is an age-specific effect modifier for papillary cancers of the thyroid gland. *Cancer Epidemiol. Biomark. Prev.* **2009**, *18*, 1092–1100. [CrossRef] [PubMed]
10. Tofe, S.; Arguelles, I.; Forteza, A.; Alvarez, C.; Repetto, A.; Masmiquel, L.; Rodriguez, I.; Losada, E.; Sukunza, N.; Cabrer, M.; et al. Age-standardized incidence, mortality rate, and trend changes of thyroid cancer in the Balearic Islands during the 2000–2020 period: A population-based study. *Eur. Thyroid J.* **2023**, *12*, e220183. [CrossRef]
11. Jegerlehner, S.; Bulliard, J.L.; Aujesky, D.; Rodondi, N.; Germann, S.; Konzelmann, I.; Chiolero, A.; Group, N.W. Overdiagnosis and overtreatment of thyroid cancer: A population-based temporal trend study. *PLoS ONE* **2017**, *12*, e0179387. [CrossRef]
12. Lamartina, L.; Leboulleux, S.; Terroir, M.; Hartl, D.; Schlumberger, M. An update on the management of low-risk differentiated thyroid cancer. *Endocr. Relat. Cancer* **2019**, *26*, R597–R610. [CrossRef]
13. Bouayed Abdelmoula, N.; Abdelmoula, B.; Masmoudi, I.; Aloulou, S. Review Histopathological-molecular classifications of papillary thyroid cancers: Challenges in genetic practice settings. *Biomed. Healthc. Res.* **2024**, *2*, 2–11. [CrossRef]
14. Lam, A.K. Papillary Thyroid Carcinoma: Current Position in Epidemiology, Genomics, and Classification. In *Papillary Thyroid Carcinoma*; Methods in Molecular Biology; Humana: New York, NY, USA, 2022; Volume 2534, pp. 1–15. [CrossRef]
15. Steinberg, E.; Dimitstein, O.; Morand, G.B.; Forest, V.I.; da Silva, S.D.; Pusztaszeri, M.; Alohali, S.; Payne, R.J. Clinical and Histopathological Features of Thyroid Cancer with TERT Promoter Molecular Alterations in Isolation Versus with Concurrent Molecular Alterations: A Multicenter Retrospective Study. *Cancers* **2024**, *16*, 3446. [CrossRef] [PubMed]
16. Gilliland, F.D.; Hunt, W.C.; Morris, D.M.; Key, C.R. Prognostic factors for thyroid carcinoma. A population-based study of 15,698 cases from the Surveillance, Epidemiology and End Results (SEER) program 1973–1991. *Cancer* **1997**, *79*, 564–573. [CrossRef]
17. Kauffmann, R.M.; Hamner, J.B.; Ituarte, P.H.G.; Yim, J.H. Age greater than 60 years portends a worse prognosis in patients with papillary thyroid cancer: Should there be three age categories for staging? *BMC Cancer* **2018**, *18*, 316. [CrossRef] [PubMed]
18. Milano, A.F. Thyroid Cancer: 20-Year Comparative Mortality and Survival Analysis of Six Thyroid Cancer Histologic Subtypes by Age, Sex, Race, Stage, Cohort Entry Time-Period and Disease Duration (SEER*Stat 8.3.2) A Systematic Review of 145,457 Cases for Diagnosis Years 1993–2013. *J. Insur. Med.* **2018**, *47*, 143–158. [CrossRef] [PubMed]
19. Marongiu, A.; Nuvoli, S.; De Vito, A.; Mura, A.; Vargiu, S.; Spanu, A.; Madeddu, G. The Role of Risk Factors for the Progression of Patients with T1b-T2 Papillary Thyroid Carcinoma (PC) during Long-Term Follow-Up. *J. Clin. Med.* **2024**, *13*, 5373. [CrossRef] [PubMed]
20. Cabanillas, M.E.; Dadu, R.; Ferrarotto, R.; Gule-Monroe, M.; Liu, S.; Fellman, B.; Williams, M.D.; Zafereo, M.; Wang, J.R.; Lu, C.; et al. Anti-Programmed Death Ligand 1 Plus Targeted Therapy in Anaplastic Thyroid Carcinoma: A Nonrandomized Clinical Trial. *JAMA Oncol.* **2024**, *10*, 1672–1680. [CrossRef] [PubMed]

21. Maniakas, A.; Dadu, R.; Busaidy, N.L.; Wang, J.R.; Ferrarotto, R.; Lu, C.; Williams, M.D.; Gunn, G.B.; Hofmann, M.C.; Cote, G.; et al. Evaluation of Overall Survival in Patients With Anaplastic Thyroid Carcinoma, 2000–2019. *JAMA Oncol.* **2020**, *6*, 1397–1404. [CrossRef]
22. Zhang, S.; Zhu, M.; Zhang, H.; Liu, H.; Fan, X.; Zhang, J.; Yu, F. The Effect of Radioiodine Therapy on the Prognosis of Differentiated Thyroid Cancer with Lung Metastases. *Biomedicines* **2024**, *12*, 532. [CrossRef] [PubMed]
23. About the SEER Registries. Available online: https://seer.cancer.gov/registries/ (accessed on 19 February 2025).
24. SEER Acknowledgment of Treatment Data Limitations. Available online: https://seer.cancer.gov/data-software/documentation/seerstat/nov2023/treatment-limitations-nov2023.html (accessed on 19 February 2025).

Journal of
Clinical Medicine

MDPI

Review

Circulating Biomarkers of Thyroid Cancer: An Appraisal

Marta Codrich [1], Alessia Biasotto [1,2] and Federica D'Aurizio [1,2,*]

1 Department of Medicine (DMED), University of Udine, 33100 Udine, Italy; marta.codrich@uniud.it (M.C.); alessia.biasotto@asufc.sanita.fvg.it (A.B.)

2 Institute of Clinical Pathology, Academic Hospital "Santa Maria della Misericordia", Azienda Sanitaria Universitaria Friuli Centrale, 33100 Udine, Italy

* Correspondence: federica.daurizio@asufc.sanita.fvg.it; Tel.: +39-0432-552404

Abstract: Thyroid cancer is the most prevalent endocrine cancer. The prognosis depends on the type and stage at diagnosis. Thyroid cancer treatments involve surgery, possibly followed by additional therapeutic options such as hormone therapy, radiation therapy, targeted therapy and chemotherapy. Besides the well-known thyroid tumor biomarkers, new circulating biomarkers are now emerging. Advances in genomic, transcriptomic and proteomic technologies have allowed the development of novel tumor biomarkers. This review explores the current literature data to critically analyze the benefits and limitations of routinely measured circulating biomarkers for the diagnosis and monitoring of thyroid cancer. The review also sheds light on new circulating biomarkers, focusing on the challenges of their use in the clinical management of thyroid cancer, underlining the need for the identification of a new generation of circulating biomarkers.

Keywords: circulating biomarkers; thyroid cancer; circulating tumor cells; circulating tumor nucleic acids; circulating tumor DNAs; circulating tumor RNAs

1. Introduction

The first use of blood biomarkers to detect and manage malignant thyroid tumors was dated almost 50 years ago [1,2]. Over the years, several circulating biomarkers have been identified and routinely used in clinical practice for the management of thyroid cancer, especially after primary treatment, to identify timely residual disease and recurrent or distant metastasis. Circulating biomarkers of thyroid cancer mainly include peptides and proteins, expressed on the cell surface or secreted into the bloodstream [3]. Recent approaches, due to the advent of new technologies such as genomics, transcriptomics and proteomics, have greatly expanded the range of blood biomarkers, considering also circulating tumor cells and circulating tumor nucleic acids, including cell-free and cell-derived exosome DNA and RNA, released from cancer cells into the bloodstream [3–5]. These markers mirror the tumor-specific characteristics, monitoring the development of the cancer disease [4,5]. This review focuses on blood biomarkers used in the clinical management of patients with thyroid cancer. In detail, we aim to both describe the advantages and limitations of circulating biomarkers commonly used in routine and highlight the challenges of new potential circulating biomarkers arising from technological developments and recent discoveries in the field of cancer. For this manuscript, the literature review was performed using the bibliographic database Pubmed. The search keywords were "thyroid cancer" and "circulating biomarkers" with no time restrictions, focusing on the latest reviews and research articles as well as on included studies of the chosen publications.

2. Thyroid Cancer

Thyroid cancer is the most common endocrine neoplasm [6] and accounts for about 2.2% of all new cancer cases [7]. The risk of developing thyroid cancer is higher in females and increases with age [8]. The classification of thyroid neoplasms is based on histopathology and molecular pathogenesis according to the fifth edition of the World Health Organization (WHO) thyroid cancer categorization released in 2022 [9]. Thyroid cancer mainly includes the tumors arising from both parafollicular cells (C cells) giving rise to the medullary thyroid carcinoma (MTC), belonging to the dispersed neuroendocrine system, and from follicular epithelial cells resulting in papillary thyroid carcinoma (PTC), follicular thyroid carcinoma (FTC), oncocytic thyroid carcinoma (OTC), high-grade non-anaplastic carcinoma or anaplastic thyroid carcinoma (ATC) [9]. The transformation that occurs in thyroid cancer is caused by mutations in genes that encode mainly for molecules involved in cell proliferation and apoptosis, thus triggering aggressiveness, dedifferentiation, and decreased or no response to therapy [10]. The most common genetic modifications occur in BRAF, RAS, TERT, RET, TP53 genes and RET/PTC gene fusion with various distributions in different histotypes of thyroid cancer [10,11]. WHO 2022 classification for thyroid tumors shows a greater interest in characterizing neoplastic lesions from a molecular perspective. Histological and molecular terminology is then used for any specific microscopic morphology related to well-known genetic alterations [9].

PTC and FTC are the most common histological types [12]. PTC, FTC and OTC are collectively referred to as differentiated thyroid carcinoma (DTC) [13] because tumor cells recollect some of the properties of normal thyrocytes, in particular, the ability to respond to stimulation by thyrotropin (TSH) and absorb and store iodine [12]. PTC accounts for about 80–85% of thyroid cancer in adults and 90% in the pediatric population [12,14]. Despite its high prevalence among endocrine neoplasms, DTC has an excellent prognosis with a 5-year survival rate of 98.4% of cases [7], especially if it is detected early and treated promptly [15]. However, regular follow-up is essential to monitor for signs of recurrence [15]. DTC usually does not cause symptoms in the early stages of the disease with normal thyroid function [16] and the clinical presentation of DTC in many cases is a solitary thyroid nodule [12]. Although most thyroid nodules are benign, a thorough examination is necessary to rule out cancer patients [16]. In this respect, imaging plays a crucial role in DTC diagnostics. Undoubtedly, ultrasonography provides detailed information on the characteristics of nodules, such as size, composition and vascularity [17,18] which, considered together and never individually, support the diagnostic accuracy of the malignancy of a thyroid nodule [19]. Ultrasound-guided fine needle aspiration biopsy (FNAB) with subsequent cytological examination of the specimen can be used to determine the benign or malignant nature of nodules [18], and it is mandatory in rapidly growing nodules, especially in younger patients [12]. However, this approach has several challenges including a high rate of inadequate sampling, the presence of a lot of blood that can obscure thyrocytes due to the extensive perfusion of the thyroid, and the frequent difficulty in follicular neoplasms to distinguish benign from malignant forms [20]. Overall, indeterminate or suspected lesions account for 15–25% of cases investigated by the FNAB, with about 30% eventually being malignant [21]. This last finding was obtained in several studies that used different cytological classifications [21], Thy 3 according to British Thyroid Association Guidelines [22], Class 3 by American Association Clinical Endocrinologists/Associazione Medici Endocrinologi and European Thyroid Association guidelines [23], or Categories III–IV of the Bethesda System for Reporting Thyroid Cytopathology [24].

The knowledge of the molecular etiology of thyroid cancer has provided the basis for a better understanding of cytologically indeterminate nodules. The introduction of molecular techniques, including polymerase chain reaction (PCR) and next-generation sequencing (NGS), has allowed the detection of the driver alterations involved in thyroid cancer development directly on FNA samples. Nowadays, there are different NGS-based assays available for clinical practice. In brief, these tests can detect not only the point gene mutations, gene–gene fusions, and insertions/deletions located in the driver genes mainly associated with components of MAPK and PI3K/Akt pathways, but also copy number alterations, differentially expressed genes, and/or miRNAs linked to the various types of thyroid cancers. In detail, ThyroSeq v.3 explores 112 thyroid cancer-related genes; Afirma Gene Sequencing Classifier analyzes RNAs' expression combining machine learning algorithms; and ThyGeNEXT/ThyraMIR merges mutational panel with miRNAs' expression. These assays are mostly used to discriminate between benign and malignant thyroid nodules and have allowed a significant reduction in unnecessary thyroid surgeries for suspicious nodules [25,26]. The main treatment for DTC is surgery, which aims to remove the tumor mass and possibly nearby lymph nodes [27]. The type of surgery to be performed depends on the size of the tumor, the presence of metastases, and the histology of the subtype [27]. In Americas, Europe, and much of Australasia, (near-) total thyroidectomy is usually performed in almost all patients [6]. Only for pT1a PTC, the hemithyroidectomy is considered sufficient [28,29]; however, some authors suggest only observation without surgery resection [6]. More recently, a discussion has arisen about the need for total thyroidectomy in non-locally invasive and non-metastatic DTC with a tumor diameter of up to 4 cm [28]; however, this strategy has yet to prove its efficacy [30]. Most current guidelines recommend the post-surgical radioactive iodine (RAI) ablation as a second component of the primary treatment of DTC in most thyroidectomized patients [28]. Specifically, RAI therapy is used to target and eliminate residual cancer cells and any surviving thyroid tissue [28]. External radiation therapy is used for situations where RAI ablation and surgery are not sufficient to manage aggressive or advanced thyroid carcinomas that do not respond to standard treatments [31]. Moreover, the treatment of resistant DTC includes immune checkpoint inhibitors which stimulate the immune system against cancer cells [31,32] and drugs targeting gene abnormalities to limit the proliferation of cancer cells [33,34].

On the other hand, MTC is a rare thyroid carcinoma that accounts for approximately 1.4–5% of all thyroid malignancies [35,36]. In general, MTC is more aggressive than follicular cell-derived carcinoma with lymph node involvement and sometimes with distant metastases at the time of diagnosis [37]. Although lower than the incidence of DTC, the incidence of MTC has increased in the last three decades, from 0.14 to 0.21 per 100,000 people [38], thanks to the introduction of serum calcitonin (CT) as a screening test in multinodular goiter and to the use of high-resolution ultrasound [39,40]. MTC is inherited in 25% of cases, due to mutations in RET proto-oncogene observed in the context of multiple endocrine neoplasia (MEN) syndromes or familial medullary thyroid cancer (FMTC) [37]. Hereditary MTC is often bilateral, multicentric, and associated with C-cell hyperplasia. Patients with inherited MTC may present with systemic manifestations as a result of excessive secretion of hormones from the tumor, which includes CT and its related peptides. Patients may also present with manifestations of MEN syndromes [37]. Sporadic MTC appears as a firm, hard nodule in the mid-upper region of the thyroid lobes where C cells predominate [41]. At presentation, most patients (70%) with sporadic disease have lymph node involvement and approximately 10% of them have distant metastases [37]. Preoperative ultrasonography typically shows non-specific features of malignancy [41], and cytology is diagnostic in only 50% of cases [39]. Adequate imaging should be performed to determine the extent of the disease. Besides CT and MRI, nuclear medicine techniques, such as PET/CT with 18F-FDOPA and 18F-FDG are used in the evaluation of disease extension for pre-operative staging and post-operative follow-up [42]. The initial treatment of MTC is surgical. Total thyroidectomy is recommended due to the high incidence of multifocal and bilateral disease, especially in patients with sporadic MTC [43]. In addition to total thyroidectomy, central lymph node compartment dissection prophylaxis is performed even if no lymph node involvement and no evidence of distant metastases have been detected in pre-operative staging [35]. Conversely, total thyroidectomy with lateral and central compartment dissection is advisable in cases with preoperatively confirmed cervical lymph node involvement [35]. In patients with basal CT levels greater than 200 ng/L with no evidence of distant metastasis, it is recommended to complete the intervention with prophylactic dissection of uninvolved contralateral neck compartments [35].

Finally, an essential part of postoperative treatment for both DTC and MTC is thyroid hormone replacement therapy. As thyroidectomy causes loss of thyroid function, patients should take thyroid hormone supplements to restore euthyroidism and to suppress TSH for cancer control [44].

3. Blood Biomarkers in Thyroid Cancer: State of Art

3.1. Thyroglobulin

Thyroglobulin (TG) is a glycoprotein of 660 kDa produced by thyroid follicular cells, and it provides the substrate for the synthesis of thyroid hormones, which are T4 and T3. TG is produced by both normal and tumor thyroid cells, thus indicating the presence of thyroid tissue [45]. In DTC, although not useful as a diagnostic marker, TG is considered the most reliable marker for the identification of disease persistence or recurrence after thyroidectomy and adjuvant administration of RAI ablation [28]. Indeed, the serum concentration of TG, usually measured with continued T4 treatment (onT4-TG) should be undetectable upon tumor thyroid tissue removal as indicated by the follow-up algorithms of the American Thyroid Association [28]. In clinical practice, the measurement of serum TG is based on immunometric assays (IMAs) starting from the first radio immunoassay (RIA) and immunoradiometric assay (IRMA) based on radioactive labeled TG, continuing with immunoluminometric assay (ILMA), chemiluminescence enzyme immunoassay (CLEIA) and chemiluminescence assays (CLIA) based on light emission, fluoroimmunoassay (FIA), fluorescence enzyme immunoassay (FEIA) and enzyme-linked fluorescence assay (ELFA) based on fluorescence emission, only to end with electrochemiluminescence assays (ECLIA), based on chemiluminescent reaction after applying a voltage and Time Resolved Amplified Cryptate Emission (TRACE) technology based on energy transferring [46,47]. The implementations of commercial TG assays with high analytical sensitivity (hsTG) have allowed an increase in their performance [48].

False-negative results may occur in the presence of extremely high levels of TG due to hook effect [48]. Specifically, two-site non-competitive IMAs are subject to the hook effect, as a result of a massive excess of analyte (antigen) that depletes the binding capacity of the capture antibody, leading to inappropriately normal or low values of analyte [45]. In the case of TG, a falsely low serum value may have important clinical consequences. Currently, commercially available TG assays are very resistant to this type of analytical interference, but it can still occasionally occur in patients with high-load metastatic disease (i.e., serum TG up to 1000 μg/L). Dilution of serum may be used to detect hook effects in suspicious cases [49]. In general, the concentration at which the hook effect can be excluded should be determined by the manufacturers and verified locally by each laboratory [48]. In addition, IMAs may be affected by paraproteins, heterophilic antibodies and high biotin serum concentration especially in streptavidin-biotin coupling assays [47]. The existence of antithyroglobulin antibodies (ATG) interferes with TG measurement, altering antigen-antibody complex formation resulting in a false-negative test in current IMAs [47]. The monitoring of both TG and ATG is fundamental during the follow-up of thyroid cancer patients [47] since 25% of DTC patients were positive for ATG [50]. Variations in serum ATG concentrations, determined longitudinally employing the same IMA, may be used as a surrogate tumor marker for residual or progressive thyroid cancer [48]. The trend of ATG levels is more important than the absolute level; indeed, a reduction in serum ATG concentrations is an indication of a disease-free condition. Conversely, the persistence or increase of ATG concentrations should suggest suspicion of persistent disease or recurrence [48]. Interestingly, liquid chromatography coupled to tandem mass spectrometry (LC-MS/MS) methods are less affected by the presence of autoantibodies. Thus, some authors suggest the use of LC-MS/MS for measuring TG serum levels in ATG-positive patients [51]. The use of trypsin digestion before the measurement results in the cleavage of all proteins, thus eliminating autoantibodies [52]. However, there is still much to be done towards the harmonization of LC-MS/MS [53]. In particular, LC-MS/MS still shows variances in the choice of the calibrator, although the latest methods show good agreement of results. For this reason, nowadays it is not the first-line test but is used only in selected cases [48].

Since the release of TG from both non-malignant thyrocytes and DTC cells is generally dependent on TSH, serum TG determination under TSH stimulation has long been considered the gold standard for ensuring remission 6–18 months after ablation of the malignant cells in addition to being recommended in many guidelines [22,28]. TSH stimulation can be achieved by T4 withdrawal (endogenous stimulation) or by recombinant human TSH (rhTSH) administration (exogenous stimulation). Both approaches provide high serum TSH concentration (>30 mIU/L) [54]. At such TSH levels, an unmeasurable TG suggests a very low risk of recurrence. Conversely, TG concentrations higher than 1–2 μg/L have to be considered suggestive of disease persistence or recurrence [54]. In recent years, the introduction of hsTG IMAs has reduced the need for stimulation of TSH to measure TG concentrations during initial and long-term follow-ups of patients with DTC [48,55,56]. In this regard, several studies were published on the role of basal hsTG versus rhTSH-stimulated hsTG showing that unstimulated serum TG concentrations lower than 0.2 μg/L ruled out additional stimulation tests in most cases [55,57–61]. Conversely, little is known about the role of basal hsTG versus endogenous stimulated hsTG [62,63]. In this respect, Trimboli et al. demonstrated that TG levels lower than 0.23 μg/L after T4 withdrawal, in low- and high-risk DTC patients, is an accurate marker of disease freedom [54]. In addition to its prognostic and predictive role of disease recurrence after total ablation, there has been an increased focus on the role of TG also in the time interval between surgery and RAI [64,65]. The value of TG as a predictive factor before treatment with ^{131}I is controversial due to several factors including the existence of residual thyroid tissue after surgery [66,67], TSH concentration, and individual risk of loco-regional or remote metastases [68,69]. In addition, the correct timing for post-operative measurement of TG and its stimulated or suppressed cut-off postoperatively, which can confirm or exclude the presence of lesions, has not yet been identified [70]. In this context, in a recent study by Signori et al., hsTG was measured at three different time points in a selected population of patients operated for PTC [71], specifically after thyroidectomy but before RAI ablation (in euthyroidism, 40 days after surgery), at the time of RAI ablation (in hypothyroidism) and after RAI ablation (in euthyroidism). After a three-year follow-up, the results showed that the determination of hsTG before RAI therapy (first-time point) was a reliable prognostic indicator to predict future nodal or distant disease recurrence, useful to guide patient management.

3.2. Calcitonin

Human calcitonin (CT) is a 32-amino acid polypeptide hormone secreted mainly by the parafollicular cells of the thyroid gland and it is involved in calcium–phosphorous metabolism. Other tissues can produce CT including lungs, parathyroid glands, bladder, small intestine, liver and thymus [72].

CT was described for the first time in 1962 by Copp and Cheney as a modulator of calcium tone [73]. CT is synthesized as part of a larger prohormone, called procalcitonin (ProCT), a precursor peptide derived from pre-procalcitonin and, its secretion is primarily regulated by calcium and gastrin levels in serum [72].

In healthy subjects, CT levels are influenced by several factors including gender and age (slightly higher in men than in women and in the pediatric population than in adults), body mass index (BMI) and smoking [74]. Based on the method employed, at least 90% of healthy adults show serum CT concentrations below 10 ng/L and, among them, more than 50% below the limit of detection (LOD) of current IMAs [74,75].

Elevated serum CT levels are highly sensitive for the diagnosis of MTC in patients with nodular/multinodular goiter, but lack strong specificity [76]. In fact, several drugs can stimulate CT secretion, i.e., proton pump inhibitors (PPIs) and beta-blockers and, as with most tumor biomarkers, the blood concentration of CT may also increase in other pathological conditions such as chronic renal failure, autoimmune thyroiditis, hypergastrinemia, sepsis, type 1A pseudohypoparathyroidism and mastocytosis [76]. In addition, several types of neoplasms, including breast cancer and neuroendocrine neoplasms (NENs), may present with an ectopic CT secretion [77]. Therefore, the identification of a reliable cut-off for basal CT in order to support a more accurate initial diagnostic evaluation of thyroid nodules is still missing [78]. Giannetta et al., in an extensive review of the literature, suggested 100 ng/L as cut-off to strongly suspect thyroid malignancy, with a positive predictive value (PPV) for MTC reaching 100%, whereas in subjects showing moderately high values (10–100 ng/L) diagnostic accuracy could be enhanced by performing a stimulation test (e.g., Calcium test) [79]. Over the years, several authors have proposed various cut-offs for basal CT, generally below 100 ng/L with differences between females and males [78,80,81]. The discrepancies between the cut-offs in different studies can, at least in part, be attributed to the different population inclusion criteria and the different methods used for CT measurement [78]. Similarly, cut-offs for CT after stimulation vary in the different studies published with a distinction between females and males [78]. A slight CT increase is observed in C-cell hyperplasia (CCH), with concentrations setting between 10 and 20 ng/L. However, it is reported in a Cochrane systematic review that only 0.32% of patients with thyroid nodules were diagnosed with MTC, showing a low prevalence of the disease and opening a debate for routine CT measurement in these patients [82]. In the preoperative setting, basal CT levels are indicative of tumor burden, metastatic potential and lymph node invasion and extent [83]. Postoperatively, CT concentrations are of great prognostic value; basal CT should be measured 3 months after surgery and monitored every 6–12 months as suggested in the ATA guidelines [35].

Several analytical methods have been used to measure serum CT levels over the decades. They were first revealed by RIA, whose inaccuracy was attributable to the use of polyclonal antibodies that detected both mature and immature monomers of CT, as well as other circulating forms (precursors and degradation products) [84]. RIA was replaced by two-sided IRMA, whose improved specificity was derived from the implementation of two monoclonal antibodies, capable of binding to two different specific epitopes within the CT molecule [85]. The LOD reached 1 ng/L following the introduction of IMAs based on fluorescence and chemiluminescence, which were more sensitive and specific for CT in their architecture. Currently, the employment of an ECLIA based on streptavidin–biotin technology has shortened testing time and lowered the LOD to less than 1 ng/L [86].

The introduction of more accurate cut-offs would be helpful in the differential diagnosis between CCH and micro-MTC and the exclusion of ectopic CT production by various NENs [83]. CT levels measured with different commercial assays may vary widely, and it is of primary importance that each laboratory establishes and maintains its reference intervals and cut-offs; patients' follow-up should be performed using the same method, and re-baseline is required in case of method changeover [87].

3.3. Carcinoembryonic Antigen

Carcinoembryonic antigen (CEA) is an intercellular adhesion glycoprotein, with a molecular weight of 200 kDa, initially detected in human tissue of colorectal cancer in 1965 by Gold and Freedman [88]. CEA is expressed in normal tissue and a broad range of epithelial neoplasms (e.g., colorectal cancer, lung cancer, pancreatic cancer, etc.) [89]. Since CEA is released into the bloodstream, the measurement of circulating CEA is used as a tool for early diagnosis, monitoring of cancer recurrence and treatment efficacy [90]. In healthy subjects, the blood concentration of CEA generally ranges from 2.5 to 5 ng/mL, with higher values in men than in women. CEA values greater than 5 ng/mL may indicate the presence of malignant tumors. However, as in the majority of tumor biomarkers, blood levels of CEA may also increase in non-neoplastic diseases such as ulcerative colitis, pancreatitis, liver cirrhosis, hepatitis, renal insufficiency and in heavy smokers [91]. In addition to cancer diagnosis and monitoring, there are currently several therapeutic approaches targeting this biomarker, such as in metastatic colorectal and lung carcinomas that are CEA-positive [92].

Literature reports that 60–70% of MTC patients have elevated serum CEA levels [93]. Although not specific, CEA can have a role as a marker of tumor progression and invasion, especially in MTC with low or no production of CT, as its blood levels are associated with tumor size, lymph node involvement and also distant metastases [93,94]. CEA is also useful for the evaluation of response to initial therapy in MTC patients [93]. Some studies have considered CEA as a marker of dedifferentiation in MTC follow-up. In detail, in cases of decreased levels of postoperative CT, increased levels of CEA may be an indication of dedifferentiation [95]. A fraction of MTC shows no immunohistochemical expression of CT and low or negative serum levels of both CT and CEA. This subset of MTC enters into differential diagnosis of thyroid high-grade NENs, which are also negative for CT and CEA both at tissue and blood levels [96].

Currently, the detection of CEA is performed by automated CLIA which has almost completely displaced RIA and enzyme-linked immunosorbent assay (ELISA) [97,98]. Although the International Reference Preparation (IRP) has been in use for several decades, numerous studies have reported the persistence of method- and/or manufacturer-dependent differences for CEA [99–101]. Over the years, there has been a clear improvement in the maximum bias among manufacturers, from 85% in 2005 [102] to less than 50% in 2023 [103]. There was also an improvement within the same method with intra-assay coefficients of variation (CV) less than 10% [103]. However, despite technological improvements over the last two decades, a very recent study comparing six immunoassays has shown that there is still no full harmonization for CEA determination [98]. The lack of inter-method comparability may be due to several factors [103]. Firstly, structural aspects (i.e., high molecular weight, significant carbohydrate content, several isoforms and numerous possible epitopes) may influence the definition of specific peptide epitopes suitable for antibody binding in IMAs [103]. Secondly, antigen–antibody binding affinity may vary depending on the antibodies used in the assay as well as the conformation and glycosylation of their epitopes [104,105]. Finally, the characteristics of antibodies may affect the specificity of the binding, which is probably lower for polyclonal than monoclonal antibodies [106]. Therefore, in the absence of a reference method and complete harmonization between IMAs, each laboratory must establish its reference intervals/cut-offs to reflect the situation of its specific population. Moreover, the results of the CEA have to be always evaluated together with the patient's medical history, clinical examination and imaging information [98].

3.4. Carbohydrate Antigen 19-9

Recently, carbohydrate antigen 19-9 (Ca 19-9) has emerged as a potentially useful prognostic predictor in both MTC and advanced DTC [107]. Ca 19-9 is a 36 kDa glycolipid belonging to the mucin family. Mucins are highly glycosylated proteins, abundantly distributed on the surface of epithelial cells that present alterations in their expression and structure in numerous pre-neoplastic and neoplastic lesions [108]. Serum levels of Ca 19-9 are high in carcinomas of the digestive tract, especially pancreatic, but also in lung, ovarian and uterine tumors [109,110]. Unfortunately, the lack of satisfactory sensitivity and especially specificity does not allow its measurement for early diagnosis of cancer [108,111]. Currently, it is used in the follow-up phase, particularly in the monitoring of pancreatic cancer [109].

Several studies, published in the last 10–15 years, have identified Ca 19-9 as a marker of MTC, expressed both at tissue and blood levels [112,113]. Overall, these results showed that increased serum Ca 19-9 levels are an adverse prognostic factor in patients with advanced MTC, especially in cases with a higher risk of short-term mortality [114,115]. Similarly, Alencar et al. reported that serum Ca 19-9 may have a role as a prognostic factor in patients with MTC [116]. On the other hand, the precise relationship between PTC and Ca 19-9 in tissues and serum has not been well established. Some studies have shown positivity for Ca 19-9 immunohistochemical staining in tumor tissue [117–119]. Little detailed information is available on serum Ca 19-9 levels in patients with PTC. Kihara et al. reported a case of hepatic metastasis in PTC patients after several years from thyroidectomy accompanied by elevated serological levels of Ca 19-9. After partial liver resection, a significant decrease in serum concentrations of Ca 19-9 was observed [120]. In addition, Yamaguchi et al. described a case of elevated serum levels of Ca 19-9 in a patient with PTC-related lung metastasis diagnosed 15 years after thyroidectomy [118]. Finally, very recently, Kihara et al. have retrospectively analyzed 196 patients with PTC (maximum diameter 2 cm). For each patient, serum Ca 19-9 values were determined before and after the surgery. Elevated serum levels of Ca 19-9 before thyroidectomy were observed in 6.1% of patients. After the surgical procedure, serum levels of Ca 19-9 in all patients decreased back to the normal range. Although further studies with longer follow-up are needed, the authors suggested serum Ca 19-9 levels as a tumor marker for PTC [121].

To date, most IMAs for quantitative detection of Ca 19-9 use a sandwich format and depend on the use of the monoclonal antibody 1116-NS-19-9, called Centocor, which recognizes the sialyl Lewis A glycan motif, a member of the Lewis family of blood group antigens involved in the binding of glycans, lipids and proteins [122,123]. Although extensive research has been conducted on the determination of Ca 19-9, challenges remain in achieving standardization and harmonization between methods. Recent automation of IMAs has certainly improved accuracy, but it has not yet succeeded in reducing the discrepancy between results obtained from the same samples using different methods [124–127]. In this respect, the Society for Promoting Quality Assurance in Medical Laboratories (INSTAND, Germany) observed a manufacturer-dependent bias of up to 194% for Ca 19-9 as part of the results of the external quality assessment (EQA) in 2005 [102]. Significant variations have also been reported in clinical trials comparing different manufacturers [128]. Recently, Kremser et al. conducted a longitudinal re-evaluation of EQA data for some cancer markers including Ca 19-9 [129]. The authors compared intra- and inter-method variations between participants using the most common analytical platforms and tested their adherence to EQA limits [129]. They concluded that the intra-method precision of most analytical platforms has become accepted for Ca 19-9 (CV less than 16% for each individual collective) [129]. Conversely, the variability between different methods remains significant [129]. Potential causes of these differences may include the use of monoclonal antibodies with different antigen-binding sites, antigen modifications and different assay architectures/formulations [129].

Finally, tissue expression dependence and circulating levels of sLeA in Lewis blood group also influence the sensitivity of Ca 19-9 assay. False negative results were found in subjects with a negative Lewis genotype, which represents 5–10% of the Caucasian population, while no data are available on other ethnicities [110]. Interestingly, low or medium levels of Ca 19-9 (approximately 100 kU/l) have been reported in some patients with negative Lewis genotype and advanced pancreatic cancer [122,130,131].

The above-cited biomarkers are summarized in Table 1.

Table 1. List of well-known circulating biomarkers for the management of thyroid tumor disease. TG, thyroglobulin; CT, calcitonin; CEA, carcinoembryonic antigen; Ca 19-9, cancer antigen 19-9; DTC, differentiated thyroid carcinoma; MTC, medullary thyroid carcinoma; IMAs, immunoassays; LC-MS/MS, liquid chromatography coupled to tandem mass spectrometry.

Biomarker	Thyroid Tumor	Biological Matrix	Currently Available Methods	Clinical Use	Limitations	References
TG	DTC	Plasma, Serum	IMAs, LC-MS/MS	Prediction of tumor relapses after treatment (surgery, RAI ablation); estimation of tumor burden.	Elevations in non-neoplastic disorders; analytical interferences.	[28,47–52,54,64–70]
CT	MTC	Plasma, Serum	IMAs	Preoperative MTC identification (most sensitive marker); estimation of tumor burden; prognostic predictor; evaluation of response to therapy.	Elevations in non-neoplastic disorders; lack of a univocal cut-off for basal CT; analytical interferences.	[35,74,76–78,80,81,83]
CEA	MTC	Plasma, Serum	IMAs	Prognostic predictor; marker of tumor dedifferentiation, progression and invasion; evaluation of response to therapy.	Elevations in non-neoplastic disorders; lack of specificity for thyroid cancer (other neoplasms such as colon, breast, ...); analytical interferences.	[89–95,97,98]
Ca 19-9	DTC, MTC	Plasma, Serum	IMAs	Prognostic predictor; marker of MTC dedifferentiation and disease aggressiveness.	Elevations in non-neoplastic disorders; lack of specificity for thyroid cancer (other neoplasms such as pancreas); lack of a univocal cut-off to distinguish between benign and malignant disease; analytical interferences.	[107–116,121]

4. Emerging Blood Biomarkers in Thyroid Cancer

Besides the well-known thyroid tumor biomarkers, new circulating biomarkers are now emerging. Advances in genomic, transcriptomic and proteomic technologies have allowed the development of novel tumor biomarkers. Liquid biopsy is a minimally invasive laboratory test that permits the detection and analysis of circulating tumor cells (CTCs) and circulating tumor nucleic acids (ctNAs) in the peripheral blood and other body fluids of patients with cancer, offering real-time information on tumor diagnosis, progression and therapeutic response. In this section, we have reviewed the recent discoveries on thyroid biomarkers presenting promising clinical uses for diagnosing and following up on thyroid disease (Figure 1).

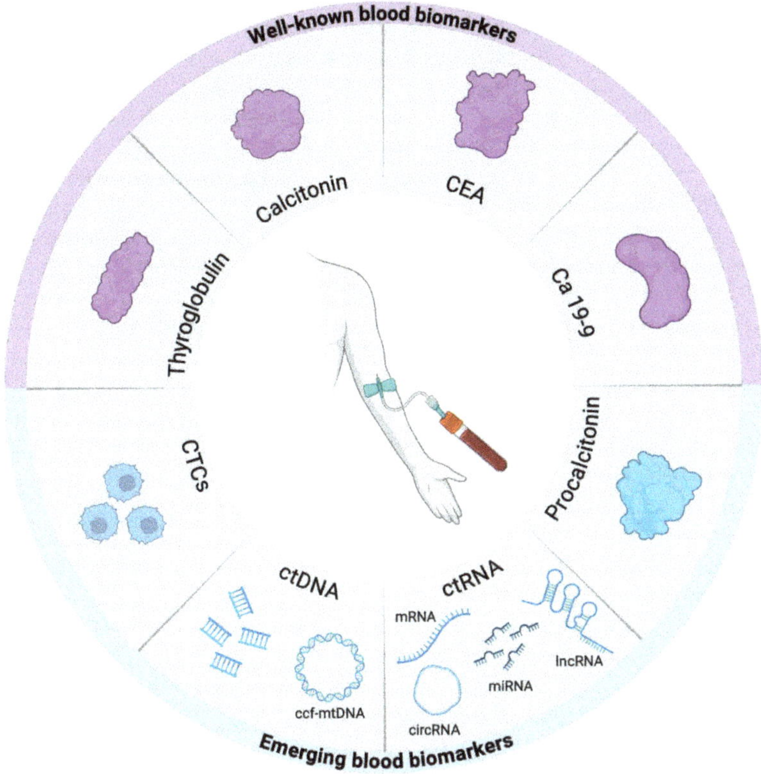

Figure 1. Overview of blood biomarkers in thyroid cancer. Schematic representation of well-known and emerging biomarkers for thyroid tumors. CEA, carcinoembryonic antigen; Ca 19-9, cancer antigen 19-9; CTCs, circulating tumor cells; ctDNA, circulating tumor DNA; ccf-mtDNA, circulating cell-free mitochondrial DNA; ctRNA, circulating tumor RNA; mRNA, messenger RNA; miRNA, microRNA, lncRNA, long non-coding RNA; circRNA, circular RNA. Created with BioRender.com accessed on 16 February 2025.

4.1. Circulating Tumor Cells

CTCs are tumor cells derived from the primary solid tumor that extravasate into and circulate mainly in the bloodstream [132]. CTCs possess significant metastatic potential thanks to their capability to reach other sites easily since their presence in the blood [133]. However, only a small percentage of CTCs can metastasize, suggesting that escaping the immune system and interacting with the specific microenvironment in the secondary loci are required [134,135].

With the development of molecular technologies, CTCs isolation and enrichment have allowed a detailed investigation into CTCs biology, thus providing greater details about tumor gene mutations and heterogeneity. Nowadays, CTCs isolation and identification are based on antigen-dependent (such as epithelial marker, e.g., EpCAM) [136] or antigen-independent approaches combined with molecular techniques [137]. Indeed, thanks to single-cell sequencing technology, CTCs genome and transcriptome have been extensively investigated [138,139]. Importantly, CTCs may facilitate clinical practice. Indeed, many clinical trials have been carried out focusing mainly on the usage of CTCs in breast and prostate cancer considering clinical prognosis and therapy response [140]. Recent data have highlighted their potential not only in early cancer detection [141,142], but also in the minimal residual disease and the relapse of the tumor [143].

Few studies have been conducted to point out new potential alternative biomarkers for clinical application in thyroid cancer patients considering the diagnostic value of CTCs. Li et al. demonstrated a higher detection of CTCs in patients affected by PTC and by FTC associated with a shorter overall survival. Moreover, the authors showed that increased CD133 levels were associated with the differentiation grades of thyroid cancers [144]. A clear correlation was found between the number of CTCs and the tumor stage in PTC, FTC, and MTC patients. Moreover, compared to the control subjects, CTCs were detectable in patients with DTC after complete thyroidectomy in the absence of serum TG and no evidence of tumor recurrence. Furthermore, the number of CTCs correlated to the radioiodine therapy in PTC patients. The authors suggest that PTC patients need a restrictive follow-up due to the increased numbers of CTCs even in a remission condition [133]. A similar result has been obtained by Sriramareddy et al., who demonstrated the presence of CT-positive CTCs in the bloodstream of MTC patients following complete thyroidectomy although serum CT was not detectable. The authors encourage a strict follow-up for these patients since the number of CTCs was correlated with the probability of tumor relapse [145]. Indeed, Weng et al. demonstrated a positive correlation between the detection of CTCs and the metastasis rates in patients with PTC and with FTC correlated with poor progress-free survival [146]. Furthermore, Xu et al. proved a negative association between the overall survival and the number of CTCs in patients with metastatic MTC [147]. Additionally, a prospective study demonstrated the increased detection of CTCs mainly in patients with DTC, especially in those with metastases compared to healthy subjects [148]. However, a retrospective study concluded that the efficacy of CTCs in diagnosing thyroid cancer is still limited considering the number of CTCs and the antibodies against thyroid peroxidase (ATPO) values in a cohort of thyroid tumor patients divided into malignant and benign groups [149]. Nevertheless, a recent meta-analysis showed that CTCs expressing thyroid-stimulating hormone receptor (TSHR), rather than EpCAM, are a reliable marker for the diagnosis of patients with thyroid cancer recurrence or metastasis [150].

Interestingly, a recent study considered Survivin gene expression among different markers of malignancy. An increased Survivin mRNA isolated from mononuclear cells is indicative of low differentiation grades of thyroid cancers [146]. Similar results were reported by Li et al. In detail, CTCs were detected and CK19, Survivin and TG mRNAs were analyzed. The authors demonstrated that CTCs were increased in PTC patients with distant metastasis and highlighted the role of CTCs signature Survivin as a potential marker of PTC diagnosis [151].

4.2. ctNAs

On the other hand, ctNAs are cell-free nucleic acids, comprising circulating tumor DNA (ctDNA) and RNA (ctRNA), that originate from tumor cells and are shed into the blood circulation [152]. ctNAs can be released directly from the primary tumor, CTCs or tumor extracellular vesicles, thus harboring the mutational status of the original tumor [153–155]. ctDNAs are fragmented DNA [156], while ctRNAs include messenger RNA (mRNA) and non-coding RNAs (ncRNAs), such as microRNA (miRNAs), circular RNA (circRNA), and long non-coding RNA (lncRNA) [157]. The ncRNAs are functional RNA molecules that are not translated into a protein and play a key regulatory role in multiple biological functions. Indeed, their dysregulations have been implicated in multiple diseases including tumorigenesis acting as oncogenic molecules or tumor suppressors [158,159]. CtNAs analysis consists of the extraction of cell-free nucleic acids mainly from a blood sample, avoiding invasive procedures. Thus, the evaluation of ctNAs provides important information about the mutational spectrum of the tumor. As with CTCs, the development of NGS techniques and molecular technologies for the isolation of ctNAs have allowed us to deepen our knowledge of the characteristics of blood ctNA markers for the diagnosis, monitoring and prognosis of cancer [160]. However, there are some limitations, such as the low signal-to-noise ratio and the short bioavailability [152]. Therefore, the current challenge aims to improve the current expertise in using ctNAs as blood clinical markers as a tumor screening tool and for the detection of minimal residual disease.

4.2.1. ctDNAs

The analysis of ctDNAs can detect the mutations and epigenetic changes useful for diagnosis and treatment strategy choice. In the thyroid cancer field, recent evidence observed the presence of ctDNA containing BRAFV600E mutation, the most frequent genetic event in DTC, in patients affected by PTC compared to those with benign nodules [161]. Moreover, a hypermethylation state of SLC5A8 and SLC26A4, associated with BRAFV600E mutation, was found in PTC patients [162]. Interestingly, the level of circulating BRAFV600E has been observed to dramatically decrease after surgery in PTC patients [161]. In addition, the detection of residual circulating BRAFV600E post-surgery is suggestive of recurrence in patients with PTC [163]. Circulating RETM918T mutation was detectable in the plasma of patients affected by MTC, suggesting a worse outcome [164]. However, it has been shown that there is a very low concordance in BRAF, KRAS, NRAS and TERT promoter mutations between primary or metastatic thyroid tissues and plasma ctDNAs in early stage thyroid cancer patients [165]. Nevertheless, through NGS analysis on ctDNAs extracted from blood samples of patients affected by different thyroid tumor types, it has been observed that the large majority of patients presented one or more genomic alterations and TP53 mutation was the most frequent in all thyroid tumor types, followed by BRAFV600E, RAS, RET, ALK and NTRK with variable frequency according to the type of tumors taken into account [166].

A mention of mitochondrial DNA (mtDNA) deserves to be discussed. The mtDNA is a double-stranded circular chromosome located in the mitochondria organelles in a tissue-specific number of copies [167]. The mitochondrial genome consists of 16 kb and contains genes that encode for its tRNAs and rRNAs and proteins involved in oxidative phosphorylation [168]. The involvement of mtDNA in the pathogenesis of several diseases including cancer has been demonstrated [169]. Indeed, tumors exhibit an altered bioenergetic process due to gene copy numbers or gene expression modifications [169]. For instance, an aberrant accumulation of mitochondria due to mtDNA mutations is characteristic of the oncocytic phenotype in thyroid gland tumors [170]. Moreover, an increased tissue mtDNA copy number is associated with carcinogenesis in PTC [171]. The altered presence of circulating cell-free mtDNA (ccf-mtDNA) is indicative of mitochondrial dysfunction and thus of a pathological condition [172]. A lower content in plasma ccf-mtDNA has been shown in patients with PTC compared with healthy subjects [173]. Thus, the ccf-mtDNA may be a valid alternative to ctDNA as it is easily detectable due to its abundance compared to ctDNA in the bloodstream and especially due to its strict correlation with tumor progression.

4.2.2. ctRNAs

In the last decade, ncRNAs have yielded great interest as potential circulating biomarkers, particularly in cancer research. In contrast to ctDNAs, circulating ncRNAs can be easily quantified in the blood, especially miRNAs. Indeed, miRNAs reflect the clinical features of the tumor and their blood levels can be associated with treatment response and patient outcome [174]. To date, certain studies have been conducted on the expression profile and clinical significance of circulating miRNAs in thyroid cancer.

Using a microarray approach, Romeo et al. identified miR-375 as the most upregulated miRNA in C cells and plasma of MTC patients compared to healthy controls and subjects in remission, associating miR-375 with reduced overall survival and poor prognosis [175]. The same results were obtained by Censi et al., who showed serum miR-375 overexpression in pre-surgical MTC patients compared to controls and patients affected by different diseases. Unfortunately, no correlation was identified between serum and tissue. However, a concordance was observed between serum miR-375 and CT [176]. This data was also confirmed by Melone et al., who identified a serum molecular signature in MTC patients applying miRNome profiling. The authors reported an upregulation of miR-375, miR-144-3p, miR-7-5p and miR-335-5p [177]. MiR-144 was also detected by Shabani et al. Indeed, increased plasma levels of miR-144 and miR-34a were observed in MTC patients compared to controls. Interestingly, MTC patients carrying RET mutation presented a much higher expression of miR-144 and miR-34a than wild-type RET MTC patients [178]. Among miRNAs identified using miRNA arrays, plasma miR-26b-5p and miR-451a were observed to be highly expressed in a cohort of MTC patients. Interestingly, their expression decreased after surgery [179]. Furthermore, serum levels of miR-222-3p and miR-17-5p were found significantly increased in MTC patients compared to benign nodule and control groups. In the same study, the authors observed also a trend for patients affected by PTC. In detail, miR-222-3p, miR-17-5p, and miR-451a were shown to increase, whereas miR-146a-5p, miR-132-3p, and miR-183-3p were decreased in the serum of PTC patients and those with benign nodules compared to the control group [180]. Similar findings have resulted from using miRNA profiling that identified serum miR-221-3p, miR-222-3p, miR-146a-5p, miR-146b-5p, miR-24-3p, miR-191-5p, miR-103-3p and miR-28-3p as upregulated in PTC patients compared to healthy subjects. Among these miRNAs, miR-146a-5p, miR-221-3p and miR-222-3p markedly decreased after tumor excision in PTC patients. Moreover, levels of miR-146a-5p and miR-221-3p correlated with serum TG levels [181]. Yu et al. also demonstrated that the expression of serum miR-222, miR-151-5p and let-7e was higher in PTC patients compared to benign cases and healthy controls. In addition, a lower expression of miR-151-5p and miR-222 was shown in a subset of PTC patients after thyroidectomy [182]. Equally, plasma miR-222 and miR-146b were increased in pre-surgery PTC patients in comparison with healthy volunteers and after thyroidectomy. Importantly, Lee et al. demonstrated that miR-222 and miR-146b are associated with PTC recurrence [183]. Razei et al. evaluated miRNAs pre- and post-surgery and showed a decreased expression of plasma miR-222 and miR-181a in PTC patients after thyroidectomy. In addition, miR-181a and miR-146a distinguished between cancerous and benign cases. Moreover, the levels of miR-181a were associated with increasing tumor size in PTC cases. Interestingly, there was a correlation between miR-222 and BRAFV600E mutation in PTC patients [184]. Likewise, serum miR-221, miR-222, miR-31, and miR-151-5p were observed to decrease in PTC after surgery compared to PTC pre-surgery patients. Moreover, the serum amount of miR-222, miR-31, miR-151-5p and let-7 was revealed to increase, whereas miR-21 was decreased in PTC patients relative to controls and patients affected by benign nodules [185]. Graham et al. showed an mRNA profiling to distinguish PTC from benign nodules. Particularly, serum miR-146a-5p and miR-199b-3p were downregulated, whereas let7b-5p and miR-10a-5p were upregulated in PTC serum samples than benign tumor [186]. The level of serum miR-579, miR-95, miR-29b, and miR-190 were lower in PTC patients respect to controls and patients with nodular goiters, among which miR-95 and miR-190 resulted the most promising [187]. An increased expression of plasma miR-25-3p, miR-451a, miR-140-3p and let-7i was observed in PTC cases compared to benign nodules or healthy controls. Importantly, miR-25-3p and miR-451a decreased after tumor excision. Moreover, the plasma levels of miR-25-3p and miR-451a were correlated with those expressed in thyroid tissues from PTC patients [188].

In summary, miR-375 and miR-144 turned out to be the most interesting miRNAs dysregulated in plasma and serum of MTC patients, whereas miR-222, miR-221, miR-146a, miR-151, miR-31, and miR-21 in PTC cases. Thus, these miRNAs are promising circulating biomarkers for the management of thyroid tumor disease (Table 2).

In the literature, there is very little evidence of the presence of lncRNAs in the blood of thyroid cancer patients. For instance, Jiang et al. identified 6 lncRNAs (CCAT1, SYNPR, SFTA1P, HOTAIR, HCG22, and CLDN10) in the plasma of PTC patients. Furthermore, all these lncRNAs correlate with overall survival affecting progression and invasion in thyroid tumors. Moreover, CCAT1, SYNPR, SFTA1P, HOTAIR, and HCG22 were found to be upregulated in PTC tumor tissue except for CLDN10, which was downregulated (Table 2) [189]. Other authors demonstrated the involvement of lncRNAs in thyroid cancer tissue, but not their presence in the bloodstream. Nevertheless, the lncRNAs MALAT1 [190], HOTAIR [191], and BANCR [192] are encouraging candidates for circulating thyroid cancer blood markers.

Nothing is known about circulating circRNAs' implication in thyroid tumors. However, circRNAs are emerging as promising biomarkers for thyroid cancer. Indeed, there is evidence of the involvement of circRNAs in the onco-pathogenesis of the thyroid. For instance, it has been demonstrated that the impairment of circ-ITCH/miR--22-3p/CBL/β-catenin axis in PTC development and progression. In detail, circ-ITCH competes with miR--22-3p to upregulate the expression of CBL, thus inactivating the Wnt/β-catenin pathway and consequently attenuating PTC progression [193]. Yao et al. identified circ0058124 as a novel driver for PTC tumorigenesis by regulating NUMB through binding to miR-218-5p, thus repressing NOTCH3/GATAD2A signaling [194]. Likewise, circZFR plays a role in PTC cell proliferation, migration and invasion by miR-1261/C8orf4 axis [195] and circNUP214 acts as an oncogene and sponges miR-145 and its target ZEB2 in PTC cells [196]. Finally, circ-0004458 was found to be overexpressed in PTC tissues and cells. Circ-0004458 silencing induced cell cycle arrest and apoptosis by miR-885-5p/RAC1 pathway [197].

Regarding coding RNAs, Yang et al. have developed a multiplex approach for the quantification of circulating transcripts in thyroid tumor patients, identifying 4 circulating RNAs (thyroid peroxidase TPO, TG, glial cell line-derived neurotrophic factor family receptor alpha-2 GFRA2, and iodotyrosine deiodinase IYD) in the plasma of thyroid cancer patients, among which TPO transcript resulted in the most promising marker to estimate residual disease [198]. Similar results were obtained in two different studies whereby the levels of TG mRNA were estimated in the peripheral blood of thyroid tumor patients [199,200]. In detail, it has been demonstrated that the presence of TG transcript in blood samples of subjects affected by PTC [200] and in all metastatic DTC cases [199]. Nevertheless, TG mRNA was detectable in patients with benign thyroid nodules as well as in healthy subjects [199], potentially derived from lymphocytes and renal cells besides circulating thyrocytes [201,202]. Among well-known thyroid-associated markers, it has been suggested that the detection of TSHR mRNA in patients with thyroid lesions be used not only as a marker of recurrence but also as a marker of diagnosis and aggressiveness [203–207]. Likewise, it has been demonstrated that the levels of blood CT-related polypeptide alpha transcript (CT-CALCA) correlated with serum CT in MTC patients, including RET mutation carriers [208]. Finally, Lubitz et al. demonstrated the detection of BRAFV600E mutation in reverse-transcribed RNA isolated from peripheral blood lymphocytes of PTC patients [209].

Extracellular vesicles (EVs) deserve specific attention, in particular the well-characterized exosomes. Over the last years, many authors have reported the involvement of exosomes in tumor progression and metastasis processes. In detail, exosomes are extracellular vesicles secreted from cells carrying nucleic acids (such as miRNAs, circRNAs and lncRNAs), proteins, lipids, and metabolites [210]. Recently, evidence highlighted the dysregulation of exosome content in the pathogenesis of thyroid cancer, revealing their potential as biomarkers in tumor diagnosis and clinical prognosis. Among the different exosomal miRNAs, miR24-3p, miR146a-5p, miR181a-5p and miR382-5p were found to be downregulated, whereas miR127-3p and miR376a-3p were upregulated in the serum of PTC patients compared to healthy subjects. Interestingly, exosomal miR24-3p was positively correlated with the same circulating miRNA free of any encapsulation [211]. Similarly, Liang et al. observed a lower expression of plasma exosomal miR-16-2-3p, miR-34c-5p, miR-182-5p, miR-146b-5p, miR-223-3p and miR-223-5p in nodular goitres and PTC patients compared to controls. Moreover, the authors proposed miR-16-2-3p and miR-223-5p as biomarkers to be utilized to distinguish between benign and malignant nodules [212]. A decreased serum exosomal miR-29a was also identified in PTC subjects relative to controls [213]. Conversely, increased expression of plasma or serum EVs-derived miR-1-3p, miR-206, miR-221-3p [214], miR-10a-5p, miR-34a-5p, miR-346 [215], miR-145 [216], miR-376a-3p, miR-485-3p, miR4306 and miR-4433a-5p [217] well-differentiated PTC patients from controls [214–217], benign thyroid nodules from malignant ones [217] and after surgery [214]. Besides PTC cases, Samsonov et al. observed overexpression of miR-21, miR-31, miR146a, miR-181a, and miR-221 in plasma exosomes of different thyroid tumor cases compared to normal subjects. Interestingly, miR-21, miR126, and miR145 distinguish between PTC and benign tumor patients, whereas miR-31 between FTC and adenomas. In the same study, miR-21 and miR-181a were able to differentiate between FTC and PTC patients [218]. Regarding the possibility of improving prognosis, plasma exosomal miR146b-5p and miR222-3p were identified as upregulated in PTC patients with lymph node metastasis (LNM) compared to those without invasion [219]. Similar results were obtained by Chen et al., who identified plasma exosomal miR-6774-3p and miR-6879-5p as discriminants among PTC patients with and without LNM [220]. In addition to miRNAs, other ncRNAs are found to be dysregulated in thyroid patients' exosomes. Within circRNAs, circ-007293 [221,222], circ-031752 and circ-020135 [222] were upregulated in PTC patients' serum, whereas among lncRNAs, DOCK9-AS2 was enriched in exosomes derived from PTC patients' plasma [223]. Interestingly, some authors provided evidence that exosome-derived proteins are dysregulated in thyroid cancer as well as ncRNAs. Indeed, through mass spectrometry, a different pattern of ITGB2, TLN1, CAPNS1 and SRC in exosome-derived serum from PTC patients has been identified, correlating their increased expression with LNM [224]. Furthermore, using the same approach, bone marrow stromal cell antigen 2 (BST2) was found to be well associated with PTMC progression [225]. An enhanced expression was also shown for chaperone proteins Hsp27, Hsp60, and Hsp90 in thyroid tissue and plasma exosomes of PTC patients as compared with benign goitre and after thyroidectomy [226]. Finally, a recent multi-omics analysis pointed out a transcriptomic and proteomic signature for indeterminate thyroid nodules. In detail, the authors revealed an enhanced expression of EV-derived CXCR7, CD147, SDC4 and EpCAM in the plasma of patients with indeterminate thyroid nodules compared with healthy controls. Additionally, mir-195-3p was found to be upregulated and mir-3176, mir-205-5p, novel-hsa-mir-208-3p, mir-3529-3p and let-7i-3p downregulated [227]. Thus, exosomes are key players in thyroid cancer pathogenesis and therefore can be considered promising tumor biomarkers on a par with ctNAs (Table 2).

Table 2. List of promising extracellular vesicles-derived and free circulating ncRNAs for the management of thyroid tumor disease with potential diagnostic and prognostic significance. In the table, the expression level is indicated as follows: upregulated ↑ and downregulated ↓. PTC, papillary thyroid carcinoma; FTC, follicular thyroid carcinoma; MTC, medullary thyroid carcinoma.

Circulating ncRNA	Thyroid Tumor	Expression Level	Biological Matrix	References
miR-1	PTC	↑	Plasma-derived exosomes	[214]
miR-7	MTC	↑	Serum	[177]
miR-10	PTC	↑	Serum, Plasma-derived exosomes	[186,215]
miR-16	PTC	↓	Plasma-derived exosomes	[180]
miR-17	MTC, PTC	↑	Serum	[180]
miR-21	FTC, PTC	↑↓	Serum, Plasma-derived exosomes	[185,218]
miR-24	PTC	↑↓	Serum, Serum-derived exosomes	[181,211]
miR-25	PTC	↑	Plasma	[188]
miR-26	MTC	↑	Plasma	[179]
miR-28	PTC	↑	Serum	[181]
miR-29	PTC	↓	Serum, Serum-derived exosomes	[187,213]
miR-31	FTC, PTC	↑	Serum, Plasma-derived exosomes	[185,218]
miR-34	MTC, PTC	↑↓	Plasma, Plasma-derived exosomes	[178,212,215]
miR-95	PTC	↓	Serum	[187]
miR-103	PTC	↑	Serum	[181]
miR-126	PTC	↑	Plasma-derived exosomes	[218]
miR127	PTC	↑	Serum-derived exosomes	[211]
miR-132	PTC	↓	Serum	[180]
miR-140	PTC	↑	Plasma	[188]
miR-144	MTC	↑	Plasma, Serum	[177,178]
miR-145	PTC	↑	Plasma/Serum-derived exosomes	[216,218]
miR-146 family	PTC	↑↓	Plasma, Serum, Plasma/Serum-derived exosomes	[180,181,183,184,186, 211,212,218,219]
miR-151	PTC	↑	Serum	[182,185]
miR-181	FTC, PTC	↑↓	Plasma, Plasma/Serum-derived exosomes	[184,211,218]
miR-182	PTC	↓	Plasma-derived exosomes	[212]
miR-183	PTC	↓	Serum	[180]
miR-190	PTC	↓	Serum	[187]
miR-191	PTC	↑	Serum	[181]
miR-199	PTC	↓	Serum	[186]
miR-206	PTC	↑	Plasma-derived exosomes	[214]
miR-221	PTC	↑	Serum, Plasma-derived exosomes/EVs	[181,185,214,218]
miR-222	MTC, PTC	↑	Plasma, Serum	[180–185,219]
miR-223	PTC	↓	Plasma-derived exosomes	[212]
miR-335	MTC	↑	Serum	[177]
miR-346	PTC	↑	Plasma-derived exosomes	[186,215]
miR-375	MTC	↑	Plasma, Serum	[175,176]
miR376	PTC	↑	Plasma/Serum-derived exosomes	[211,217]
miR382	PTC	↓	Serum-derived exosomes	[211]
miR-451	MTC, PTC	↑	Plasma, Serum	[179,180,188]
miR485	PTC	↑	Plasma-derived exosomes	[217]
miR-579	PTC	↓	Serum	[187]
miR4306	PTC	↑	Plasma-derived exosomes	[217]
miR4433	PTC	↑	Plasma-derived exosomes	[217]
miR6774	PTC	↑	Plasma-derived exosomes	[220]
miR6879	PTC	↑	Plasma-derived exosomes	[220]
let-7 family	PTC	↑	Plasma, Serum	[182,185,186,188]
circ-007293	PTC	↑	Serum-derived exosomes	[221,222]
circ-031752	PTC	↑	Serum-derived exosomes	[222]
circ-020135	PTC	↑	Serum-derived exosomes	[222]

Table 2. *Cont.*

Circulating ncRNA	Thyroid Tumor	Expression Level	Biological Matrix	References
CCAT1	PTC	↑	Plasma	[189]
SYNPR	PTC	↑	Plasma	[189]
SFTA1P	PTC	↑	Plasma	[189]
HOTAIR	PTC	↑	Plasma	[189]
HCG22	PTC	↑	Plasma	[189]
CLDN10	PTC	↓	Plasma	[189]
DOCK9-AS2	PTC	↓	Plasma-derived exosomes	[223]

4.3. Procalcitonin

Procalcitonin (ProCT) is the peptide precursor of CT, a hormone synthesized by the parafollicular C cells of the thyroid and involved in calcium homeostasis [228]. ProCT is also released by the neuroendocrine cells of the lung and intestine in response to inflammatory stimuli [228]. ProCT was first described as a marker of sepsis (differentiating bacterial from non-bacterial infection) and multiple organ failure as well as to manage antibiotic therapy [229]. Besides CT as a well-known marker for MTC, there has been a shift in focus on ProCT as an emerging blood biomarker [230,231]. Indeed, ProCT has a half-life of 24 h and is less influenced by circadian rhythm compared to CT [232–234]. Moreover, ProCT is more stable at room temperature than CT and presents a comparable measurement between different current commercial IMAs [93]. However, ProCT is influenced by trauma and the inflammatory state of the patient, thus limiting its use in clinical practice in the case of inflammatory conditions. For instance, similarities between ProCT and CT values have been observed reflecting the clinical states of patients with MTC using Roche ECLIA for CT measurement and Roche, PES, Abbott for ProCT [235]. Similar results were obtained in other studies [236–239], demonstrating that ProCT presents an equivalent or even superior alternative to CT for the follow-up of MTC patients. A recent meta-analysis showed how serum ProCT can be considered a highly accurate test for MTC management, in terms of diagnosis and disease monitoring, thanks to its higher sensitivity and specificity [240]. In particular, using a fully automated homogeneous TRACE immunometric fluorescent assay on the Kryptor® system, a cut-off value of ProCT > 0.1 ng/mL is considered a good marker for the diagnosis of MTC since it resulted in a sensitivity of 100%, specificity of 99.9%, PPV of 77.8%, and NPV of 100% [241]. Furthermore, the same authors suggest measuring ProCT to detect false hypercalcitoninemia due to heterophilic antibody interference [242]. Moreover, a study conducted by Kratzsch et al. demonstrated the usage of ProCT as an alternative method to CT to overcome false hypercalcitonemic conditions, in this case associated with PPIs therapy, chronic kidney disease and Hashimoto's thyroiditis. In this study, CT was tested using two fully automated assays (IMMULITE, Siemens Healthineers and Liaison, Diasorin) and one nonautomated assay (IRMA, Medipan), and ProCT using Brahms Kryptor (ThermoFisher Scientific) [243]. Furthermore, the possibility to measure both CT and ProCT markers on the same automated platform facilitates the interpretation of the laboratory results by matching reflex strategies.

5. Discussion

This review explores the current literature data to critically analyze the benefits and limitations of routinely measured circulating biomarkers for the diagnosis and/or monitoring of DTC and MTC. The review also sheds light on new circulating biomarkers, focusing on the challenges of their use in the clinical management of thyroid cancer.

Thyroid cancer is the most frequent endocrine neoplasm. Its incidence rate is rapidly increasing worldwide [7], representing a potential threat to public health [244]. In fact, although having a good prognosis in a large percentage of cases, thyroid cancer can evolve negatively with lymph node invasion and distant metastasis [245].

CT and TG were the first two biomarkers discovered almost 50 years ago [1,2,246]. TG is the best available tumor marker for DTC after (near-) total thyroidectomy and subsequent RAI ablation of the remaining thyroid tissue [31]. Its periodic measurement provides crucial information on the patient's response to treatment and the patient's status regarding a possible recurrence of the disease after successful treatment [31], in association with the use of proper imaging procedures [247]. However, the determination of TG, as described before, is affected by the presence of antibodies against TG that negatively interfere with the measurement. Not being affected by the presence of any interfering antibodies, LC-MS/MS has been suggested as a second-line test in some selected cases. In addition, very recently, the estimation of TG transcript levels in peripheral blood has also been proposed as an innovative approach for overcoming antibody-mediated interference [173,174]. However, the presence of transcript variants, the mRNA expression from other sources, and the setting up of the PCR (such as primer design and number of amplification cycles) need to be improved. All these aspects can lead to false-negative or false-positive screening results. On the other hand, CT is used as a screening test in multinodular goiter allowing earlier MTC diagnosis and thus earlier intervention and higher cure rates of the disease [35]. Despite these observations, international scientific societies do not recommend either for or against serum CT determination as a screening test [17,28] since concerns related to cost-effectiveness and the association of high CT serum levels with diseases other than MTC continue to be discussed [41]. For example, CCH is a common cause of marginally elevated CT preceding tumor development in familial MTC. However, increased CT is also found in PTC, autoimmune thyroiditis, chronic renal failure, and non-thyroid-related conditions such as smoking or the use of PPIs. Finally, CT may also be elevated in patients with NENs [41]. Moreover, CT-negative tumors with aggressive biological behavior have been described [36]. In these cases, other markers such as ProCT and CEA may be useful [35].

Currently, serum levels of TG, CT, ATG, CEA and Ca 19-9 are measured mainly by IMAs, which are based on antigen-antibody reactions. Although they display numerous advantages, IMAs are sensitive to analytical interferences such as heterophile antibodies, human anti-animal antibodies (HAMA), anti-analyte autoantibodies, matrix effect, hook effect, biotin, etc., which can cause false-positive or false-negative results [248]. Difficulties in interpreting data may also be due to frequent variability between methods. The lack of standardization and harmonization causes differences among the results obtained from the same samples by different IMAs, as well as discrepancies in reference intervals and cut-offs [249]. The scientific community, regulatory agencies, manufacturers and clinical laboratories should work together in order to minimize manufacturer-specific differences and optimize analytical performance [250]. To overcome these issues, in the last decades, other molecules have been studied such as Cyfra 21.1 [47]. Although some studies have shown their potential clinical application in ATC, overall they are not as useful as the well-known biomarkers widely used in routine [31]. However, current circulating tumor biomarkers for thyroid cancer are not always able to distinguish between benign and malignant neoplasms or between low-risk and high-risk malignant lesions in the preoperative phase [17]. In addition, they are not specific since they can be high even in non-neoplastic conditions [249].

In this context, the post-analytical phase, which concerns the reporting and the interpretation of the result, is fundamental. Indeed, the choice of the appropriate reference interval and/or the clinical decision limit (cut-off) of the biomarker is crucial [251]. The reference interval is a statistical calculation based on the determination of 2.5 and 97.5 percentiles obtained in a sample of unaffected subjects selected from the general population for a given biomarker [252]. The reference interval is defined by laboratory experts according to a well-defined consensus [251]. The clinical cut-off is quite different. It addresses a decision about a clinical condition in a precise clinical patient group. The clinical cut-off derives from clinical outcome studies, guidelines and consensus values, predictive values and ROC (receiver-operating characteristic) curves [251]. The optimal cut-off value for detecting cancer with 100% sensitivity and 100% specificity does not exist because for many cancer biomarkers, the values of the two groups of individuals often overlap [253]. This is even more difficult if cancer patients need to be distinguished from the group of patients with organ-related non-malignant diseases [253]. Therefore, the identification of a specific cut-off for thyroid tumor biomarkers is essential for the correct diagnosis of patients.

Another important aspect is the improvement of the technology that has allowed the development of genomic, transcriptomic and proteomic assays enabling the identification of a multitude of biomarkers which reflect a high signature of the molecular profile for each type of tumor [254]. The general aim is to identify novel circulating biomarkers that can supplement information from the currently used biomarkers. Regarding this aspect, CTCs and EVs-derived and free ctNAs offer a great possibility to assess genotypic features of cancer, besides observing cancer progression and treatment response, without the need for invasive biopsy thanks to their presence in the peripheral blood. Indeed, the evidence of the existence of ctDNAs and ctRNAs and the dysregulation of ccf-mtDNA, mRNAs, miRNAs, lncRNAs and circRNAs as well as proteins in several types of thyroid neoplasms offer the possibility of their potential use in clinical practice. The combination of high-throughput assays aimed at identifying the common mutations such as BRAF, RET, and RAS and at evaluating ctNAs can provide important information about the mutational spectrum of the tumor and guide the selection of appropriate targeted therapy. Indeed, the development of molecular technologies and NGS techniques allows us to characterize blood ctNA markers more deeply for the diagnosis, monitoring and prognosis of cancer [160]. Here, we have listed plenty of potential biomarkers sorted into different types of thyroid tumors. However, the literature data show limitations in their possible practical use. Firstly, most of them are general cancer markers. For instance, among miRNAs, miR-375 and miR-144, miR-221, miR-222, and miR-21 are found to be dysregulated in glioblastomas, breast, prostate, lung, colorectal, stomach, pancreatic, hepatic and neuroendocrine tumors [175,255–257]. In addition, the data currently available in the literature are derived from experimental studies or small-scale clinical trials in specific patient cohorts. Therefore, large-scale studies are required to confirm and validate their use in clinical practice. Furthermore, the current clinical use of CTCs and ctNAs is limited and still requires a complete integration of ctNAs as tumor-derived liquid biopsy markers. Thereby, several studies are needed to carefully identify circulating biomarkers and to design a panel of dysregulated ctNAs specific for thyroid cancer able to discriminate between malignant and benign nodules and, in case, between the different types of thyroid cancer. Moreover, combining several kinds of circulating markers (e.g., the well-known thyroid tumor proteins, CTCs, and ctNAs) in a single diagnostic panel may probably be helpful. Thus, the current challenge aims to improve the current expertise in using ctNAs as blood clinical markers to screen for thyroid neoplasms and detect minimal residual disease.

6. Conclusions and Future Perspectives

Recent findings in the field of tumors are paving the way for a new era of personalized and precision medicine by improving prognosis and quality of life for individuals. The discovery of new biomarkers of thyroid cancer can contribute to early disease detection, careful follow-up and personalized treatments by maximizing therapeutic results [31]. Furthermore, early diagnosis of thyroid cancer allows for less invasive surgery with consequent lower risks for the patient and may also avoid RAI ablation. Moreover, the ability to distinguish between benign and malignant lesions could help in choosing the most appropriate approach. Tailored to the specific needs of each patient and type of cancer, a targeted therapeutic regimen requires medical supervision to prevent adverse effects and maintain maximum effectiveness and quality of life. In thyroid cancer, personalized treatment can interfere with the development and multiplication of cancer cells by using specialized means to identify the molecules involved in the growth of cancer [258]. Tyrosine kinase inhibitors, immunotherapy and gene-targeted therapy are some of the main targeted treatments for thyroid cancer [31] that currently play a supporting role to the well-established surgical therapy and RAI ablation in advanced or treatment-refractory thyroid tumors [259]. Despite progress in recent years, much remains to be explored in the field of cancer and in particular in thyroid cancer to overcome current obstacles to the clinical application of new biomarkers [260]. In particular, future research should focus on the following areas: (1) development of standardized protocols for the validation of biomarkers to demonstrate reliability and reproducibility of assays in different conditions [261]; (2) support for collaborative multi-centre research initiatives that allow for the expansion of study sample numbers, resulting in faster and more convincing data on thyroid cancer [31]; (3) integration of genomic, transcriptomic, proteomic and metabolomic data to increase the sensitivity and specificity of biomarkers [3]; (4) advancement of bioinformatics tools and machine learning algorithms to better understand new biomarker models [262]; and (5) study of potential combinations of biomarkers with consolidated therapeutic strategies to ensure treatment efficacy and to predict treatment response [260].

Author Contributions: Conceptualization, M.C. and F.D.; writing—original draft preparation, M.C., A.B. and F.D.; writing—review and editing, M.C., A.B. and F.D. All authors have read and agreed to the published version of the manuscript.

Funding: This research received no external funding.

Data Availability Statement: No new data were created or analyzed in this study. Data sharing is not applicable to this article.

Conflicts of Interest: The authors declare no conflicts of interest.

Abbreviations

The following abbreviations are used in this manuscript:

ATC	Anaplastic thyroid carcinoma
ATG	Anti-thyroglobulin antibodies
ATPO	Antibodies against thyroid peroxidase
BMI	Body mass index
BST2	Bone marrow stromal cell antigen 2
Ca 19-9	Carbohydrate antigen 19-9
CCH	C-cell hyperplasia
ccf-mtDNA	Cell-free mtDNA
CEA	Carcinoembryonic antigen
circRNAs	Circular RNAs
CLEIA	Chemiluminescence enzyme immunoassay
CLIA	Chemiluminescence assays
CT	Calcitonin
CT-CALCA	CT-related polypeptide alpha transcript

CTCs	Circulating tumor cells
ctDNAs	Circulating tumor DNAs
ctNAs	Circulating tumor nucleic acids
ctRNAs	Circulating tumor RNAs
CV	Coefficients of variation
DTC	Differentiated thyroid carcinoma
ECLIA	Electrochemiluminescence assays
ELISA	Enzyme-linked immunosorbent assay
ELFA	Enzyme-linked fluorescence assay
EQA	External quality assessment
EVs	Extracellular vesicles
FIA	Fluoroimmunoassay
FEIA	Fluorescence enzyme immunoassay
FMTC	Familial medullary thyroid cancer
FNAB	Fine needle aspiration biopsy
FTC	Follicular thyroid carcinoma
GFRA2	Glial cell line-derived neurotrophic factor family receptor alpha-2
HAMA	Human anti-animal antibodies
hsTG	TG assays with high analytical sensitivity
IYD	Iodotyrosine deiodinase
ILMA	Immunoluminometric assay
IMAs	Immunoassays
IRMA	Immunoradiometric assay
IRP	International Reference Preparation
LC-MS/MS	Liquid chromatography coupled to tandem mass spectrometry
lncRNAs	Long non-coding RNAs
LNM	Lymph node metastasis
LOD	Limit of detection
MEN	Multiple endocrine neoplasia
mRNAs	Messenger RNAs
miRNAs	MicroRNAs
MTC	Medullary thyroid carcinoma
mtDNA	Mitochondrial DNA
ncRNAs	Non-coding RNAs
NENs	Neuroendocrine neoplasms
NGS	Next-generation sequencing
OTC	Oncocytic thyroid carcinoma
PPIs	Proton pump inhibitors
PPV	Positive predictive value
ProCT	Procalcitonin
PTC	Papillary thyroid carcinoma
PTMC	Papillary microcarcinoma
RAI	Radioactive iodine
rhTSH	Recombinant human TSH
RIA	Radio immunoassay
ROC	Receiver-operating characteristic
TG	Thyroglobulin
T3	Triiodothyronine
T4	Thyroxine
TPO	Thyroid peroxidase
TRACE	Time Resolved Amplified Cryptate Emission
TSH	Thyrotropin
TSHR	Thyroid-stimulating hormone receptor

References

1. Melvin, K.E.; Miller, H.H.; Tashjian, A.H. Early Diagnosis of Medullary Carcinoma of the Thyroid Gland by Means of Calcitonin Assay. *N. Engl. J. Med.* **1971**, *285*, 1115–1120. [CrossRef] [PubMed]
2. Milhaud, G.; Calmette, C.; Taboulet, J.; Julienne, A.; Moukhtar, M.S. Letter: Hypersecretion of Calcitonin in Neoplastic Conditions. *Lancet* **1974**, *1*, 462–463. [CrossRef] [PubMed]
3. Fang, B. Introduction to This Special Issue: "Biomarker Discovery and Precision Medicine". *J. Cancer Metastasis Treat.* **2020**, *6*, 1. [CrossRef] [PubMed]
4. Wang, Y.; Xu, F.; Zhong, J.-Y.; Lin, X.; Shan, S.-K.; Guo, B.; Zheng, M.-H.; Yuan, L.-Q. Exosomes as Mediators of Cell-to-Cell Communication in Thyroid Disease. *Int. J. Endocrinol.* **2020**, *2020*, 4378345. [CrossRef] [PubMed]
5. Feng, K.; Ma, R.; Zhang, L.; Li, H.; Tang, Y.; Du, G.; Niu, D.; Yin, D. The Role of Exosomes in Thyroid Cancer and Their Potential Clinical Application. *Front. Oncol.* **2020**, *10*, 596132. [CrossRef]
6. Boucai, L.; Zafereo, M.; Cabanillas, M.E. Thyroid Cancer: A Review. *JAMA* **2024**, *331*, 425–435. [CrossRef]
7. Cancer of the Thyroid-Cancer Stat Facts. Available online: https://seer.cancer.gov/statfacts/html/thyro.html (accessed on 8 January 2025).
8. Cao, J.; He, X.; Li, X.; Sun, Y.; Zhang, W.; Li, Y.; Zhu, X. The Potential Association of Peripheral Inflammatory Biomarkers in Patients with Papillary Thyroid Cancer before Radioiodine Therapy to Clinical Outcomes. *Front. Endocrinol.* **2023**, *14*, 1253394. [CrossRef]
9. WHO Classification of Tumours Online. Available online: https://tumourclassification.iarc.who.int/welcome/ (accessed on 8 January 2025).
10. Hlozek, J.; Pekova, B.; Rotnágl, J.; Holý, R.; Astl, J. Genetic Changes in Thyroid Cancers and the Importance of Their Preoperative Detection in Relation to the General Treatment and Determination of the Extent of Surgical Intervention—A Review. *Biomedicines* **2022**, *10*, 1515. [CrossRef]
11. Prete, A.; Borges de Souza, P.; Censi, S.; Muzza, M.; Nucci, N.; Sponziello, M. Update on Fundamental Mechanisms of Thyroid Cancer. *Front. Endocrinol.* **2020**, *11*, 102. [CrossRef]
12. Verburg, F.A. Differentiated Thyroid Cancer: Diagnosis, Therapy, and Follow-Up. In *Atlas of Thyroid and Neuroendocrine Tumor Markers*; Giovanella, L., Ed.; Springer International Publishing: Cham, Switzerland, 2018; pp. 51–64. ISBN 978-3-319-62506-5.
13. Conzo, G.; Avenia, N.; Bellastella, G.; Candela, G.; de Bellis, A.; Esposito, K.; Pasquali, D.; Polistena, A.; Santini, L.; Sinisi, A.A. The Role of Surgery in the Current Management of Differentiated Thyroid Cancer. *Endocrine* **2014**, *47*, 380–388. [CrossRef]
14. Kitahara, C.M.; Sosa, J.A. Understanding the Ever-Changing Incidence of Thyroid Cancer. *Nat. Rev. Endocrinol.* **2020**, *16*, 617–618. [CrossRef] [PubMed]
15. Liang, N.; Zhang, H.; Sui, C.; Du, R.; Li, C.; Li, J.; Dionigi, G.; Zhang, D.; Sun, H. Surgical Resection of Recurrent Differentiated Thyroid Cancer: Patterns, Detection, Staging, and Treatment of 683 Patients. *Front. Endocrinol.* **2023**, *14*, 1301620. [CrossRef] [PubMed]
16. Chen, D.W.; Lang, B.H.H.; McLeod, D.S.A.; Newbold, K.; Haymart, M.R. Thyroid Cancer. *Lancet* **2023**, *401*, 1531–1544. [CrossRef]
17. Gharib, H.; Papini, E.; Garber, J.R.; Duick, D.S.; Harrell, R.M.; Hegedüs, L.; Paschke, R.; Valcavi, R.; Vitti, P. American association of clinical endocrinologists, american college of endocrinology, and associazione medici endocrinologi medical guidelines for clinical practice for the diagnosis and management of thyroid nodules—2016 update. *Endocr. Pract.* **2016**, *22*, 622–639. [CrossRef] [PubMed]
18. Kang, Y.J.; Stybayeva, G.; Hwang, S.H. Surgical Completeness and Safety of Minimally Invasive Thyroidectomy in Patients with Thyroid Cancer: A Network Meta-Analysis. *Surgery* **2023**, *173*, 1381–1390. [CrossRef] [PubMed]
19. Alfuraih, A.M.; Alotaibi, A.M.; Alshammari, A.K.; Alrashied, B.F.; Mashhor, Y.M.; Mahmoud, M.; Alsaadi, M.J. Evaluating Diagnostic Accuracy and Agreement of TI-RADS Scoring in Thyroid Nodules: A Comparative Analysis between Sonographers and Radiologists. *PLoS ONE* **2024**, *19*, e0312121. [CrossRef]
20. Alexander, E.K.; Kennedy, G.C.; Baloch, Z.W.; Cibas, E.S.; Chudova, D.; Diggans, J.; Friedman, L.; Kloos, R.T.; LiVolsi, V.A.; Mandel, S.J.; et al. Preoperative Diagnosis of Benign Thyroid Nodules with Indeterminate Cytology. *N. Engl. J. Med.* **2012**, *367*, 705–715. [CrossRef]
21. Trimboli, P.; Treglia, G.; Guidobaldi, L.; Saggiorato, E.; Nigri, G.; Crescenzi, A.; Romanelli, F.; Orlandi, F.; Valabrega, S.; Sadeghi, R.; et al. Clinical Characteristics as Predictors of Malignancy in Patients with Indeterminate Thyroid Cytology: A Meta-Analysis. *Endocrine* **2014**, *46*, 52–59. [CrossRef]
22. Perros, P.; Boelaert, K.; Colley, S.; Evans, C.; Evans, R.M.; Gerrard Ba, G.; Gilbert, J.; Harrison, B.; Johnson, S.J.; Giles, T.E.; et al. Guidelines for the Management of Thyroid Cancer. *Clin. Endocrinol.* **2014**, *81* (Suppl 1), 1–122. [CrossRef]
23. Gharib, H.; Papini, E.; Paschke, R.; Duick, D.S.; Valcavi, R.; Hegedüs, L.; Vitti, P.; et al. American Association of Clinical Endocrinologists, Associazione Medici Endocrinologi, and European Thyroid Association Medical Guidelines for Clinical Practice for the Diagnosis and Management of Thyroid Nodules: Executive Summary of Recommendations. *Endocr. Pract.* **2010**, *16*, 468–475. [CrossRef]

24. Cibas, E.S.; Ali, S.Z. The Bethesda System for Reporting Thyroid Cytopathology. *Thyroid Off. J. Am. Thyroid Assoc.* **2009**, *19*, 1159–1165. [CrossRef] [PubMed]
25. Alzahrani, A.S. Clinical Use of Molecular Data in Thyroid Nodules and Cancer. *J. Clin. Endocrinol. Metab.* **2023**, *108*, 2759–2771. [CrossRef]
26. Fumagalli, C.; Serio, G. Molecular Testing in Indeterminate Thyroid Nodules: An Additional Tool for Clinical Decision-Making. *Pathol.-J. Ital. Soc. Anat. Pathol. Diagn. Cytopathol.* **2023**, *115*, 205–216. [CrossRef] [PubMed]
27. He, J.; Sun, P.; Lin, J.; Shen, J.; Lin, H.; Jiang, H.; Qiu, R.; Lin, E.; Lu, Y. Application of Carbon Nanoparticles in Endoscopic Thyroid Cancer Surgery: A Systematic Review and Meta-Analysis. *Front. Surg.* **2023**, *10*, 1283573. [CrossRef]
28. Haugen, B.R.; Alexander, E.K.; Bible, K.C.; Doherty, G.M.; Mandel, S.J.; Nikiforov, Y.E.; Pacini, F.; Randolph, G.W.; Sawka, A.M.; Schlumberger, M.; et al. 2015 American Thyroid Association Management Guidelines for Adult Patients with Thyroid Nodules and Differentiated Thyroid Cancer: The American Thyroid Association Guidelines Task Force on Thyroid Nodules and Differentiated Thyroid Cancer. *Thyroid* **2016**, *26*, 1–133. [CrossRef]
29. Vaisman, F.; Shaha, A.; Fish, S.; Michael Tuttle, R. Initial Therapy with Either Thyroid Lobectomy or Total Thyroidectomy without Radioactive Iodine Remnant Ablation Is Associated with Very Low Rates of Structural Disease Recurrence in Properly Selected Patients with Differentiated Thyroid Cancer. *Clin. Endocrinol.* **2011**, *75*, 112–119. [CrossRef]
30. Addasi, N.; Fingeret, A.; Goldner, W. Hemithyroidectomy for Thyroid Cancer: A Review. *Med. Kaunas Lith.* **2020**, *56*, 586. [CrossRef]
31. Guo, M.; Sun, Y.; Wei, Y.; Xu, J.; Zhang, C. Advances in Targeted Therapy and Biomarker Research in Thyroid Cancer. *Front. Endocrinol.* **2024**, *15*, 1372553. [CrossRef]
32. Tao, Y.; Li, P.; Feng, C.; Cao, Y. New Insights into Immune Cells and Immunotherapy for Thyroid Cancer. *Immunol. Investig.* **2023**, *52*, 1039–1064. [CrossRef]
33. Li, J.; Li, Z.; Zhao, P. Diagnosis and Prognosis of Thyroid Cancer by Immune-Related Genes. *Am. J. Clin. Oncol.* **2024**, *47*, 1–10. [CrossRef]
34. Drugs Approved for Thyroid Cancer-NCI. Available online: https://www.cancer.gov/about-cancer/treatment/drugs/thyroid (accessed on 8 January 2025).
35. Wells, S.A.; Asa, S.L.; Dralle, H.; Elisei, R.; Evans, D.B.; Gagel, R.F.; Lee, N.; Machens, A.; Moley, J.F.; Pacini, F.; et al. Revised American Thyroid Association Guidelines for the Management of Medullary Thyroid Carcinoma. *Thyroid Off. J. Am. Thyroid Assoc.* **2015**, *25*, 567–610. [CrossRef] [PubMed]
36. Trimboli, P.; Giovanella, L. Serum Calcitonin Negative Medullary Thyroid Carcinoma: A Systematic Review of the Literature. *Clin. Chem. Lab. Med.* **2015**, *53*, 1507–1514. [CrossRef] [PubMed]
37. Jayasinghe, R.; Basnayake, O.; Jayarajah, U.; Seneviratne, S. Management of Medullary Carcinoma of the Thyroid: A Review. *J. Int. Med. Res.* **2022**, *50*, 3000605221110698. [CrossRef] [PubMed]
38. Bartz-Kurycki, M.A.; Oluwo, O.E.; Morris-Wiseman, L.F. Medullary Thyroid Carcinoma: Recent Advances in Identification, Treatment, and Prognosis. *Ther. Adv. Endocrinol. Metab.* **2021**, *12*, 20420188211049611. [CrossRef] [PubMed]
39. Elisei, R.; Bottici, V.; Luchetti, F.; Di Coscio, G.; Romei, C.; Grasso, L.; Miccoli, P.; Iacconi, P.; Basolo, F.; Pinchera, A.; et al. Impact of Routine Measurement of Serum Calcitonin on the Diagnosis and Outcome of Medullary Thyroid Cancer: Experience in 10,864 Patients with Nodular Thyroid Disorders. *J. Clin. Endocrinol. Metab.* **2004**, *89*, 163–168. [CrossRef]
40. Alevizaki, M.; Saltiki, K.; Rentziou, G.; Papathoma, A.; Sarika, L.; Vasileiou, V.; Anastasiou, E. Medullary Thyroid Carcinoma: The Influence of Policy Changing in Clinical Characteristics and Disease Progression. *Eur. J. Endocrinol.* **2012**, *167*, 799–808. [CrossRef]
41. Alevizaki, M.; Saltiki, K.; Simeakis, G.; Pappa, T. Medullary Thyroid Carcinoma (MTC): Diagnosis, Treatment and Follow-Up. In *Atlas of Thyroid and Neuroendocrine Tumor Markers*; Giovanella, L., Ed.; Springer International Publishing: Cham, Switzerland, 2018; pp. 119–132. ISBN 978-3-319-62506-5.
42. Kushchayev, S.V.; Kushchayeva, Y.S.; Tella, S.H.; Glushko, T.; Pacak, K.; Teytelboym, O.M. Medullary Thyroid Carcinoma: An Update on Imaging. *J. Thyroid Res.* **2019**, *2019*, 1893047. [CrossRef]
43. Essig, G.F.; Porter, K.; Schneider, D.; Arpaia, D.; Lindsey, S.C.; Busonero, G.; Fineberg, D.; Fruci, B.; Boelaert, K.; Smit, J.W.; et al. Multifocality in Sporadic Medullary Thyroid Carcinoma: An International Multicenter Study. *Thyroid Off. J. Am. Thyroid Assoc.* **2016**, *26*, 1563–1572. [CrossRef]
44. Yang, G.; Pu, J.; Zhu, S.; Shi, Y.; Yang, Y.; Mao, J.; Sun, Y.; Zhao, B. Optimizing Levothyroxine Replacement: A Precision Dosage Model for Post-Thyroidectomy Patients. *Int. J. Gen. Med.* **2024**, *17*, 377–386. [CrossRef]
45. Giovanella, L.; Feldt-Rasmussen, U.; Verburg, F.A.; Grebe, S.K.; Plebani, M.; Clark, P.M. Thyroglobulin Measurement by Highly Sensitive Assays: Focus on Laboratory Challenges. *Clin. Chem. Lab. Med. CCLM* **2015**, *53*, 1301–1314. [CrossRef]
46. Mater, A.; Boelen, A.; Heijboer, A.C.; Hillebrand, J.J. Thyroglobulin and Calcitonin Measurements: Pitfalls and Future Perspectives. *J. Endocrinol.* **2024**, *264*, JOE-24-0156. [CrossRef] [PubMed]
47. Giovanella, L. (Ed.) *Atlas of Thyroid and Neuroendocrine Tumor Markers*; Springer International Publishing: Cham, Switzerland, 2018; ISBN 978-3-319-62505-8.

48. Giovanella, L.; D'Aurizio, F.; Algeciras-Schimnich, A.; Görges, R.; Petranovic Ovcaricek, P.; Tuttle, R.M.; Visser, W.E.; Verburg, F.A.; hsTg; TgAb Consensus Working Group. Thyroglobulin and Thyroglobulin Antibody: An Updated Clinical and Laboratory Expert Consensus. *Eur. J. Endocrinol.* **2023**, *189*, R11–R27. [CrossRef] [PubMed]
49. Ward, G.; Simpson, A.; Boscato, L.; Hickman, P.E. The Investigation of Interferences in Immunoassay. *Clin. Biochem.* **2017**, *50*, 1306–1311. [CrossRef] [PubMed]
50. Rosario, P.W.; Côrtes, M.C.S.; Mourão, G.F. Follow-up of Patients with Thyroid Cancer and Antithyroglobulin Antibodies: A Review for Clinicians. *Endocr. Relat. Cancer* **2021**, *28*, R111–R119. [CrossRef]
51. Jin, Y.; Zhai, T.; Wang, Y.; Li, J.; Wang, T.; Huang, J. Recent Advances in Liquid Chromatography-Tandem Mass Spectrometry for the Detection of Thyroid Hormones and Thyroglobulin in Clinical Samples: A Review. *J. Sep. Sci.* **2024**, *47*, e2400466. [CrossRef]
52. Giovanella, L.; D'Aurizio, F.; Petranović Ovčariček, P.; Görges, R. Diagnostic, Theranostic and Prognostic Value of Thyroglobulin in Thyroid Cancer. *J. Clin. Med.* **2024**, *13*, 2463. [CrossRef]
53. Netzel, B.C.; Grant, R.P.; Hoofnagle, A.N.; Rockwood, A.L.; Shuford, C.M.; Grebe, S.K.G. First Steps toward Harmonization of LC-MS/MS Thyroglobulin Assays. *Clin. Chem.* **2016**, *62*, 297–299. [CrossRef]
54. Trimboli, P.; La Torre, D.; Ceriani, L.; Condorelli, E.; Laurenti, O.; Romanelli, F.; Ventura, C.; Signore, A.; Valabrega, S.; Giovanella, L. High Sensitive Thyroglobulin Assay on Thyroxine Therapy: Can It Avoid Stimulation Test in Low and High Risk Differentiated Thyroid Carcinoma Patients? *Horm. Metab. Res. Horm. Stoffwechselforschung Horm. Metab.* **2013**, *45*, 664–668. [CrossRef]
55. Giovanella, L.; Treglia, G.; Sadeghi, R.; Trimboli, P.; Ceriani, L.; Verburg, F.A. Unstimulated Highly Sensitive Thyroglobulin in Follow-up of Differentiated Thyroid Cancer Patients: A Meta-Analysis. *J. Clin. Endocrinol. Metab.* **2014**, *99*, 440–447. [CrossRef]
56. Giovanella, L.; Castellana, M.; Trimboli, P. Unstimulated High-Sensitive Thyroglobulin Is a Powerful Prognostic Predictor in Patients with Thyroid Cancer. *Clin. Chem. Lab. Med.* **2019**, *58*, 130–137. [CrossRef]
57. Spencer, C.; Fatemi, S.; Singer, P.; Nicoloff, J.; Lopresti, J. Serum Basal Thyroglobulin Measured by a Second-Generation Assay Correlates with the Recombinant Human Thyrotropin-Stimulated Thyroglobulin Response in Patients Treated for Differentiated Thyroid Cancer. *Thyroid Off. J. Am. Thyroid Assoc.* **2010**, *20*, 587–595. [CrossRef] [PubMed]
58. Malandrino, P.; Latina, A.; Marescalco, S.; Spadaro, A.; Regalbuto, C.; Fulco, R.A.; Scollo, C.; Vigneri, R.; Pellegriti, G. Risk-Adapted Management of Differentiated Thyroid Cancer Assessed by a Sensitive Measurement of Basal Serum Thyroglobulin. *J. Clin. Endocrinol. Metab.* **2011**, *96*, 1703–1709. [CrossRef] [PubMed]
59. Chindris, A.M.; Diehl, N.N.; Crook, J.E.; Fatourechi, V.; Smallridge, R.C. Undetectable Sensitive Serum Thyroglobulin (<0.1 Ng/Ml) in 163 Patients with Follicular Cell-Derived Thyroid Cancer: Results of rhTSH Stimulation and Neck Ultrasonography and Long-Term Biochemical and Clinical Follow-Up. *J. Clin. Endocrinol. Metab.* **2012**, *97*, 2714–2723. [CrossRef]
60. Castagna, M.G.; Tala Jury, H.P.; Cipri, C.; Belardini, V.; Fioravanti, C.; Pasqui, L.; Sestini, F.; Theodoropoulou, A.; Pacini, F. The Use of Ultrasensitive Thyroglobulin Assays Reduces but Does Not Abolish the Need for TSH Stimulation in Patients with Differentiated Thyroid Carcinoma. *J. Endocrinol. Investig.* **2011**, *34*, e219–e223. [CrossRef]
61. Spencer, C.; LoPresti, J.; Fatemi, S. How Sensitive (Second-Generation) Thyroglobulin Measurement Is Changing Paradigms for Monitoring Patients with Differentiated Thyroid Cancer, in the Absence or Presence of Thyroglobulin Autoantibodies. *Curr. Opin. Endocrinol. Diabetes Obes.* **2014**, *21*, 394–404. [CrossRef]
62. Smallridge, R.C.; Meek, S.E.; Morgan, M.A.; Gates, G.S.; Fox, T.P.; Grebe, S.; Fatourechi, V. Monitoring Thyroglobulin in a Sensitive Immunoassay Has Comparable Sensitivity to Recombinant Human Tsh-Stimulated Thyroglobulin in Follow-up of Thyroid Cancer Patients. *J. Clin. Endocrinol. Metab.* **2007**, *92*, 82–87. [CrossRef]
63. Rosario, P.W.; Purisch, S. Does a Highly Sensitive Thyroglobulin (Tg) Assay Change the Clinical Management of Low-Risk Patients with Thyroid Cancer with Tg on T4 < 1 Ng/Ml Determined by Traditional Assays? *Clin. Endocrinol.* **2008**, *68*, 338–342. [CrossRef]
64. Lamartina, L.; Durante, C.; Filetti, S.; Cooper, D.S. Low-Risk Differentiated Thyroid Cancer and Radioiodine Remnant Ablation: A Systematic Review of the Literature. *J. Clin. Endocrinol. Metab.* **2015**, *100*, 1748–1761. [CrossRef]
65. Schlumberger, M.; Leboulleux, S.; Catargi, B.; Deandreis, D.; Zerdoud, S.; Bardet, S.; Rusu, D.; Godbert, Y.; Buffet, C.; Schvartz, C.; et al. Outcome after Ablation in Patients with Low-Risk Thyroid Cancer (ESTIMABL1): 5-Year Follow-up Results of a Randomised, Phase 3, Equivalence Trial. *Lancet Diabetes Endocrinol.* **2018**, *6*, 618–626. [CrossRef]
66. Makarewicz, J.; Adamczewski, Z.; Knapska-Kucharska, M.; Lewiński, A. Evaluation of the Diagnostic Value of the First Thyroglobulin Determination in Detecting Metastases after Differentiated Thyroid Carcinoma Surgery. *Exp. Clin. Endocrinol. Diabetes Off. J. Ger. Soc. Endocrinol. Ger. Diabetes Assoc.* **2006**, *114*, 485–489. [CrossRef]
67. Salvatori, M.; Raffaelli, M.; Castaldi, P.; Treglia, G.; Rufini, V.; Perotti, G.; Lombardi, C.P.; Rubello, D.; Ardito, G.; Bellantone, R. Evaluation of the Surgical Completeness after Total Thyroidectomy for Differentiated Thyroid Carcinoma. *Eur. J. Surg. Oncol. J. Eur. Soc. Surg. Oncol. Br. Assoc. Surg. Oncol.* **2007**, *33*, 648–654. [CrossRef] [PubMed]

68. McLeod, D.S.A.; Cooper, D.S.; Ladenson, P.W.; Ain, K.B.; Brierley, J.D.; Fein, H.G.; Haugen, B.R.; Jonklaas, J.; Magner, J.; Ross, D.S.; et al. Prognosis of Differentiated Thyroid Cancer in Relation to Serum Thyrotropin and Thyroglobulin Antibody Status at Time of Diagnosis. *Thyroid Off. J. Am. Thyroid Assoc.* **2014**, *24*, 35–42. [CrossRef] [PubMed]
69. Husseini, M.A.E. Implication of Different Clinical and Pathological Variables in Patients with Differentiated Thyroid Cancer on Successful Ablation for 3700 MBq (131)I: A Single Egyptian Institutional Experience over 14 Years. *Ann. Nucl. Med.* **2016**, *30*, 468–476. [CrossRef] [PubMed]
70. Zhao, T.; Liang, J.; Li, T.; Gao, W.; Lin, Y. Serial Stimulated Thyroglobulin Measurements Are More Specific for Detecting Distant Metastatic Differentiated Thyroid Cancer before Radioiodine Therapy. *Chin. J. Cancer Res. Chung-Kuo Yen Cheng Yen Chiu* **2017**, *29*, 213–222. [CrossRef]
71. Signore, A.; Lauri, C.; Di Paolo, A.; Stati, V.; Santolamazza, G.; Capriotti, G.; Prosperi, D.; Tofani, A.; Valabrega, S.; Campagna, G. Predictive Role of Serum Thyroglobulin after Surgery and before Radioactive Iodine Therapy in Patients with Thyroid Carcinoma. *Cancers* **2023**, *15*, 2976. [CrossRef]
72. Nozières, C.; Chardon, L.; Goichot, B.; Borson-Chazot, F.; Hervieu, V.; Chikh, K.; Lombard-Bohas, C.; Walter, T. Neuroendocrine Tumors Producing Calcitonin: Characteristics, Prognosis and Potential Interest of Calcitonin Monitoring during Follow-Up. *Eur. J. Endocrinol.* **2016**, *174*, 335–341. [CrossRef]
73. Copp, D.H.; Cheney, B. Calcitonin—A Hormone from the Parathyroid Which Lowers the Calcium-Level of the Blood. *Nature* **1962**, *193*, 381–382. [CrossRef]
74. d'Herbomez, M.; Caron, P.; Bauters, C.; Do Cao, C.; Schlienger, J.-L.; Sapin, R.; Baldet, L.; Carnaille, B.; Wémeau, J.-L.; French Group GTE (Groupe des Tumeurs Endocrines). Reference Range of Serum Calcitonin Levels in Humans: Influence of Calcitonin Assays, Sex, Age, and Cigarette Smoking. *Eur. J. Endocrinol.* **2007**, *157*, 749–755. [CrossRef]
75. Kahaly, G.J.; Algeciras-Schimnich, A.; Davis, T.E.; Diana, T.; Feldkamp, J.; Karger, S.; König, J.; Lupo, M.A.; Raue, F.; Ringel, M.D.; et al. United States and European Multicenter Prospective Study for the Analytical Performance and Clinical Validation of a Novel Sensitive Fully Automated Immunoassay for Calcitonin. *Clin. Chem.* **2017**, *63*, 1489–1496. [CrossRef]
76. Vardarli, I.; Weber, M.; Weidemann, F.; Führer, D.; Herrmann, K.; Görges, R. Diagnostic Accuracy of Routine Calcitonin Measurement for the Detection of Medullary Thyroid Carcinoma in the Management of Patients with Nodular Thyroid Disease: A Meta-Analysis. *Endocr. Connect.* **2021**, *10*, 358–370. [CrossRef]
77. Costante, G.; Durante, C.; Francis, Z.; Schlumberger, M.; Filetti, S. Determination of Calcitonin Levels in C-Cell Disease: Clinical Interest and Potential Pitfalls. *Nat. Clin. Pract. Endocrinol. Metab.* **2009**, *5*, 35–44. [CrossRef] [PubMed]
78. Fugazzola, L.; Di Stefano, M.; Censi, S.; Repaci, A.; Colombo, C.; Grimaldi, F.; Magri, F.; Pagotto, U.; Iacobone, M.; Persani, L.; et al. Basal and Stimulated Calcitonin for the Diagnosis of Medullary Thyroid Cancer: Updated Thresholds and Safety Assessment. *J. Endocrinol. Investig.* **2021**, *44*, 587–597. [CrossRef] [PubMed]
79. Giannetta, E.; Guarnotta, V.; Altieri, B.; Sciammarella, C.; Guadagno, E.; Malandrino, P.; Puliani, G.; Feola, T.; Isidori, A.M.; Colao, A.A.L.; et al. ENDOCRINE TUMOURS: Calcitonin in Thyroid and Extra-Thyroid Neuroendocrine Neoplasms: The Two-Faced Janus. *Eur. J. Endocrinol.* **2020**, *183*, R197–R215. [CrossRef] [PubMed]
80. Allelein, S.; Ehlers, M.; Morneau, C.; Schwartz, K.; Goretzki, P.E.; Seppel, T.; Feldkamp, J.; Krieg, A.; Knoefel, W.T.; Kuebart, A.; et al. Measurement of Basal Serum Calcitonin for the Diagnosis of Medullary Thyroid Cancer. *Horm. Metab. Res. Horm. Stoffwechselforschung Horm. Metab.* **2018**, *50*, 23–28. [CrossRef]
81. Niederle, M.B.; Scheuba, C.; Riss, P.; Selberherr, A.; Koperek, O.; Niederle, B. Early Diagnosis of Medullary Thyroid Cancer: Are Calcitonin Stimulation Tests Still Indicated in the Era of Highly Sensitive Calcitonin Immunoassays? *Thyroid Off. J. Am. Thyroid Assoc.* **2020**, *30*, 974–984. [CrossRef]
82. Verbeek, H.H.; de Groot, J.W.B.; Sluiter, W.J.; Muller Kobold, A.C.; van den Heuvel, E.R.; Plukker, J.T.; Links, T.P. Calcitonin Testing for Detection of Medullary Thyroid Cancer in People with Thyroid Nodules. *Cochrane Database Syst. Rev.* **2020**, *3*, CD010159. [CrossRef]
83. Kiriakopoulos, A.; Giannakis, P.; Menenakos, E. Calcitonin: Current Concepts and Differential Diagnosis. *Ther. Adv. Endocrinol. Metab.* **2022**, *13*, 20420188221099344. [CrossRef]
84. Tobler, P.H.; Tschopp, F.A.; Dambacher, M.A.; Born, W.; Fischer, J.A. Identification and Characterization of Calcitonin Forms in Plasma and Urine of Normal Subjects and Medullary Carcinoma Patients. *J. Clin. Endocrinol. Metab.* **1983**, *57*, 749–754. [CrossRef]
85. Motté, P.; Vauzelle, P.; Gardet, P.; Ghillani, P.; Caillou, B.; Parmentier, C.; Bohuon, C.; Bellet, D. Construction and Clinical Validation of a Sensitive and Specific Assay for Serum Mature Calcitonin Using Monoclonal Anti-Peptide Antibodies. *Clin. Chim. Acta Int. J. Clin. Chem.* **1988**, *174*, 35–54. [CrossRef]
86. Schiettecatte, J.; Strasser, O.; Anckaert, E.; Smitz, J. Performance Evaluation of an Automated Electrochemiluminescent Calcitonin (CT) Immunoassay in Diagnosis of Medullary Thyroid Carcinoma. *Clin. Biochem.* **2016**, *49*, 929–931. [CrossRef]
87. Costante, G.; Lalami, Y.; Jungels, C.; Awada, A. Calcitonin and Carcinoembryonic Antigen for the Diagnosis and Management of Medullary Thyroid Carcinoma. In *Atlas of Thyroid and Neuroendocrine Tumor Markers*; Giovanella, L., Ed.; Springer International Publishing: Cham, Switzerland, 2018; pp. 133–150. ISBN 978-3-319-62506-5.

88. Gold, P.; Freedman, S.O. Demonstration of tumor-specific antigens in human colonic carcinomata by immunological tolerance and absorption techniques. *J. Exp. Med.* **1965**, *121*, 439–462. [CrossRef] [PubMed]
89. Jansen, K.; Kornfeld, L.; Lennartz, M.; Dwertmann Rico, S.; Kind, S.; Reiswich, V.; Viehweger, F.; Bawahab, A.A.; Fraune, C.; Gorbokon, N.; et al. Carcinoembryonic Antigen Expression in Human Tumors: A Tissue Microarray Study on 13,725 Tumors. *Cancers* **2024**, *16*, 4052. [CrossRef] [PubMed]
90. Nicholson, B.D.; Shinkins, B.; Pathiraja, I.; Roberts, N.W.; James, T.J.; Mallett, S.; Perera, R.; Primrose, J.N.; Mant, D. Blood CEA Levels for Detecting Recurrent Colorectal Cancer. *Cochrane Database Syst. Rev.* **2015**, *2015*, CD011134. [CrossRef] [PubMed]
91. Hall, C.; Clarke, L.; Pal, A.; Buchwald, P.; Eglinton, T.; Wakeman, C.; Frizelle, F. A Review of the Role of Carcinoembryonic Antigen in Clinical Practice. *Ann. Coloproctology* **2019**, *35*, 294–305. [CrossRef]
92. Bhagat, A.; Lyerly, H.K.; Morse, M.A.; Hartman, Z.C. CEA Vaccines. *Hum. Vaccines Immunother.* **2023**, *19*, 2291857. [CrossRef]
93. Liu, S.; Zhao, H.; Li, X. Serum Biochemical Markers for Medullary Thyroid Carcinoma: An Update. *Cancer Manag. Res.* **2024**, *16*, 299. [CrossRef]
94. Fan, W.; Xiao, C.; Wu, F. Analysis of Risk Factors for Cervical Lymph Node Metastases in Patients with Sporadic Medullary Thyroid Carcinoma. *J. Int. Med. Res.* **2018**, *46*, 1982–1989. [CrossRef]
95. Wang, B.; Huang, J.; Chen, L. Management of Medullary Thyroid Cancer Based on Variation of Carcinoembryonic Antigen and Calcitonin. *Front. Endocrinol.* **2024**, *15*, 1418657. [CrossRef]
96. Cameselle-Teijeiro, J.M.; Eloy, C.; Sobrinho-Simões, M. Pitfalls in Challenging Thyroid Tumors: Emphasis on Differential Diagnosis and Ancillary Biomarkers. *Endocr. Pathol.* **2020**, *31*, 197–217. [CrossRef]
97. Park, J.; Lee, S.; Kim, Y.; Choi, A.; Lee, H.; Lim, J.; Kim, Y.; Han, K.; Oh, E.J. Comparison of Four Automated Carcinoembryonic Antigen Immunoassays: ADVIA Centaur XP, ARCHITECT I2000sr, Elecsys E170, and Unicel Dxi800. *Ann. Lab. Med.* **2018**, *38*, 355–361. [CrossRef]
98. Fu, W.; Yue, Y.; Song, Y.; Zhang, S.; Shi, J.; Zhao, R.; Wang, Q.; Zhang, R. Comparable Analysis of Six Immunoassays for Carcinoembryonic Antigen Detection. *Heliyon* **2024**, *10*, e25158. [CrossRef] [PubMed]
99. Börmer, O.P. Standardization, Specificity, and Diagnostic Sensitivity of Four Immunoassays for Carcinoembryonic Antigen. *Clin. Chem.* **1991**, *37*, 231–236. [CrossRef] [PubMed]
100. Dominici, R.; Cabrini, E.; Cattozzo, G.; Ceriotti, F.; Grazioli, V.; Scapellato, L.; Franzini, C. Intermethod Variation in Serum Carcinoembryonic Antigen (CEA) Measurement. Fresh Serum Pools and Control Materials Compared. *Clin. Chem. Lab. Med.* **2002**, *40*, 167–173. [CrossRef] [PubMed]
101. Taylor, R.N.; Fulford, K.M.; Huong, A.Y. Results of a Nationwide Proficiency Test for Carcinoembryonic Antigen. *J. Clin. Microbiol.* **1977**, *5*, 433–438. [CrossRef]
102. Reinauer, H.; Wood, W.G. External Quality Assessment of Tumour Marker Analysis: State of the Art and Consequences for Estimating Diagnostic Sensitivity and Specificity. *Ger. Med. Sci. GMS E-J.* **2005**, *3*, Doc02.
103. Wojtalewicz, N.; Vierbaum, L.; Kaufmann, A.; Schellenberg, I.; Holdenrieder, S. Longitudinal Evaluation of AFP and CEA External Proficiency Testing Reveals Need for Method Harmonization. *Diagnostics* **2023**, *13*, 2019. [CrossRef]
104. Bjerner, J.; Lebedin, Y.; Bellanger, L.; Kuroki, M.; Shively, J.E.; Varaas, T.; Nustad, K.; Hammarström, S.; Børmer, O.P. Protein Epitopes in Carcinoembryonic Antigen. Report of the ISOBM TD8 Workshop. *Tumour Biol. J. Int. Soc. Oncodevelopmental Biol. Med.* **2002**, *23*, 249–262. [CrossRef]
105. Zeng, X.; Shen, Z.; Mernaugh, R. Recombinant Antibodies and Their Use in Biosensors. *Anal. Bioanal. Chem.* **2012**, *402*, 3027–3038. [CrossRef]
106. Ascoli, C.A.; Aggeler, B. Overlooked Benefits of Using Polyclonal Antibodies. *BioTechniques* **2018**, *65*, 127–136. [CrossRef]
107. Giovanella, L.; D'Aurizio, F.; Tozzoli, R. *Circulating Mucins and Cytokeratins in Aggressive Thyroid Cancers*; Giovanella, L., Ed.; Springer International Publishing: Cham, Switzerland, 2018; pp. 175–189.
108. Luo, G.; Jin, K.; Deng, S.; Cheng, H.; Fan, Z.; Gong, Y.; Qian, Y.; Huang, Q.; Ni, Q.; Liu, C.; et al. Roles of CA19-9 in Pancreatic Cancer: Biomarker, Predictor and Promoter. *Biochim. Biophys. Acta Rev. Cancer* **2021**, *1875*, 188409. [CrossRef]
109. Plebani, M.; Basso, D.; Panozzo, M.P.; Fogar, P.; Del Favero, G.; Naccarato, R. Tumor Markers in the Diagnosis, Monitoring and Therapy of Pancreatic Cancer: State of the Art. *Int. J. Biol. Markers* **1995**, *10*, 189–199. [CrossRef] [PubMed]
110. Duffy, M.J.; Sturgeon, C.; Lamerz, R.; Haglund, C.; Holubec, V.L.; Klapdor, R.; Nicolini, A.; Topolcan, O.; Heinemann, V. Tumor Markers in Pancreatic Cancer: A European Group on Tumor Markers (EGTM) Status Report. *Ann. Oncol. Off. J. Eur. Soc. Med. Oncol.* **2010**, *21*, 441–447. [CrossRef] [PubMed]
111. Galli, C.; Basso, D.; Plebani, M. CA 19-9: Handle with Care. *Clin. Chem. Lab. Med.* **2013**, *51*, 1369–1383. [CrossRef] [PubMed]
112. Milman, S.; Whitney, K.D.; Fleischer, N. Metastatic Medullary Thyroid Cancer Presenting with Elevated Levels of CA 19-9 and CA 125. *Thyroid Off. J. Am. Thyroid Assoc.* **2011**, *21*, 913–916. [CrossRef]
113. Elisei, R.; Lorusso, L.; Romei, C.; Bottici, V.; Mazzeo, S.; Giani, C.; Fiore, E.; Torregrossa, L.; Insilla, A.C.; Basolo, F.; et al. Medullary Thyroid Cancer Secreting Carbohydrate Antigen 19-9 (Ca 19-9): A Fatal Case Report. *J. Clin. Endocrinol. Metab.* **2013**, *98*, 3550–3554. [CrossRef]

114. Elisei, R.; Lorusso, L.; Piaggi, P.; Torregrossa, L.; Pellegrini, G.; Molinaro, E.; Agate, L.; Bottici, V.; Pani, F.; Cacciato Insilla, A.; et al. Elevated Level of Serum Carbohydrate Antigen 19.9 as Predictor of Mortality in Patients with Advanced Medullary Thyroid Cancer. *Eur. J. Endocrinol.* **2015**, *173*, 297–304. [CrossRef]
115. Lorusso, L.; Romei, C.; Piaggi, P.; Fustini, C.; Molinaro, E.; Agate, L.; Bottici, V.; Viola, D.; Pellegrini, G.; Elisei, R. Ca19.9 Positivity and Doubling Time Are Prognostic Factors of Mortality in Patients with Advanced Medullary Thyroid Cancer with No Evidence of Structural Disease Progression According to Response Evaluation Criteria in Solid Tumors. *Thyroid Off. J. Am. Thyroid Assoc.* **2021**, *31*, 1050–1055. [CrossRef]
116. Alencar, R.; Kendler, D.B.; Andrade, F.; Nava, C.; Bulzico, D.; Cordeiro de Noronha Pessoa, C.; Corbo, R.; Vaisman, F. CA19-9 as a Predictor of Worse Clinical Outcome in Medullary Thyroid Carcinoma. *Eur. Thyroid J.* **2019**, *8*, 186–191. [CrossRef]
117. Hashimoto, T.; Matsubara, F.; Mizukami, Y.; Miyazaki, I.; Michigishi, T.; Yanaihara, N. Tumor Markers and Oncogene Expression in Thyroid Cancer Using Biochemical and Immunohistochemical Studies. *Endocrinol. Jpn.* **1990**, *37*, 247–254. [CrossRef]
118. Yamaguchi, E.; Makino, Y.; Sato, T.; Uchida, M.; Harada, Y.; Maruyama, R. CA19-9-Producing Lung Metastasis after Surgery for Papillary Thyroid Carcinoma: Report of a Case. *Surg. Today* **2014**, *44*, 2157–2161. [CrossRef]
119. Vierbuchen, M.; Schröder, S.; Uhlenbruck, G.; Ortmann, M.; Fischer, R. CA 50 and CA 19-9 Antigen Expression in Normal, Hyperplastic, and Neoplastic Thyroid Tissue. *Lab. Investig. J. Tech. Methods Pathol.* **1989**, *60*, 726–732.
120. Kihara, M.; Miyauchi, A.; Hirokawa, M.; Fujishima, M.; Masuoka, H.; Higashiyama, T.; Onoda, N.; Ito, Y.; Miya, A. Metastatic Papillary Thyroid Carcinoma Presenting with Elevated Serum Levels of Carbohydrate Antigen 19-9 (CA19-9): A Case Report. *Surg. Case Rep.* **2022**, *8*, 45. [CrossRef] [PubMed]
121. Kihara, M.; Miyauchi, A.; Hirokawa, M.; Suzuki, A.; Akamizu, T. Availability of Serum Levels of Carbohydrate Antigen 19-9 (CA19-9) as a Surrogate Tumor Marker for Papillary Thyroid Carcinoma. *JMA J.* **2024**, *7*, 250–257. [CrossRef]
122. Munkley, J. The Glycosylation Landscape of Pancreatic Cancer. *Oncol. Lett.* **2019**, *17*, 2569–2575. [CrossRef]
123. Partyka, K.; Maupin, K.A.; Brand, R.E.; Haab, B.B. Diverse Monoclonal Antibodies against the CA 19-9 Antigen Show Variation in Binding Specificity with Consequences for Clinical Interpretation. *Proteomics* **2012**, *12*, 2212–2220. [CrossRef]
124. Passerini, R.; Riggio, D.; Salvatici, M.; Zorzino, L.; Radice, D.; Sandri, M.T. Interchangeability of Measurements of CA 19-9 in Serum with Four Frequently Used Assays: An Update. *Clin. Chem. Lab. Med.* **2007**, *45*, 100–104. [CrossRef]
125. La'ulu, S.L.; Roberts, W.L. Performance Characteristics of Five Automated CA 19-9 Assays. *Am. J. Clin. Pathol.* **2007**, *127*, 436–440. [CrossRef]
126. Hotakainen, K.; Tanner, P.; Alfthan, H.; Haglund, C.; Stenman, U.-H. Comparison of Three Immunoassays for CA 19-9. *Clin. Chim. Acta Int. J. Clin. Chem.* **2009**, *400*, 123–127. [CrossRef]
127. Deinzer, M.; Faissner, R.; Metzger, T.; Kaminski, W.E.; Löhr, M.; Neumaier, M.; Brinkmann, T. Comparison of Two Different Methods for CA19-9 Antigen Determination. *Clin. Lab.* **2010**, *56*, 319–325.
128. Stieber, P.; Molina, R.; Gion, M.; Gressner, A.; Troalen, F.; Holdenrieder, S.; Auge, J.M.; Zancan, M.; Wycislo, M.; Jarrige, V. Alternative Antibody for the Detection of CA19-9 Antigen: A European Multicenter Study for the Evaluation of the Analytical and Clinical Performance of the Access GI Monitor Assay on the UniCel Dxl 800 Immunoassay System. *Clin. Chem. Lab. Med.* **2008**, *46*, 600–611. [CrossRef]
129. Kremser, M.; Weiss, N.; Kaufmann-Stoeck, A.; Vierbaum, L.; Schmitz, A.; Schellenberg, I.; Holdenrieder, S. Longitudinal Evaluation of External Quality Assessment Results for CA 15-3, CA 19-9, and CA 125. *Front. Mol. Biosci.* **2024**, *11*, 1401619. [CrossRef] [PubMed]
130. Hamada, E.; Taniguchi, T.; Baba, S.; Maekawa, M. Investigation of Unexpected Serum CA19-9 Elevation in Lewis-Negative Cancer Patients. *Ann. Clin. Biochem.* **2012**, *49*, 266–272. [CrossRef] [PubMed]
131. Luo, G.; Jin, K.; Guo, M.; Cheng, H.; Liu, Z.; Xiao, Z.; Lu, Y.; Long, J.; Liu, L.; Xu, J.; et al. Patients with Normal-Range CA19-9 Levels Represent a Distinct Subgroup of Pancreatic Cancer Patients. *Oncol. Lett.* **2017**, *13*, 881–886. [CrossRef] [PubMed]
132. Lin, D.; Shen, L.; Luo, M.; Zhang, K.; Li, J.; Yang, Q.; Zhu, F.; Zhou, D.; Zheng, S.; Chen, Y.; et al. Circulating Tumor Cells: Biology and Clinical Significance. *Signal Transduct. Target. Ther.* **2021**, *6*, 1–24. [CrossRef]
133. Capuozzo, M.; Ferrara, F.; Santorsola, M.; Zovi, A.; Ottaiano, A. Circulating Tumor Cells as Predictive and Prognostic Biomarkers in Solid Tumors. *Cells* **2023**, *12*, 2590. [CrossRef]
134. Chambers, A.F.; Groom, A.C.; MacDonald, I.C. Dissemination and Growth of Cancer Cells in Metastatic Sites. *Nat. Rev. Cancer* **2002**, *2*, 563–572. [CrossRef]
135. Kanwar, N.; Balde, Z.; Nair, R.; Dawe, M.; Chen, S.; Maganti, M.; Atenafu, E.G.; Manolescu, S.; Wei, C.; Mao, A.; et al. Heterogeneity of Circulating Tumor Cell-Associated Genomic Gains in Breast Cancer and Its Association with the Host Immune Response. *Cancer Res.* **2021**, *81*, 6196–6206. [CrossRef]
136. Racila, E.; Euhus, D.; Weiss, A.J.; Rao, C.; McConnell, J.; Terstappen, L.W.M.M.; Uhr, J.W. Detection and Characterization of Carcinoma Cells in the Blood. *Proc. Natl. Acad. Sci. USA* **1998**, *95*, 4589–4594. [CrossRef]
137. Yoon, H.J.; Kozminsky, M.; Nagrath, S. Emerging Role of Nanomaterials in Circulating Tumor Cell Isolation and Analysis. *ACS Nano* **2014**, *8*, 1995–2017. [CrossRef]

138. Lim, S.B.; Lim, C.T.; Lim, W.-T. Single-Cell Analysis of Circulating Tumor Cells: Why Heterogeneity Matters. *Cancers* **2019**, *11*, 1595. [CrossRef]
139. Orrapin, S.; Thongkumkoon, P.; Udomruk, S.; Moonmuang, S.; Sutthitthasakul, S.; Yongpitakwattana, P.; Pruksakorn, D.; Chaiyawat, P. Deciphering the Biology of Circulating Tumor Cells through Single-Cell RNA Sequencing: Implications for Precision Medicine in Cancer. *Int. J. Mol. Sci.* **2023**, *24*, 12337. [CrossRef] [PubMed]
140. Theil, G.; Fornara, P.; Bialek, J. Position of Circulating Tumor Cells in the Clinical Routine in Prostate Cancer and Breast Cancer Patients. *Cancers* **2020**, *12*, 3782. [CrossRef] [PubMed]
141. Lawrence, R.; Watters, M.; Davies, C.R.; Pantel, K.; Lu, Y.-J. Circulating Tumour Cells for Early Detection of Clinically Relevant Cancer. *Nat. Rev. Clin. Oncol.* **2023**, *20*, 487–500. [CrossRef] [PubMed]
142. Ring, A.; Nguyen-Sträuli, B.D.; Wicki, A.; Aceto, N. Biology, Vulnerabilities and Clinical Applications of Circulating Tumour Cells. *Nat. Rev. Cancer* **2023**, *23*, 95–111. [CrossRef]
143. Liu, M.C.; Shields, P.G.; Warren, R.D.; Cohen, P.; Wilkinson, M.; Ottaviano, Y.L.; Rao, S.B.; Eng-Wong, J.; Seillier-Moiseiwitsch, F.; Noone, A.-M.; et al. Circulating Tumor Cells: A Useful Predictor of Treatment Efficacy in Metastatic Breast Cancer. *J. Clin. Oncol.* **2009**, *27*, 5153. [CrossRef]
144. Li, D.; Li, N.; Ding, Y. Epithelial-to-Mesenchymal Transition of Circulating Tumor Cells and CD133 Expression on Predicting Prognosis of Thyroid Cancer Patients. *Mol. Clin. Oncol.* **2022**, *17*, 141. [CrossRef]
145. Sriramareddy, S.N.; Hamoir, E.; Chavez, M.; Louis, R.; Beckers, A.; Willems, L. Tumor Cells May Circulate in Medullary Thyroid Cancer Patients Independently of Serum Calcitonin. *Endocr. Relat. Cancer* **2018**, *25*, ERC-18-0180. [CrossRef]
146. Weng, X.; YangYang; Cai, Y. Clinical Significance of Circulating Tumor Cells (CTCs) and Survivin on Predicting Prognosis in Thyroid Cancer Patients. *Dis. Markers* **2022**, *2022*, 5188006. [CrossRef]
147. Xu, J.Y.; Handy, B.; Michaelis, C.L.; Waguespack, S.G.; Hu, M.I.; Busaidy, N.; Jimenez, C.; Cabanillas, M.E.; Fritsche, H.A., Jr.; Cote, G.J.; et al. Detection and Prognostic Significance of Circulating Tumor Cells in Patients With Metastatic Thyroid Cancer. *J. Clin. Endocrinol. Metab.* **2016**, *101*, 4461. [CrossRef]
148. Qiu, Z.-L.; Wei, W.-J.; Sun, Z.-K.; Shen, C.-T.; Song, H.-J.; Zhang, X.-Y.; Zhang, G.-Q.; Chen, X.-Y.; Luo, Q.-Y. Circulating Tumor Cells Correlate with Clinicopathological Features and Outcomes in Differentiated Thyroid Cancer. *Cell. Physiol. Biochem.* **2018**, *48*, 718–730. [CrossRef]
149. Zeng, Q.; Zhong, H.; Rao, H.; Wang, Y. Diagnostic Value of Circulating Tumor Cells in Patients with Thyroid Cancer: A Retrospective Study of 1478 Patients. *Discov. Oncol.* **2024**, *15*, 114. [CrossRef] [PubMed]
150. Liang, M.-X.; Fei, Y.-J.; Yang, K.; Tang, W.-J.; Cao, X.-H.; Tang, J.-H. Potential Values of Circulating Tumor Cell for Detection of Recurrence in Patients of Thyroid Cancer: A Diagnostic Meta-Analysis. *BMC Cancer* **2022**, *22*, 954. [CrossRef] [PubMed]
151. Xu, S.; Cheng, J.; Wei, B.; Zhang, Y.; Li, Y.; Zhang, Z.; Liu, Y.; Zhang, Y.; Zhang, R.; Wang, K.; et al. Development and Validation of Circulating Tumor Cells Signatures for Papillary Thyroid Cancer Diagnosis: A Prospective, Blinded, Multicenter Study. *Clin. Transl. Med.* **2020**, *10*, e142. [CrossRef] [PubMed]
152. Stejskal, P.; Goodarzi, H.; Srovnal, J.; Hajdúch, M.; van 't Veer, L.J.; Magbanua, M.J.M. Circulating Tumor Nucleic Acids: Biology, Release Mechanisms, and Clinical Relevance. *Mol. Cancer* **2023**, *22*, 15. [CrossRef]
153. Cui, M.; Wang, H.; Yao, X.; Zhang, D.; Xie, Y.; Cui, R.; Zhang, X. Circulating MicroRNAs in Cancer: Potential and Challenge. *Front. Genet.* **2019**, *10*, 626. [CrossRef]
154. Gold, B.; Cankovic, M.; Furtado, L.V.; Meier, F.; Gocke, C.D. Do Circulating Tumor Cells, Exosomes, and Circulating Tumor Nucleic Acids Have Clinical Utility? A Report of the Association for Molecular Pathology. *J. Mol. Diagn. JMD* **2015**, *17*, 209–224. [CrossRef]
155. Sadik, N.; Cruz, L.; Gurtner, A.; Rodosthenous, R.S.; Dusoswa, S.A.; Ziegler, O.; Solinge, T.S.V.; Wei, Z.; Salvador-Garicano, A.M.; Gyorgy, B.; et al. Extracellular RNAs: A New Awareness of Old Perspectives. *Methods Mol. Biol. Clifton NJ* **2018**, *1740*, 1. [CrossRef]
156. Cheng, F.; Su, L.; Qian, C. Circulating Tumor DNA: A Promising Biomarker in the Liquid Biopsy of Cancer. *Oncotarget* **2016**, *7*, 48832. [CrossRef]
157. Kan, C.-M.; Pei, X.M.; Yeung, M.H.Y.; Jin, N.; Ng, S.S.M.; Tsang, H.F.; Cho, W.C.S.; Yim, A.K.-Y.; Yu, A.C.-S.; Wong, S.C.C. Exploring the Role of Circulating Cell-Free RNA in the Development of Colorectal Cancer. *Int. J. Mol. Sci.* **2023**, *24*, 11026. [CrossRef]
158. Nemeth, K.; Bayraktar, R.; Ferracin, M.; Calin, G.A. Non-Coding RNAs in Disease: From Mechanisms to Therapeutics. *Nat. Rev. Genet.* **2024**, *25*, 211–232. [CrossRef]
159. Slack, F.J.; Chinnaiyan, A.M. The Role of Non-Coding RNAs in Oncology. *Cell* **2019**, *179*, 1033–1055. [CrossRef] [PubMed]
160. Liu, S.-C. Circulating Tumor DNA in Liquid Biopsy: Current Diagnostic Limitation. *World J. Gastroenterol.* **2024**, *30*, 2175. [CrossRef] [PubMed]

161. Pupilli, C.; Pinzani, P.; Salvianti, F.; Fibbi, B.; Rossi, M.; Petrone, L.; Perigli, G.; De Feo, M.L.; Vezzosi, V.; Pazzagli, M.; et al. Circulating BRAFV600E in the Diagnosis and Follow-Up of Differentiated Papillary Thyroid Carcinoma. *J. Clin. Endocrinol. Metab.* **2013**, *98*, 3359–3365. [CrossRef]
162. Zane, M.; Agostini, M.; Enzo, M.V.; Casal Ide, E.; Del Bianco, P.; Torresan, F.; Merante Boschin, I.; Pennelli, G.; Saccani, A.; Rubello, D.; et al. Circulating Cell-Free DNA, *SLC5A8* and *SLC26A4* Hypermethylation, *BRAFV600E*: A Non-Invasive Tool Panel for Early Detection of Thyroid Cancer. *Biomed. Pharmacother.* **2013**, *67*, 723–730. [CrossRef]
163. Sato, A.; Tanabe, M.; Tsuboi, Y.; Niwa, T.; Shinozaki-Ushiku, A.; Seto, Y.; Murakami, Y. Circulating Tumor DNA Harboring the BRAFV600E Mutation May Predict Poor Outcomes of Primary Papillary Thyroid Cancer Patients. *Thyroid Off. J. Am. Thyroid Assoc.* **2021**, *31*, 1822–1828. [CrossRef]
164. Cote, G.J.; Evers, C.; Hu, M.I.; Grubbs, E.G.; Williams, M.D.; Hai, T.; Duose, D.Y.; Houston, M.R.; Bui, J.H.; Mehrotra, M.; et al. Prognostic Significance of Circulating RET M918T Mutated Tumor DNA in Patients With Advanced Medullary Thyroid Carcinoma. *J. Clin. Endocrinol. Metab.* **2017**, *102*, 3591. [CrossRef]
165. Suh, Y.J.; Kwon, M.J.; Noh, H.-M.; Lee, H.K.; Ra, Y.J.; Kim, N.Y. Limited Clinical and Diagnostic Utility of Circulating Tumor DNA Detection in Patients with Early-Stage Well-Differentiated Thyroid Cancer: Comparison with Benign Thyroid Nodules and Healthy Individuals. *Healthcare* **2021**, *9*, 386. [CrossRef]
166. Tarasova, V.D.; Tsai, J.; Masannat, J.; Hernandez Prera, J.C.; Hallanger Johnson, J.; Veloski, C.; Agosto Salgado, S.; McIver, B.; Drusbosky, L.M.; Chung, C.H. Characterization of the Thyroid Cancer Genomic Landscape by Plasma-Based Circulating Tumor DNA Next-Generation Sequencing. *Thyroid Off. J. Am. Thyroid Assoc.* **2024**, *34*, 197–205. [CrossRef]
167. Shokolenko, I.N.; Alexeyev, M.F. Mitochondrial DNA: A Disposable Genome? *Biochim. Biophys. Acta BBA-Mol. Basis Dis.* **2015**, *1852*, 1805–1809. [CrossRef]
168. Tan, B.G.; Gustafsson, C.M.; Falkenberg, M. Mechanisms and Regulation of Human Mitochondrial Transcription. *Nat. Rev. Mol. Cell Biol.* **2024**, *25*, 119–132. [CrossRef]
169. Kopinski, P.K.; Singh, L.N.; Zhang, S.; Lott, M.T.; Wallace, D.C. Mitochondrial DNA Variation and Cancer. *Nat. Rev. Cancer* **2021**, *21*, 431–445. [CrossRef] [PubMed]
170. Gasparre, G.; Porcelli, A.M.; Bonora, E.; Pennisi, L.F.; Toller, M.; Iommarini, L.; Ghelli, A.; Moretti, M.; Betts, C.M.; Martinelli, G.N.; et al. Disruptive Mitochondrial DNA Mutations in Complex I Subunits Are Markers of Oncocytic Phenotype in Thyroid Tumors. *Proc. Natl. Acad. Sci. USA* **2007**, *104*, 9001–9006. [CrossRef] [PubMed]
171. Alwehaidah, M.S.; Al-Awadhi, R.; Roomy, M.A.; Baqer, T.A. Mitochondrial DNA Copy Number and Risk of Papillary Thyroid Carcinoma. *BMC Endocr. Disord.* **2024**, *24*, 138. [CrossRef] [PubMed]
172. Cabané, P.; Correa, C.; Bode, I.; Aguilar, R.; Elorza, A.A. Biomarkers in Thyroid Cancer: Emerging Opportunities from Non-Coding RNAs and Mitochondrial Space. *Int. J. Mol. Sci.* **2024**, *25*, 6719. [CrossRef]
173. Perdas, E.; Stawski, R.; Kaczka, K.; Nowak, D.; Zubrzycka, M. Altered Levels of Circulating Nuclear and Mitochondrial DNA in Patients with Papillary Thyroid Cancer. *Sci. Rep.* **2019**, *9*, 14438. [CrossRef]
174. Ricci, C.; Salvemini, A.; Dalmiglio, C.; Castagna, M.G.; Cantara, S. From Circulating Tumor Cells to Mirna: New Challenges in the Diagnosis and Prognosis of Medullary Thyroid Cancer. *Cancers* **2023**, *15*, 4009. [CrossRef]
175. Romeo, P.; Colombo, C.; Granata, R.; Calareso, G.; Gualeni, A.V.; Dugo, M.; De Cecco, L.; Rizzetti, M.G.; Zanframundo, A.; Aiello, A.; et al. Circulating miR-375 as a Novel Prognostic Marker for Metastatic Medullary Thyroid Cancer Patients. *Endocr. Relat. Cancer* **2018**, *25*, 217–231. [CrossRef]
176. Censi, S.; Bertazza, L.; Piva, I.; Manso, J.; Benna, C.; Iacobone, M.; Mondin, A.; Plebani, M.; Faggian, D.; Galuppini, F.; et al. Serum miR-375 for Diagnostic and Prognostic Purposes in Medullary Thyroid Carcinoma. *Front. Endocrinol.* **2021**, *12*, 647369. [CrossRef]
177. Melone, V.; Salvati, A.; Palumbo, D.; Giurato, G.; Nassa, G.; Rizzo, F.; Palo, L.; Giordano, A.; Incoronato, M.; Vitale, M.; et al. Identification of Functional Pathways and Molecular Signatures in Neuroendocrine Neoplasms by Multi-Omics Analysis. *J. Transl. Med.* **2022**, *20*, 306. [CrossRef]
178. Shabani, N.; Sheikholeslami, S.; Paryan, M.; Zarif Yeganeh, M.; Tavangar, S.M.; Azizi, F.; Mohammadi-Yeganeh, S.; Hedayati, M. An Investigation on the Expression of miRNAs Including miR-144 and miR-34a in Plasma Samples of RET-Positive and RET-Negative Medullar Thyroid Carcinoma Patients. *J. Cell. Physiol.* **2020**, *235*, 1366–1373. [CrossRef]
179. Besharat, Z.M.; Trocchianesi, S.; Verrienti, A.; Ciampi, R.; Cantara, S.; Romei, C.; Sabato, C.; Noviello, T.M.R.; Po, A.; Citarella, A.; et al. Circulating miR-26b-5p and miR-451a as Diagnostic Biomarkers in Medullary Thyroid Carcinoma Patients. *J. Endocrinol. Investig.* **2023**, *46*, 2583. [CrossRef] [PubMed]
180. Zhang, A.; Wang, C.; Lu, H.; Chen, X.; Ba, Y.; Zhang, C.; Zhang, C.-Y. Altered Serum MicroRNA Profile May Serve as an Auxiliary Tool for Discriminating Aggressive Thyroid Carcinoma from Nonaggressive Thyroid Cancer and Benign Thyroid Nodules. *Dis. Markers* **2019**, *2019*, 3717683. [CrossRef] [PubMed]
181. Rosignolo, F.; Sponziello, M.; Giacomelli, L.; Russo, D.; Pecce, V.; Biffoni, M.; Bellantone, R.; Lombardi, C.P.; Lamartina, L.; Grani, G.; et al. Identification of Thyroid-Associated Serum microRNA Profiles and Their Potential Use in Thyroid Cancer Follow-Up. *J. Endocr. Soc.* **2017**, *1*, 3. [CrossRef] [PubMed]

182. Yu, S.; Liu, Y.; Wang, J.; Guo, Z.; Zhang, Q.; Yu, F.; Zhang, Y.; Huang, K.; Li, Y.; Song, E.; et al. Circulating MicroRNA Profiles as Potential Biomarkers for Diagnosis of Papillary Thyroid Carcinoma. *J. Clin. Endocrinol. Metab.* **2012**, *97*, 2084–2092. [CrossRef]
183. Lee, J.C.; Zhao, J.T.; Clifton-Bligh, R.J.; Gill, A.; Gundara, J.S.; Ip, J.C.; Glover, A.; Sywak, M.S.; Delbridge, L.W.; Robinson, B.G.; et al. MicroRNA-222 and microRNA-146b Are Tissue and Circulating Biomarkers of Recurrent Papillary Thyroid Cancer. *Cancer* **2013**, *119*, 4358–4365. [CrossRef]
184. Rezaei, M.; Khamaneh, A.M.; Zarghami, N.; Vosoughi, A.; Hashemzadeh, S. Evaluating Pre- and Post-Operation Plasma miRNAs of Papillary Thyroid Carcinoma (PTC) Patients in Comparison to Benign Nodules. *BMC Cancer* **2019**, *19*, 690. [CrossRef]
185. Yoruker, E.E.; Terzioglu, D.; Teksoz, S.; Uslu, F.E.; Gezer, U.; Dalay, N. MicroRNA Expression Profiles in Papillary Thyroid Carcinoma, Benign Thyroid Nodules and Healthy Controls. *J. Cancer* **2016**, *7*, 803. [CrossRef]
186. Graham, M.E.R.; Hart, R.D.; Douglas, S.; Makki, F.M.; Pinto, D.; Butler, A.L.; Bullock, M.; Rigby, M.H.; Trites, J.R.B.; Taylor, S.M.; et al. Serum microRNA Profiling to Distinguish Papillary Thyroid Cancer from Benign Thyroid Masses. *J. Otolaryngol.-Head Neck Surg. J. Oto-Rhino-Laryngol. Chir. Cervico-Faciale* **2015**, *44*, 33. [CrossRef]
187. Cantara, S.; Pilli, T.; Sebastiani, G.; Cevenini, G.; Busonero, G.; Cardinale, S.; Dotta, F.; Pacini, F. Circulating miRNA95 and miRNA190 Are Sensitive Markers for the Differential Diagnosis of Thyroid Nodules in a Caucasian Population. *J. Clin. Endocrinol. Metab.* **2014**, *99*, 4190–4198. [CrossRef]
188. Li, M.; Song, Q.; Li, H.; Lou, Y.; Wang, L. Circulating miR-25-3p and miR-451a May Be Potential Biomarkers for the Diagnosis of Papillary Thyroid Carcinoma. *PLoS ONE* **2015**, *10*, e0132403. [CrossRef]
189. Jiang, Y.; Wang, J.; Chen, J.; Wang, J.; Xu, J. Construction and Analysis of an Aberrant lncRNA-miRNA-mRNA Network Associated with Papillary Thyroid Cancer. *Medicine* **2020**, *99*, e22705. [CrossRef] [PubMed]
190. Gou, L.; Zou, H.; Li, B. Long Noncoding RNA MALAT1 Knockdown Inhibits Progression of Anaplastic Thyroid Carcinoma by Regulating miR-200a-3p/FOXA1. *Cancer Biol. Ther.* **2019**, *20*, 1355–1365. [CrossRef] [PubMed]
191. Wu, L.; Shi, Y.; Liu, B.; Zhao, M. Expression of lncRNA-HOTAIR in the Serum of Patients with Lymph Node Metastasis of Papillary Thyroid Carcinoma and Its Impact. *Oncol. Lett.* **2020**, *20*, 907–913. [CrossRef] [PubMed]
192. Wang, Y.; Lin, X.; Fu, X.; Yan, W.; Lin, F.; Kuang, P.; Luo, Y.; Lin, E.; Hong, X.; Wu, G. Long Non-Coding RNA BANCR Regulates Cancer Stem Cell Markers in Papillary Thyroid Cancer via the RAF/MEK/ERK Signaling Pathway. *Oncol. Rep.* **2018**, *40*, 859–866. [CrossRef] [PubMed]
193. Wang, M.; Chen, B.; Ru, Z.; Cong, L. CircRNA Circ-ITCH Suppresses Papillary Thyroid Cancer Progression through miR-22-3p/CBL/β-Catenin Pathway. *Biochem. Biophys. Res. Commun.* **2018**, *504*, 283–288. [CrossRef]
194. Yao, Y.; Chen, X.; Yang, H.; Chen, W.; Qian, Y.; Yan, Z.; Liao, T.; Yao, W.; Wu, W.; Yu, T.; et al. Hsa_circ_0058124 Promotes Papillary Thyroid Cancer Tumorigenesis and Invasiveness through the NOTCH3/GATAD2A Axis. *J. Exp. Clin. Cancer Res.* **2019**, *38*, 318. [CrossRef]
195. Wei, H.; Pan, L.; Tao, D.; Li, R. Circular RNA circZFR Contributes to Papillary Thyroid Cancer Cell Proliferation and Invasion by Sponging miR-1261 and Facilitating C8orf4 Expression. *Biochem. Biophys. Res. Commun.* **2018**, *503*, 56–61. [CrossRef]
196. Li, X.; Tian, Y.; Hu, Y.; Yang, Z.; Zhang, L.; Luo, J. CircNUP214 Sponges miR-145 to Promote the Expression of ZEB2 in Thyroid Cancer Cells. *Biochem. Biophys. Res. Commun.* **2018**, *507*, 168–172. [CrossRef]
197. Jin, X.; Wang, Z.; Pang, W.; Zhou, J.; Liang, Y.; Yang, J.; Yang, L.; Zhang, Q. Upregulated Hsa_circ_0004458 Contributes to Progression of Papillary Thyroid Carcinoma by Inhibition of miR-885-5p and Activation of RAC1. *Med. Sci. Monit. Int. Med. J. Exp. Clin. Res.* **2018**, *24*, 5488. [CrossRef]
198. Yang, S.P.; Koh, L.C.W.; Kong, K.W.; Parameswaran, R.; Loke, K.S.H.; Ngiam, K.Y.; Tan, W.B.; Loh, T.; Ng, D.C.E.; Goh, B.C.; et al. A Multiplex Thyroid-Specific Assay for Quantification of Circulating Thyroid Cell-Free RNA in Plasma of Thyroid Cancer Patients. *Front. Genet.* **2021**, *12*, 721832. [CrossRef]
199. Ringel, M.D.; Ladenson, P.W.; Levine, M.A. Molecular Diagnosis of Residual and Recurrent Thyroid Cancer by Amplification of Thyroglobulin Messenger Ribonucleic Acid in Peripheral Blood. *J. Clin. Endocrinol. Metab.* **1998**, *83*, 4435–4442. [CrossRef] [PubMed]
200. Bellantone, R.; Lombardi, C.P.; Bossola, M.; Ferrante, A.; Princi, P.; Boscherini, M.; Maussier, L.; Salvatori, M.; Rufini, V.; Reale, F.; et al. Validity of Thyroglobulin mRNA Assay in Peripheral Blood of Postoperative Thyroid Carcinoma Patients in Predicting Tumor Recurrences Varies According to the Histologic Type: Results of a Prospective Study. *Cancer* **2001**, *92*, 2273–2279. [CrossRef]
201. Amakawa, M.; Kato, R.; Kameko, F.; Maruyama, M.; Tajiri, J. Thyroglobulin mRNA Expression in Peripheral Blood Lymphocytes of Healthy Subjects and Patients with Thyroid Disease. *Clin. Chim. Acta Int. J. Clin. Chem.* **2008**, *390*, 97–103. [CrossRef] [PubMed]
202. Sellitti, D.F.; Akamizu, T.; Doi, S.Q.; Kim, G.H.; Kariyil, J.T.; Kopchik, J.J.; Koshiyama, H. Renal Expression of Two "thyroid-Specific" Genes: Thyrotropin Receptor and Thyroglobulin. *Exp. Nephrol.* **2000**, *8*, 235–243. [CrossRef]
203. Aliyev, A.; Gupta, M.; Nasr, C.; Hatipoglu, B.; Milas, M.; Siperstein, A.; Berber, E. Circulating thyroid-stimulating hormone receptor messenger rna as a marker of tumor aggressiveness in patients with papillary thyroid microcarcinoma. *Endocr. Pract. Off. J. Am. Coll. Endocrinol. Am. Assoc. Clin. Endocrinol.* **2015**, *21*, 777–781. [CrossRef] [PubMed]

204. Aliyev, A.; Patel, J.; Brainard, J.; Gupta, M.; Nasr, C.; Hatipoglu, B.; Siperstein, A.; Berber, E. Diagnostic Accuracy of Circulating Thyrotropin Receptor Messenger RNA Combined with Neck Ultrasonography in Patients with Bethesda III-V Thyroid Cytology. *Surgery* **2016**, *159*, 113–117. [CrossRef]
205. Chia, S.-Y.; Milas, M.; Reddy, S.K.; Siperstein, A.; Skugor, M.; Brainard, J.; Gupta, M.K. Thyroid-Stimulating Hormone Receptor Messenger Ribonucleic Acid Measurement in Blood as a Marker for Circulating Thyroid Cancer Cells and Its Role in the Preoperative Diagnosis of Thyroid Cancer. *J. Clin. Endocrinol. Metab.* **2007**, *92*, 468–475. [CrossRef]
206. Chinnappa, P.; Taguba, L.; Arciaga, R.; Faiman, C.; Siperstein, A.; Mehta, A.E.; Reddy, S.K.; Nasr, C.; Gupta, M.K. Detection of Thyrotropin-Receptor Messenger Ribonucleic Acid (mRNA) and Thyroglobulin mRNA Transcripts in Peripheral Blood of Patients with Thyroid Disease: Sensitive and Specific Markers for Thyroid Cancer. *J. Clin. Endocrinol. Metab.* **2004**, *89*, 3705–3709. [CrossRef]
207. Savagner, F.; Rodien, P.; Reynier, P.; Rohmer, V.; Bigorgne, J.-C.; Malthiery, Y. Analysis of Tg Transcripts by Real-Time RT-PCR in the Blood of Thyroid Cancer Patients. *J. Clin. Endocrinol. Metab.* **2002**, *87*, 635–639. [CrossRef]
208. Camacho, C.P.; Lindsey, S.C.; Melo, M.C.C.; Yang, J.H.; Germano-Neto, F.; de Valente, O.F.; Lima, T.R.; Biscolla, R.P.M.; Vieira, J.G.; Cerutti, J.M.; et al. Measurement of Calcitonin and Calcitonin Gene–Related Peptide mRNA Refines the Management of Patients with Medullary Thyroid Cancer and May Replace Calcitonin-Stimulation Tests. *Thyroid* **2013**, *23*, 308. [CrossRef]
209. Lubitz, C.C.; Parangi, S.; Holm, T.M.; Bernasconi, M.J.; Schalck, A.P.; Suh, H.; Economopoulos, K.P.; Gunda, V.; Donovan, S.E.; Sadow, P.M.; et al. Detection of Circulating BRAFV600E in Patients with Papillary Thyroid Carcinoma. *J. Mol. Diagn. JMD* **2016**, *18*, 100. [CrossRef] [PubMed]
210. Yokoi, A.; Ochiya, T. Exosomes and Extracellular Vesicles: Rethinking the Essential Values in Cancer Biology. *Semin. Cancer Biol.* **2021**, *74*, 79–91. [CrossRef] [PubMed]
211. Capriglione, F.; Verrienti, A.; Celano, M.; Maggisano, V.; Sponziello, M.; Pecce, V.; Gagliardi, A.; Giacomelli, L.; Aceti, V.; Durante, C.; et al. Analysis of Serum microRNA in Exosomal Vehicles of Papillary Thyroid Cancer. *Endocrine* **2022**, *75*, 185–193. [CrossRef] [PubMed]
212. Liang, M.; Yu, S.; Tang, S.; Bai, L.; Cheng, J.; Gu, Y.; Li, S.; Zheng, X.; Duan, L.; Wang, L.; et al. A Panel of Plasma Exosomal miRNAs as Potential Biomarkers for Differential Diagnosis of Thyroid Nodules. *Front. Genet.* **2020**, *11*, 449. [CrossRef]
213. Wen, Q.; Wang, Y.; Li, X.; Jin, X.; Wang, G. Decreased Serum Exosomal miR-29a Expression and Its Clinical Significance in Papillary Thyroid Carcinoma. *J. Clin. Lab. Anal.* **2021**, *35*, e23560. [CrossRef]
214. D'Amico, G.; Santonocito, R.; Grech, G.; Graceffa, G.; Cipolla, C.; Scalia, F.; Raccosta, S.; Manno, M.; Conway de Macario, E.; Macario, A.J.L.; et al. MiRNAs in Extracellular Vesicles as Biomarkers in Plasma of Papillary Thyroid Cancer Patients: A Proof-of-Concept Study. *Biology* **2024**, *13*, 743. [CrossRef]
215. Wang, Z.; Lv, J.; Zou, X.; Huang, Z.; Zhang, H.; Liu, Q.; Jiang, L.; Zhou, X.; Zhu, W. A Three Plasma microRNA Signature for Papillary Thyroid Carcinoma Diagnosis in Chinese Patients. *Gene* **2019**, *693*, 37–45. [CrossRef]
216. Boufraqech, M.; Zhang, L.; Jain, M.; Patel, D.; Ellis, R.; Xiong, Y.; He, M.; Nilubol, N.; Merino, M.J.; Kebebew, E. miR-145 Suppresses Thyroid Cancer Growth and Metastasis and Targets AKT3. *Endocr. Relat. Cancer* **2014**, *21*, 517–531. [CrossRef]
217. Dai, D.; Tan, Y.; Guo, L.; Tang, A.; Zhao, Y. Identification of Exosomal miRNA Biomarkers for Diagnosis of Papillary Thyroid Cancer by Small RNA Sequencing. *Eur. J. Endocrinol.* **2020**, *182*, 111–121. [CrossRef]
218. Samsonov, R.; Burdakov, V.; Shtam, T.; Radzhabova, Z.; Vasilyev, D.; Tsyrlina, E.; Titov, S.; Ivanov, M.; Berstein, L.; Filatov, M.; et al. Plasma Exosomal miR-21 and miR-181a Differentiates Follicular from Papillary Thyroid Cancer. *Tumour Biol. J. Int. Soc. Oncodevelopmental Biol. Med.* **2016**, *37*, 12011–12021. [CrossRef]
219. Jiang, K.; Li, G.; Chen, W.; Song, L.; Wei, T.; Li, Z.; Gong, R.; Lei, J.; Shi, H.; Zhu, J. Plasma Exosomal miR-146b-5p and miR-222-3p Are Potential Biomarkers for Lymph Node Metastasis in Papillary Thyroid Carcinomas. *OncoTargets Ther.* **2020**, *13*, 1311–1319. [CrossRef] [PubMed]
220. Chen, W.; Li, G.; Li, Z.; Zhu, J.; Wei, T.; Lei, J. Evaluation of Plasma Exosomal miRNAs as Potential Diagnostic Biomarkers of Lymph Node Metastasis in Papillary Thyroid Carcinoma. *Endocrine* **2022**, *75*, 846–855. [CrossRef]
221. Lin, Q.; Qi, Q.; Hou, S.; Chen, Z.; Jiang, N.; Zhang, L.; Lin, C. Exosomal Circular RNA Hsa_circ_007293 Promotes Proliferation, Migration, Invasion, and Epithelial–Mesenchymal Transition of Papillary Thyroid Carcinoma Cells through Regulation of the microRNA-653-5p/Paired Box 6 Axis. *Bioengineered* **2021**, *12*, 10136–10149. [CrossRef] [PubMed]
222. Yang, C.; Wei, Y.; Yu, L.; Xiao, Y. Identification of Altered Circular RNA Expression in Serum Exosomes from Patients with Papillary Thyroid Carcinoma by High-Throughput Sequencing. *Med. Sci. Monit.* **2019**, *25*, 2785–2791. [CrossRef] [PubMed]
223. Dai, W.; Jin, X.; Han, L.; Huang, H.; Ji, Z.; Xu, X.; Tang, M.; Jiang, B.; Chen, W. Exosomal lncRNA DOCK9-AS2 Derived from Cancer Stem Cell-like Cells Activated Wnt/β-Catenin Pathway to Aggravate Stemness, Proliferation, Migration, and Invasion in Papillary Thyroid Carcinoma. *Cell Death Dis.* **2020**, *11*, 743. [CrossRef] [PubMed]
224. Luo, D.; Zhan, S.; Xia, W.; Huang, L.; Ge, W.; Wang, T. Proteomics Study of Serum Exosomes from Papillary Thyroid Cancer Patients. *Endocr. Relat. Cancer* **2018**, *25*, 879–891. [CrossRef]

225. Cao, Z.; Wang, Y.; Wu, J.; Tang, X.; Qian, Z.; Zhang, Z.; Liu, R.; Liu, P.; Li, Z.; Xu, X.; et al. Serum Small Extracellular Vesicles-Derived BST2 as a Biomarker for Papillary Thyroid Microcarcinoma Promotes Lymph Node Metastasis. *Cancer Gene Ther.* **2025**, *32*, 38–50. [CrossRef]
226. Caruso Bavisotto, C.; Cipolla, C.; Graceffa, G.; Barone, R.; Bucchieri, F.; Bulone, D.; Cabibi, D.; Campanella, C.; Marino Gammazza, A.; Pitruzzella, A.; et al. Immunomorphological Pattern of Molecular Chaperones in Normal and Pathological Thyroid Tissues and Circulating Exosomes: Potential Use in Clinics. *Int. J. Mol. Sci.* **2019**, *20*, 4496. [CrossRef]
227. Ahmed, N.M.; Eddama, M.M.R.; Beatson, K.; Gurung, R.; Patel, J.; Iskandar, G.; Abdel-Salam, A.; Al-Omar, A.; Cohen, R.; Abdel-Aziz, T.; et al. Circulating Large Extracellular Vesicles as Diagnostic Biomarkers of Indeterminate Thyroid Nodules: Multi-Platform Omics Analysis. *BJS Open* **2024**, *9*, zrae139. [CrossRef]
228. Zaccone, V.; Falsetti, L.; Nitti, C.; Gentili, T.; Marchetti, A.; Piersantelli, M.N.; Sampaolesi, M.; Riccomi, F.; Raponi, A.; Salvi, A. The Prognostic Role of Procalcitonin in Critically Ill Patients Admitted in a Medical Stepdown Unit: A Retrospective Cohort Study. *Sci. Rep.* **2020**, *10*, 4531. [CrossRef]
229. Azzini, A.M.; Dorizzi, R.M.; Sette, P.; Vecchi, M.; Coledan, I.; Righi, E.; Tacconelli, E. A 2020 Review on the Role of Procalcitonin in Different Clinical Settings: An Update Conducted with the Tools of the Evidence Based Laboratory Medicine. *Ann. Transl. Med.* **2020**, *8*, 610. [CrossRef] [PubMed]
230. Trimboli, P.; Seregni, E.; Treglia, G.; Alevizaki, M.; Giovanella, L. Procalcitonin for Detecting Medullary Thyroid Carcinoma: A Systematic Review. *Endocr. Relat. Cancer* **2015**, *22*, R157–R164. [CrossRef] [PubMed]
231. Karagiannis, A.K.A.; Girio-Fragkoulakis, C.; Nakouti, T. Procalcitonin: A New Biomarker for Medullary Thyroid Cancer? A Systematic Review. *Anticancer Res.* **2016**, *36*, 3803–3810. [PubMed]
232. Austin, L.A.; Heath, H. Calcitonin. *N. Engl. J. Med.* **1981**, *304*, 269–278. [CrossRef]
233. Goltzman, D.; Tischler, A.S. Characterization of the Immunochemical Forms of Calcitonin Released by a Medullary Thyroid Carcinoma in Tissue Culture. *J. Clin. Investig.* **1978**, *61*, 449–458. [CrossRef]
234. Meisner, M.; Schmidt, J.; Hüttner, H.; Tschaikowsky, K. The Natural Elimination Rate of Procalcitonin in Patients with Normal and Impaired Renal Function. *Intensive Care Med.* **2000**, *26* (Suppl. 2), S212–S216. [CrossRef]
235. Kratzsch, J.; Willenberg, A.; Frank-Raue, K.; Kempin, U.; Rocktäschel, J.; Raue, F. Procalcitonin Measured by Three Different Assays Is an Excellent Tumor Marker for the Follow-up of Patients with Medullary Thyroid Carcinoma. *Clin. Chem. Lab. Med. CCLM* **2021**, *59*, 1861–1868. [CrossRef]
236. Giovanella, L.; Verburg, F.A.; Imperiali, M.; Valabrega, S.; Trimboli, P.; Ceriani, L. Comparison of Serum Calcitonin and Procalcitonin in Detecting Medullary Thyroid Carcinoma among Patients with Thyroid Nodules. *Clin. Chem. Lab. Med.* **2013**, *51*, 1477–1481. [CrossRef]
237. Machens, A.; Lorenz, K.; Dralle, H. Utility of Serum Procalcitonin for Screening and Risk Stratification of Medullary Thyroid Cancer. *J. Clin. Endocrinol. Metab.* **2014**, *99*, 2986–2994. [CrossRef]
238. Giovanella, L.; Fontana, M.; Keller, F.; Verburg, F.A.; Ceriani, L. Clinical Performance of Calcitonin and Procalcitonin Elecsys® Immunoassays in Patients with Medullary Thyroid Carcinoma. *Clin. Chem. Lab. Med.* **2021**, *59*, 743–747. [CrossRef]
239. Censi, S.; Manso, J.; Benvenuti, T.; Piva, I.; Iacobone, M.; Mondin, A.; Torresan, F.; Basso, D.; Crivellari, G.; Zovato, S.; et al. The Role of Procalcitonin in the Follow-up of Medullary Thyroid Cancer. *Eur. Thyroid J.* **2023**, *12*, e220161. [CrossRef] [PubMed]
240. Giovanella, L.; Garo, M.L.; Ceriani, L.; Paone, G.; Campenni', A.; D'Aurizio, F. Procalcitonin as an Alternative Tumor Marker of Medullary Thyroid Carcinoma. *J. Clin. Endocrinol. Metab.* **2021**, *106*, 3634–3643. [CrossRef] [PubMed]
241. Giovanella, L.; Imperiali, M.; Piccardo, A.; Taborelli, M.; Verburg, F.A.; Daurizio, F.; Trimboli, P. Procalcitonin Measurement to Screen Medullary Thyroid Carcinoma: A Prospective Evaluation in a Series of 2705 Patients with Thyroid Nodules. *Eur. J. Clin. Investig.* **2018**, *48*, e12934. [CrossRef]
242. Giovanella, L.; Giordani, I.; Imperiali, M.; Orlandi, F.; Trimboli, P. Measuring Procalcitonin to Overcome Heterophilic-Antibody-Induced Spurious Hypercalcitoninemia. *Clin. Chem. Lab. Med. CCLM* **2018**, *56*, e191–e193. [CrossRef]
243. Kratzsch, J.; Petzold, A.; Raue, F.; Reinhardt, W.; Bröcker-Preuss, M.; Görges, R.; Mann, K.; Karges, W.; Morgenthaler, N.; Luster, M.; et al. Basal and Stimulated Calcitonin and Procalcitonin by Various Assays in Patients with and without Medullary Thyroid Cancer. *Clin. Chem.* **2011**, *57*, 467–474. [CrossRef]
244. Bytnar, J.A.; Enewold, L.; Shriver, C.D.; Zhu, K. Incidence of Papillary Thyroid Cancer: Comparison of the Military and the General Population by Race and Tumor Stage/Size. *Cancer Epidemiol.* **2024**, *89*, 102539. [CrossRef]
245. Yu, Q.; Zhang, X.; Li, L.; Zhang, C.; Huang, J.; Huang, W. Molecular Basis and Targeted Therapies for Radioiodine Refractory Thyroid Cancer. *Asia Pac. J. Clin. Oncol.* **2023**, *19*, 279–289. [CrossRef]
246. Grogan, R.H.; Mitmaker, E.J.; Clark, O.H. The Evolution of Biomarkers in Thyroid Cancer—From Mass Screening to a Personalized Biosignature. *Cancers* **2010**, *2*, 885–912. [CrossRef]

247. Avram, A.M.; Giovanella, L.; Greenspan, B.; Lawson, S.A.; Luster, M.; Van Nostrand, D.; Peacock, J.G.; Ovčariček, P.P.; Silberstein, E.; Tulchinsky, M.; et al. SNMMI Procedure Standard/EANM Practice Guideline for Nuclear Medicine Evaluation and Therapy of Differentiated Thyroid Cancer: Abbreviated Version. *J. Nucl. Med. Off. Publ. Soc. Nucl. Med.* **2022**, *63*, 15N–35N.
248. Favresse, J.; Burlacu, M.-C.; Maiter, D.; Gruson, D. Interferences With Thyroid Function Immunoassays: Clinical Implications and Detection Algorithm. *Endocr. Rev.* **2018**, *39*, 830–850. [CrossRef]
249. Garo, M.L.; Campennì, A.; Petranovic-Ovcaricek, P.; D'Aurizio, F.; Giovanella, L. Evolution of Thyroid Cancer Biomarkers: From Laboratory Test to Patients' Clinical Management. *Clin. Chem. Lab. Med.* **2023**, *61*, 935–945. [CrossRef] [PubMed]
250. Ceriotti, F. Harmonization Initiatives in Europe. *EJIFCC* **2016**, *27*, 23–29. [PubMed]
251. Ozarda, Y.; Sikaris, K.; Streichert, T.; Macri, J.; IFCC Committee on Reference intervals and Decision Limits (C-RIDL). Distinguishing Reference Intervals and Clinical Decision Limits—A Review by the IFCC Committee on Reference Intervals and Decision Limits. *Crit. Rev. Clin. Lab. Sci.* **2018**, *55*, 420–431. [CrossRef] [PubMed]
252. EP28 A3C: Define and Verify Reference Intervals in Lab. Available online: https://clsi.org/standards/products/method-evaluation/documents/ep28/ (accessed on 8 January 2025).
253. Holdenrieder, S. Circulating Biomarkers: Biological Basis, Methods, and Interpretation Criteria. In *Atlas of Thyroid and Neuroendocrine Tumor Markers*; Giovanella, L., Ed.; Springer International Publishing: Cham, Switzerland, 2018; pp. 39–48, ISBN 978-3-319-62506-5.
254. Xie, K. A Biomarker and Molecular Mechanism Investigation for Thyroid Cancer. *Cent.-Eur. J. Immunol.* **2023**, *48*, 203–218. [CrossRef]
255. Gao, Z.; Jiang, J.; Hou, L.; Zhang, B. Dysregulation of MiR-144-5p/RNF187 Axis Contributes to the Progression of Colorectal Cancer. *J. Transl. Intern. Med.* **2022**, *10*, 65–75. [CrossRef]
256. Garofalo, M.; Quintavalle, C.; Romano, G.; Croce, C.M.; Condorelli, G. miR221/222 in Cancer: Their Role in Tumor Progression and Response to Therapy. *Curr. Mol. Med.* **2012**, *12*, 27–33. [CrossRef]
257. Rhim, J.; Baek, W.; Seo, Y.; Kim, J.H. From Molecular Mechanisms to Therapeutics: Understanding MicroRNA-21 in Cancer. *Cells* **2022**, *11*, 2791. [CrossRef]
258. Capdevila, J.; Awada, A.; Führer-Sakel, D.; Leboulleux, S.; Pauwels, P. Molecular Diagnosis and Targeted Treatment of Advanced Follicular Cell-Derived Thyroid Cancer in the Precision Medicine Era. *Cancer Treat. Rev.* **2022**, *106*, 102380. [CrossRef]
259. Agarwal, S.; Bychkov, A.; Jung, C.-K. Emerging Biomarkers in Thyroid Practice and Research. *Cancers* **2021**, *14*, 204. [CrossRef]
260. Zakari, S.; Niels, N.K.; Olagunju, G.V.; Nnaji, P.C.; Ogunniyi, O.; Tebamifor, M.; Israel, E.N.; Atawodi, S.E.; Ogunlana, O.O. Emerging Biomarkers for Non-Invasive Diagnosis and Treatment of Cancer: A Systematic Review. *Front. Oncol.* **2024**, *14*, 1405267. [CrossRef]
261. D'Avó Luís, A.B.; Seo, M.K. Has the Development of Cancer Biomarkers to Guide Treatment Improved Health Outcomes? *Eur. J. Health Econ. HEPAC Health Econ. Prev. Care* **2021**, *22*, 789–810. [CrossRef]
262. Sebastian, A.M.; Peter, D. Artificial Intelligence in Cancer Research: Trends, Challenges and Future Directions. *Life* **2022**, *12*, 1991. [CrossRef]

Journal of
Clinical Medicine

MDPI

Review

Radioiodine Therapy of Graves' Disease in Women with Childbearing Potential and the Pre-Conceptional Counseling About Antithyroid Drugs

Markus Dietlein, Matthias Schmidt, Alexander Drzezga and Carsten Kobe *

Department for Nuclear Medicine, University Hospital Cologne, Kerpener Str. 62, 50937 Cologne, Germany
* Correspondence: carsten.kobe@uk-koeln.de

Abstract: Graves' disease and hyperthyroidism in women with childbearing potential are a challenge in pre-conceptional counseling. The non-surgical alternatives are radioiodine therapy or antithyroid drugs. Here, we focus on the TSH receptor antibody (TRAb) level—without or after radioiodine therapy—and the probability of fetal or neonatal hyperthyroidism. This immunological effect should be weighed against the risk of congenital malformation taking propylthiouracil during pregnancy. For up to 2 years after radioiodine therapy for Graves' disease, TRAb levels may remain above the pre-therapeutic level. The time of conception after radioiodine therapy and a high TRAb level are associated with the likelihood of neonatal hyperthyroidism: 8.8% probability if conception occurred 6–12 months after radioiodine therapy, with a 5.5% probability for 12–18 months, and 3.6% probability for 18–24 months. The TRAb value above 10 U/L in the third trimester is the main risk factor for neonatal hyperthyroidism. If a woman does not wish to postpone her family planning, the pre-conceptional counseling has to describe the risk of propylthiouracil, thiamazole, or of an uncontrolled hyperthyroidism. According to some national cohort studies (Danish, Swedish, Korean), the risk for fetal malformations (ear, urinary tract) under propylthiouracil is increased by 1.1–1.6%, in addition to the spontaneous risk for unexposed pregnant women. For thiamazole, the additional risk for fetal malformation was about 2–3%, depending on the dose of thiamazole. Propylthiouracil has posed a lower risk for congenital malformation than an uncontrolled hyperthyroidism. To minimize the risk for the newborn, women with Graves' disease and hyperthyroidism should offer a definitive therapy strategy (e.g., radioiodine therapy) long before planning a pregnancy.

Keywords: radioiodine therapy; Graves' disease; TSH receptor antibodies; fetal hyperthyroidism; propylthiouracil; thiamazole

1. Introduction

Since the 1940s, radioiodine (I-131) has been used to treat thyroid diseases. The concept of ablative radioiodine therapy for Graves' disease with hyperthyroidism (higher intended dose) and of function-optimized radioiodine therapy for toxic or non-toxic goiter (lower intended dose to the thyroid, dosimetric approach pre-therapeutically) and has remained unchanged over a long period [1]. Several subpopulations with benign thyroid diseases and specific circumstances are candidates for radioiodine therapy (Table 1) [2,3]:

I. Patients with Graves' disease (GD) are sent to radioiodine therapy when the first-line therapy has failed. The first manifestation of hyperthyroidism in Graves' disease is treated usually with carbimazole or thiamazole for 12–24 months. The individual timing to stop antithyroid medication depends on the TSH receptor antibody level (TRAb preferably <2 U/L before attempting withdrawal), the dosage of the antithyroid drug (preferably $\leq$2.5 mg carbimazole or thiamazole), and the thyroid function setting (TSH preferably $\geq$0.3 mU/L) [4]. Radioiodine therapy in Graves' disease with small goiter is the preferred option in recurrent hyperthyroidism within 2 years after withdrawal of antithyroid drugs.

II. An indication for an early radioiodine therapy in Graves' disease is the persistent TRAb value above 10 U/L after six months of antithyroid therapy. In this scenario, the success probability of conservative therapy is below 5% [5]. Radioiodine therapy can be offered first line when the risk of recurrent hyperthyroidism is high. The main risk factors are the young age at initial presentation with Graves' disease, the large goiter of >40 mL, and smoking.

III. In subclinical hyperthyroidism (TSH < 0.1 mU/L), radioiodine therapy in Graves' disease is recommended in patients >65 years old or in patients with atrial fibrillation/cardiovascular comorbidity. An individual indication for radioiodine therapy in older patients is the TSH range of 0.1–0.4 mU/L [4].

IV. Radioiodine therapy can be administered safely in adolescents, preferably those over 15 years [4,6,7]. The duration of the antithyroid medication with carbimazole or thiamazole should be longer in adolescents than in adults and can be extended to at least 3 years (up to 6 years) in adolescents [6]. Due to the increased risk of liver failure, propylthiouracil is contraindicated in adolescents.

V. In special circumstances, radioiodine therapy is an option for thyroid remnant ablation if postoperative residual thyroid tissue remains and there is an advanced florid endocrine orbitopathy ("Moleti concept"). As endogenous TSH stimulation by temporarily discontinuing thyroid medication is not considered, exogenous TSH stimulation by rhTSH is performed as "off-label use" in the usual dosage of rhTSH, followed by the administration of a fixed radioiodine activity of 1.1 GBq ^{131}I [8].

Table 1. Main features of the three available treatment strategies for hyperthyroidism due to Graves' disease or toxic goiter.

	Antithyroid Drugs	Surgery	Radioiodine
Time to initial improvement	2–4 weeks	Needs antithyroid drug pre-treatment (toxic goiter) Success immediately	Needs antithyroid drug pre-treatment; 4–8 weeks after RIT
Recurrence	90–100% (toxic goiter)	1–4%	5–10%
Use in pregnancy/ Breast feeding	Yes (First trimester: PTU)	Second trimester	No
Adverse effect on eye disease in toxic goiter	No	No	0.1% (1% risk of immune hyperthyroidism; rarely eye symptoms)
Adverse effect on eye disease in Graves' disease	Spontaneous course	Spontaneous course	Glucocorticoids in patients with Graves' ophthalomopathy
Interference with daily activities	No	Requires hospital admission	Need for radiation precautions and in many countries requires hospital admission
Key adverse effects	Rash; arthralgia; hepatitis; agranulocytosis	Surgical; vocal cord paralysis; hypoparathyroidism; hypothyroidism	Hypothyroidism (>95% with an ablative dose concept, 10% with a low-dose concept)

The immunological effects of radioiodine therapy in younger women with Graves' disease regarding family planning, pre-conceptional counseling, possible pregnancy complications (e.g., fetal or neonatal hyperthyroidism), and the teratogenic side effects of antithyroid drugs are discussed in this review [9–11]. We present the literature on TRAb after radioiodine therapy, on TRAb during pregnancy, and on antithyroid drugs during pregnancy with a search in the database of PubMed®.

2. Graves' Disease—Immunological Aspects in Women with Childbearing Potential

How can be Graves' disease in women of childbearing potential managed (Table 2)? For up to 2 years after radioiodine therapy for Graves' disease, TSH receptor antibody levels (TRAb) may remain above the pre-therapeutic level [9]. TSH receptor antibodies are going transplacentar and could lead to fetal/neonatal hyperthyroidism if the TRAb levels exceed at least 5 U/L or are increased at least by a factor of ≥3 above the upper limit in the case of stimulating TRAb in the last trimester [12–14]. However, the frequently cited TRAb level above 5 U/L is a very conservative assumption.

Table 2. Main features of the three available treatment options for Graves' disease with hyperthyroidism in women with childbearing potential. Abbreviations: ATD, antithyroid drugs; PTU, propylthiouracil; RIT, radioiodine therapy; TRAb, TSH receptor antibody.

	Antithyroid Drugs	Surgery	Radioiodine Therapy
Efficacy	Euthyroid function within 1–2 months. Thiamazole or carbimazole as standard. PTU pre-conceptional and during the first trimester of pregnancy	Euthyroid function with levothyroxine; Increase in dosage during the first and second trimester of pregnancy	Euthyroid function with levothyroxine achieved about 3–4 months after RIT
Key adverse effects in the pre-conceptional state or in pregnancy	Hepatotoxicity of PTU. Birth defects in early pregnancy with thiamazole 2–3% higher than the spontaneous risk, with PTU 1.1–1.6%	Surgical complications: vocal cord paralysis; hypoparathyroidism	TRAb elevation for up to 2 years after RIT. Fetal or neonatal hyperthyroidism, if TRAb > 10 U/L in the third trimester
Practical considerations	Pre-conceptional conseling. Change from thiamazole to PTU during the first trimester bears risk of birth defects. Low dose of PTU. Doses > 150 mg PTU induce fetal hypothyroidism	Feasible in second trimester, if refractory to ATD or adverse effects of ATD	feasible only before family planning; High TRAb levels in the third trimester require fetal monitoring

The average risk of fetal hyperthyroidism is about 1–2% of mothers with Graves' disease, manifesting beyond the 22–26 week' gestation [15]. The risk of fetal hyperthyroidism is much higher (approximately 5–20%) when the pregnancy starts with maternal TRAb levels of more than 30–40 U/L. Signs of fetal hyperthyroidism include tachycardia (>160 beats per min), goiter, oligohydramnion, growth restriction, premature bone ossification, and fetal hydrops. Fetal ultrasound surveillance is recommended in mothers with elevated TRAb above 5 U/L or with uncontrolled hyperthyroidism.

A literature review by van Dijk et al. [13] covering six cohort studies examined the individual TRAb levels of pregnant women diagnosed with fetal or neonatal hyperthyroidism. TRAb levels were measured using first to third-generation assays, so the authors related maternal TRAb levels to the upper reference limits of each assay used. As only one of the six cohort studies had consecutive patient inclusion, a selection bias limits the evidence. In the result, 31 cases of fetal/neonatal hyperthyroidism were described, with maternal TRAb levels in the six cited cohort studies being elevated by a factor of 3.7, 4, 9.2, 19.7, 26.7, and 32, respectively, above the upper limit. Inconsistent measurement times during the trimesters also limit the definition of a pre-conceptional TRAb levels requiring monitoring.

As a part of the above-mentioned review, the monocentric French study by Abeillon-du Payrat et al. is frequently cited: 47 newborns were described whose mothers had elevated TRAb levels (second-generation assay) during pregnancy [12]. Seven of these women had previously undergone radioiodine therapy. Nine of the 47 newborns had laboratory-confirmed hyperthyroidism at birth, including five newborns requiring treatment (antithyroid medication for 14–80 days, median 60 days). No neonatal hyperthyroidism was observed below a maternal TRAb level of 5.6 U/L (measured in the second trimester). The likelihood of neonatal hyperthyroidism increased with high TRAb levels. Laboratory evidence of neonatal hyperthyroidism was associated with relatively high maternal TRAb levels, with a median of 26.9 U/L (mean 62.4 U/L). Among the 35 euthyroid newborns, maternal TRAb levels ranged from 1 to >40 U/L, median 5.2 U/L, mean 8.2 U/L. Three newborns were hypothyroid, indicating blocking TSH receptor antibodies. The French authors concluded that close fetal monitoring is warranted if maternal TRAb levels exceed 5 U/L (measured in the study in the second trimester).

A monocentric Japanese study by Yoshihara et al. [14] analyzed the likelihood of neonatal hyperthyroidism if pregnancy occurred within 2 years after radioiodine therapy for Graves' disease. Despite the radioiodine therapy, 54 of the 145 pregnant women (37%) required either antithyroid medication due to persistent hyperthyroidism or high-dose iodine as another treatment concept for Graves' disease with overt hyperthyroidism in Japan. Overall, 8 of the 145 newborns showed laboratory-confirmed neonatal hyperthyroidism, corresponding to a probability of 5.5%. Four of the eight hyperthyroid newborns required antithyroid medication. Seven of the eight neonatal hyperthyroidism cases were associated with an unsuccessful ablation after radioiodine therapy in the mother before family planning. The following association was found between the time of conception after radioiodine therapy and the likelihood of neonatal hyperthyroidism: 8.8% probability if conception occurred 6–12 months after radioiodine therapy, 5.5% probability for 12–18 months, and 3.6% probability for 18–24 months (Table 3). Multivariate analysis identified only the TRAb value in the third trimester as risk factor for neonatal hyperthyroidism. In the ROC analysis, a TRAb threshold of 9.7 IU/L for the third trimester was calculated. Below a TRAb value of 9.7 IU/L (third trimester), no neonatal hyperthyroidism was observed. It is important to note that TRAb levels typically decrease during the whole duration of pregnancy. In the first trimester, maternal TRAb levels among the eight women whose newborns later had neonatal hyperthyroidism ranged from 30.6 IU/L to 40 IU/L, with seven values documented at 40 IU/L. The study also reported pre-therapeutic TRAb levels: In the 137 patients who later gave birth to euthyroid newborns, the median pre-therapeutic TRAb level was 9.95 IU/L (range 0.3–40 IU/L), while in the eight patients whose newborns later had neonatal hyperthyroidism, the median TRAb level was 40 IU/L (range 10.2–40 IU/L). Retrospective data suggest that a high TRAb level at initial diagnosis, an unsuccessful ablation after radioiodine therapy, and a short interval between radioiodine therapy and conception increase the likelihood of neonatal hyperthyroidism.

Table 3. Data from Japan on the incidence of neonatal hyperthyroidism when mothers with Graves' disease were treated with radioiodine. In the group with neonatal hyperthyroidism the mothers had a median thyroid volume of 62 mL and a median TRAb of 40 U/L when radioiodine therapy was started [14]. This is generally a negative selection with an increased probability that the first radioiodine therapy cannot eliminate hyperthyroidism. Abbreviation: TRAb, TSH receptor antibody.

Conception After Radioiodine Therapy	Incidence of Neonatal Hyperthyroidism	TRAb Values at Radioiodine Therapy in Mothers of Neonates with Hyperthyroidism
Within 6–12 months	3/34 (8.8%)	40 U/L, 40 U/L, 16.2 U/L
Within 12–18 months	3/55 (5.5%)	40 U/L, 40 U/L, 11.5 U/L
Within 18–24 months	2/56 (3.6%)	40 U/L, 10.2 U/L

In the pre-conception counseling, we should inform patients of an increase in transplacental TSH receptor antibodies within 2 years after radioiodine therapy. If TRAb levels exceed 5–6 U/L or are >3 times the upper reference limit during pregnancy, fetal monitoring (fetal sonography, fetal pulse monitoring) is advised. For newborns after a pregnancy with high maternal TRAb levels, the pediatric and endocrinological literature recommends a TRAb measurement from umbilical cord blood for risk stratification [16,17].

Ideally, women with Graves' disease and hyperthyroidism planning pregnancy would receive definitive therapy long before pregnancy [18]. If possible, radioiodine therapy should be performed early enough to delay family planning for 2 years, at least for 6 months. The treatment aim after radioiodine therapy is stable euthyroidism. There is no specific treatment to achieve normalization of TRAb pre-conception [15]. If time is pressing to get pregnant, the guidelines does not recommend a specific therapy, as alternatives like thyroidectomy or antithyroid medication with propylthiouracil also carry specific treatment risks.

3. Can Propylthiouracil Be an Alternative to Radioiodine Therapy?

A warning about the teratogenic potential has been formulated for thiamazole and carbimazole (Table 4). The teratogenic risk appears to correlate with the dosage of carbimazole or thiamazole in the first trimester; the maternal hyperthyroidism by itself is not associated with these anomalies [19]. What is the data for propylthiouracil? According to the Danish cohort study, a risk for fetal malformations of 8.3% was observed under propylthiouracil (n = 889 pregnant women) compared to a spontaneous risk for unexposed pregnant women (n = 1,159,181 pregnant women) of 6.7%. The hazard ratio for propylthiouracil was calculated at 1.17 with a 95% confidence interval of 0.91–1.49, indicating that the statistical significance for an increased risk for fetal malformations was not reached for propylthiouracil [10]. For thiamazole (n = 1574 pregnant women), the risk for fetal malformation was calculated at 9.6%, with a hazard ratio of 1.41 and a 95% confidence interval of 1.19–1.67, indicating a statistically significant risk for thiamazole compared to the spontaneous risk for fetal malformation in thyroid-healthy women without medication. In the Swedish cohort study, the spontaneous risk for birth defects was 8.04%, and the calculated risk for birth defects for pregnant women on propylthiouracil was 6.42% only [11]. However, in the Swedish cohort study, statistically increased malformations of the ear (ICD-10: Q17) and urinary tract (ICD-10: Q62) were observed in pregnant women on propylthiouracil. More evidence is needed to establish the degree of risk.

Table 4. Nationwide cohort studies on the incidence of births defects in unexposed women and after use of antithyroid drugs in early pregnancy [10,11,20]. In the Korean cohort study, the risk of congenital malformations by methimazole was dose dependent.

Cohort	Unexposed Women	Methimazole, Thiamazole Alone	Propylthiouracil Alone
Denmark 1997–2016	77,791/1,159,181 (6.7%)	151/1574 (9.6%)	74/889 (8.3%)
Sweden 2005–2014	54,827/682,343 (8.04%)	11/162 (6.79%)	14/218 (6.42%)
South Korea 2008–2014	170,716/2,872,109 (5.94%)	91/1120 (8.13%)	699/9930 (7.0%)

A Korean cohort study confirmed the estimated risk for thiamazole und propylthiouracil, based on 2,886,970 newborns, from whom 12,891 newborns were exposed to antithyroid drugs [20]. The spontaneous prevalence of congenital malformations was 5.94% without antithyroid drugs in the control group, 7.04% with propylthiouracil, 8.13% with thiamazole, and 7.98 with propylthiouracil and thiamazole. The risk difference per 1.000 birth was calculated as 8.81 under propylthiouracil, 17.05 under thiamazole, and 16.53 under propylthiouracil and thiamazole. Switching from propylthiouracil to thiamzole increased the risk of malformation significantly by the odds ratio 1.79 (Table 5). The duration and the cumulative dose of propylthiouracil were not associated with the observed risk of malformations. Prescribing thiamazol, the cumulative dose of 495 mg during the first trimester increased the risk of congenital malformations by the odds ratio 1.87 [20].

Table 5. Data from the Korean cohort study on the incidence of congenital malformations when the antithyroid drugs were switched in the period between pre-pregnancy and the first trimester [20]. Data on more accurate exposure timing will be necessary to verify the risk associated with switching antithyroid drugs. Abbreviations: MMI, methimazole; PTU, propylthiouracil.

Switch	Switch Group	Comparative Value
from methimazole to propylthiouracil	166/2079 (7.98%)	MMI continued: 70/909 (7.70%)
from propylthiouracil to methimazole	18/158 (11.39%)	PTU continued: 357/5184 (6.89%)

4. Has the Uncontrolled Hyperthyroidism a Teratogen Potential?

Larger case control studies from newborns with congenital malformations (e.g., choanal atresia) whose mothers had either uncontrolled hyperthyroidism without taking medication or whose mothers had taken antithyroid drugs indicated that hyperthyroidism is a separate risk factor [21,22]. The risk of malformations was statistically even higher for the group with an untreated hyperthyreoidism than for the group with a controlled thyroid function under methimazol [22]. The risk of choanal atresia affects the gestational weeks 9 and 10 [21]. The meta-analysis by Agrawal et al. confirmed the risk of an untreated hyperthyroidism with a risk factor of 1.04 [23]. Compared to an untreated hyperthyroidism, propylthiouracil decreased the risk of congenital malformations by the factor 0.69, whereas the risk of thiamazole did not differ significantly from the risk of an uncontrolled hyperthyroidism. The evidence of the studies is weakened by patient heterogeneity. A possible bias is the risk of birth defects in children whose mothers have taken an inappropriately high dose of antithyroid drugs with the consequence of overt hypothyroidism.

5. Timing of Radioiodine Therapy

Since radioiodine therapy is usually an elective treatment, optimal conditions should be ensured when scheduling to minimize radiation exposure. To minimize radiation exposure to the breasts, the recommended interval between the end of breastfeeding and the start of radioiodine therapy has been extended to 3 months, in line with the recommendation for radioiodine diagnostics in differentiated thyroid carcinoma [24]. The recommended interval between the administration of iodine-containing contrast media and the start of radioiodine therapy is (at least) 2 months. For the application of specific medications (amiodarone), a much longer period may be required before a successful radioiodine therapy can be performed.

6. Discussion

The association between antithyroid drugs and births defects bases on nationwide studies with larger sample sizes of exposed women (e.g., >500 women) [23]. For women on thiamazole who are planning conception soon and who require antithyroid drugs, we recommend changing to propylthiouracil pre-conception [15]. Antithyroid drug treatment carries a small risk of teratogenic side-effect in early pregnancy, especially in weeks 5–11 [18]. The recent meta-analysis by Agrawal et al. has described a high number of anomalies for exposure to both thiamazole and propylthiouracil and does not support the strategy to switch from thiamazole to propylthiouracil in the first trimester [23]. Propylthiouracil is potentially hepatotoxic, with a small risk of fulminant liver failure. Therefore, propylthiouracil is recommended as first choice only in the planning of and during pregnancy. Discontinuation of treatment with propylthiouracil may be feasible at the end of the second trimester or in the third trimester due to the disappearance of maternal TRAb [19]. Very low doses of propylthiouracil (e.g., 1/4 tablet in the morning and 1/4 tablet in the evening) have the advantage that the risk of recurrence will be minimized.

Another consideration is the risk of birth defect by hypothyroidism of the mother or the fetus. To prevent fetal hypothyroidism, the dosage of propylthiouracil should not exceed 150 mg in the third trimester [25]. If switched to thiamazole after the first trimester (despite the data of the Korean cohort study), the dosage should not exceed 10 mg thiamazole in the third trimester. These dosage recommendations are focused on the aspect of fetal hypothyroidism and were statistically determined using ROC curves, but do not cover the risk of embryopathy. A fetal hypothyroidism rarely causes fetal goiter with tracheal and esophageal compression, polyhydramnion, and complication at delivery. Therefore, the dosage of the antithyroid drugs should be as low as possible, and maternal fT4 is maintained in the high–normal range [15]. In women with mild disease, the termination of antithyroid drugs should be considered in each trimester.

What are the consequences, when a young woman with Graves' disease will ask for non-surgical treatment options under the aspect of family planning? A TRAb-induced fetal or neonatal hyperthyroidism is better to treat than a congenital malformation induced by antithyroid drugs. The probability of fetal hyperthyroidism, manifesting beyond the 22–26 week' gestation, is high (approximately 5–20%) when the pregnancy starts with maternal TRAb levels of more than 30–40 U/L. Women with childbearing potential and such high TRAb levels are not suitable candidates for radioiodine therapy. The maternal TRAb levels typically decrease during the whole duration of pregnancy. The TRAb value in the third trimester is crucial for the probability of neonatal hyperthyroidism. A close fetal monitoring is warranted if maternal TRAb levels exceed 10 U/L, measured in the third trimester. The maternal TRAb will remain in the newborns for several months, whereas the maternal antithyroid drugs are cleared from the newborns rapidly after delivery [15]. If maternal TRAb are elevated in the third trimester, neonatal TSH and fT4 should be measured at delivery, then on days 3–5, and on days 10–14 postpartum or when the newborn develops symptoms. Neonatal hyperthyroidism can be easily missed if relying on newborn screening of TSH alone, as TSH screening is optimized to screen for hypothyroidism. For a newborn with symptomatic hyperthyroidism, thiamazole is allowed, propylthiouracil has a hepatotoxic potential.

7. Conclusions

Patients with Graves' disease, small goiter, and moderately measurable TRAb levels are suitable candidates for radioiodine therapy. After a waiting period of 6 months, the risk of increased TRAb after radioiodine therapy (fetal hyperthyroidism) is no higher than the risk of propylthiouracil (congenital malformation). Prospective data from a head-to-head comparison are missing.

Funding: This research received no external funding.

Informed Consent Statement: Not applicable.

Conflicts of Interest: The authors declare no conflicts of interest.

References

1. Dietlein, M.; Grünwald, F.; Schmidt, M.; Kreissl, M.C.; Luster, M. Guideline for radioiodine therapy for benign thyroid diseases (6/2022-AWMF No. 031-003). *German. Nukl.* **2024**, *63*, 8–20.
2. Weetman, A.P. Radioiodine treatment for benign thyroid diseases. *Clin. Endocrinol.* **2007**, *66*, 757–764. [CrossRef] [PubMed]
3. Campenni, A.; Avram, A.M.; Verburg, F.A.; Iakovou, I.; Hänscheid, H.; de Keizer, B.; Ovčariček, P.P.; Giovanella, L. The EANM guideline on radioiodine therapy of benign thyroid disease. *Eur. J. Nucl. Med. Mol. Imaging* **2023**, *50*, 3324–3348. [CrossRef]
4. Kahaly, G.J.; Bartalena, L.; Hegedüs, L.; Leenhardt, L.; Poppe, K.; Pearce, S.H. 2018 European Thyroid Association guideline for the management of Graves' hyperthyroidism. *Eur. Thyroid J.* **2018**, *7*, 167–186. [CrossRef]
5. Eckstein, A.; Mann, K.; Kahaly, G.J.; Grußendorf, M.; Reiners, C.; Feldkamp, J.; Quadbeck, B.; Bockisch, A.; Schott, M. Role of TSH receptor autoantibodies for the diagnosis of Graves' disease and for the prediction of the course of hyperthyroidism and ophthalmopathy. Recommendations of the Thyroid Section of the German Society of Endocrinology. *Med. Klin.* **2009**, *104*, 343–348. [CrossRef]
6. Léger, J.; Carel, J.C. Management of endocrine disease: Arguments for the prolonged use of antithyroid drugs in children with Graves' disease. *Eur. J. Endocrinol.* **2017**, *177*, R59–R67. [CrossRef]
7. Ross, D.S.; Burch, H.B.; Cooper, D.S.; Greenlee, M.C.; Laurberg, P.; Maia, A.L.; Rivkees, S.A.; Samuels, M.; Sosa, J.A.; Stan, M.N.; et al. 2016 American Thyroid Association guidelines for diagnosis and management of hyperthyroidism and other causes of thyrotoxicosis. *Thyroid* **2016**, *26*, 1343–1421. [CrossRef]
8. Moleti, M.; Violi, M.A.; Montanini, D.; Trombetta, C.; Di Bella, B.; Sturniolo, G.; Presti, S.; Alibrandi, A.; Campennì, A.; Baldari, S.; et al. Radioiodine ablation of postsurgical thyroid remnants after treatment with recombinant human TSH (rh TSH) in patients with moderate-to-servere Graves' orbitopathy (GO): A prospective, randomized, single-blind clinical trial. *J. Clin. Endocrinol. Metab.* **2014**, *99*, 1783–1789. [CrossRef]
9. Kim, J.; Choi, M.S.; Park, J.; Park, H.; Jang, H.W.; Choe, J.-H.; Kim, J.-H.; Kim, J.S.; Cho, Y.S.; Choi, J.Y.; et al. Changes in thyrotropin receptor antibody levels following total thyroidectomy or radioiodine therapy in patients with refractory Graves' disease. *Thyroid* **2021**, *8*, 1264–1271. [CrossRef]
10. Andersen, S.L.; Knøsgaard, L.; Olsen, J.; Vestergaard, P.; Andersen, S. Maternal thyroid function, use of antithyroid drugs in early pregnancy, and birth defects. *J. Clin. Endocrinol. Metab.* **2019**, *104*, 6040–6048. [CrossRef]
11. Andersen, S.L.; Lonn, S.; Vestergaard, P.; Torring, O. Births defects after use of antithyroid drugs in early pregnancy: A Swedish nationwide study. *Eur. J. Endocrinol.* **2017**, *177*, 369–378. [CrossRef] [PubMed]
12. Abeillon-du Payrat, J.; Chikh, K.; Bossard, N.; Bretones, P.; Gaucherand, P.; Claris, O.; Charrié, A.; Raverot, V.; Orgiazzi, J.; Borson-Chazot, F.; et al. Predictive value of maternal second-generation thyroid-binding inhibitory immunoglobulin assay for neonatal autoimmune hyperthyroidism. *Eur. J. Endocrinol.* **2014**, *171*, 451–460. [CrossRef] [PubMed]
13. Van Dijk, M.M.; Smits, I.S.; Fliers, E.; Bisschop, P.H. Maternal thyrotropin receptor antibody concentration and the risk of fetal and neonatal thyrotoxicosis: A systematic review. *Thyroid* **2018**, *28*, 257–264. [CrossRef] [PubMed]
14. Yoshihara, A.; Iwaku, K.; Yoshimura Noh, Y.; Watanabe, N.; Kunii, Y.; Ohye, H.; Suzuki, M.; Matsumoto, M.; Suzuki, N.; Tadokoro, R.; et al. Incidence of neonatal hyperthyreoidism among newborns of Graves' disease patients treated with radioiodine therapy. *Thyroid* **2019**, *29*, 128–134. [CrossRef]
15. Ashkar, C.; Sztal-Mazer, S.; Topliss, D.J. How to manage Graves' disease in women of childbearing potential. *Clin. Endocrinol.* **2023**, *98*, 643–648. [CrossRef]

16. Van der Kaay, D.C.M.; Wasserman, J.D.; Palmert, M.R. Management of neonates born to mothers with Graves' disease. *Pediatrics* **2016**, *137*, e20151878. [CrossRef]
17. Besancon, A.; Beltrand, J.; Le Gac, I.; Luton, D.; Polak, M. Management of neonates born to women with Graves' disease: A cohort study. *Eur. J. Endocrinol.* **2014**, *170*, 855–862. [CrossRef]
18. Chaker, L.; Cooper, D.S.; Walsh, J.P.; Peeters, R.P. Hyperthyroidism. *Lancet* **2024**, *403*, 768–780. [CrossRef]
19. Wiersinga, W.M.; Poppe, K.G.; Effraimidis, G. Hyperthyroidism: Aetiology, pathogenesis, diagnosis, management, complications, and prognosis. *Lancet Diabetes Endocrinol.* **2023**, *11*, 282–298. [CrossRef]
20. Seo, G.H.; Kim, T.H.; Chung, J.H. Antithyroid drugs and congenital malformations. A nationwide Korean cohort study. *Ann. Intern. Med.* **2018**, *168*, 405–413. [CrossRef]
21. Barbero, P.; Valdez, R.; Rodriguez, H.; Tiscornia, C.; Mansilla, E.; Allons, A.; Coll, S.; Liascovich, R. Choanal atresia associated with maternal hyperthyroidism treated with methimazole: A case-control study. *Am. J. Med. Genet. A* **2008**, *146*, 2390–2395. [CrossRef] [PubMed]
22. Momotani, N.; Ito, K.; Hamada, N.; Ban, Y.; Nishikawa, Y.; Mimura, T. Maternal hyperthyroidism and congenital malformation in the offspring. *Clin. Endocrinol.* **1984**, *20*, 695–700. [CrossRef] [PubMed]
23. Agrawal, M.; Lewis, S.; Premawardhana, L.; Dayan, C.M.; Taylor, P.N.; Okosieme, O.E. Antithyroid drug therapy in pregnancy and risk of congenital anomalies: Systemic review and meta-analysis. *Clin. Endocrinol.* **2022**, *96*, 857–868. [CrossRef] [PubMed]
24. Verburg, F.A.; Schmidt, M.; Kreissl, M.C.; Grünwald, F.; Lassmann, M.; Hänscheid, H.; Hohberg, M.; Luster, M.; Dietlein, M. Guideline for I-131 whole body scintigraphy for differentiated thyroid cancer (AWMF No. 031-013). *German. Nukl.* **2019**, *58*, 228–241.
25. Yoshihara, A.; Yoshimura Noh, Y.; Inoue, K.; Watanabe, N.; Fukushita, M.; Matsumoto, M.; Suzuki, N.; Suzuki, A.; Kinoshita, A.; Yoshimura, R.; et al. Incidence of and risk factors for neonatal hypothyroidism among women with Graves' disease treated with antithyroid drugs until delivery. *Thyroid* **2023**, *33*, 373–379. [CrossRef]

Journal of
Clinical Medicine

MDPI

Article

Integrating Clinical Parameters into Thyroid Nodule Malignancy Risk: A Retrospective Evaluation Based on ACR TI-RADS

Nikolaos Angelopoulos [1,2], Ioannis Androulakis [2], Dimitrios P. Askitis [2], Nicolas Valvis [2], Rodis D. Paparodis [2,3,4], Valentina Petkova [2], Anastasios Boniakos [2], Dimitra Zianni [2], Andreas Rizoulis [2], Dimitra Bantouna [2], Juan Carlos Jaume [3,4] and Sarantis Livadas [2,5,*]

1 Academic Department of Nuclear Medicine, School of Medicine, AHEPA University Hospital, 546 36 Thessaloniki, Greece; drangelnick@gmail.com
2 Hellenic Endocrine Network, 105 63 Athens, Greece; i-androulakis@hen.gr (I.A.); dimitrios.askitis@gmail.com (D.P.A.); valvisnikos@yahoo.com (N.V.); rodis@paparodis.gr (R.D.P.); valiapetg@gmail.com (V.P.); anbon@otenet.gr (A.B.); dimzianni@hotmail.com (D.Z.); andreasrizoulis@hotmail.com (A.R.); dimitra.bantouna@yahoo.gr (D.B.)
3 Loyola University Medical Center, Maywood, IL 60153, USA; juan.jaume@va.gov
4 Edward Hines Jr. VA Hospital, Hines, IL 60141, USA
5 Athens Medical Centre, 117 42 Athens, Greece
* Correspondence: sarntis@gmail.com

Abstract: Background/Objectives: Thyroid nodules are commonly found through sensitive imaging methods like ultrasonography. While most nodules are benign and asymptomatic, certain characteristics may indicate malignancy, prompting fine needle aspiration biopsy. Factors like age and gender affect cancer risk, complicating ultrasound-based risk systems. We aimed to determine whether the cytological malignancy rate of thyroid nodules could be adjusted for several clinical parameters. **Methods**: Data from patients aged 18 and above with thyroid nodules assessed via fine needle aspiration (FNA) were retrospectively reviewed. Malignancy classification was based on cytopathology and histopathology results. The study examined how various clinical parameters, adjusted for the ACR TI-RADS category, affected thyroid nodule malignancy rates, including age, sex, Body Mass Index (BMI), nodule size, presence of autoimmunity, and thyroxine therapy. Additionally, we analyzed the performance of ACR TI-RADS in predicting malignant cytology across different age subgroups of thyroid nodules. **Results**: The study included 1128 thyroid nodules from 1001 adult patients, with a median age of 48 years and predominantly female (76.68%). Malignancy rates varied across ACR TI-RADS categories, with higher rates associated with larger nodules and younger age groups. Age emerged as a significant predictor of malignancy, with a consistent decrease in the odds ratio for malignant cytology with advancing age across all ACR TI-RADS categories, indicating its potential utility in risk assessment alongside nodule size and sex. **Conclusions**: Raising the size threshold for recommending FNA of TR3-3 nodules and incorporating patients' age and gender into the evaluation process could enhance the system's accuracy in assessing thyroid nodules and guiding clinical management decisions.

Keywords: thyroid nodules; malignancy; age; Thyroid Imaging Reporting and Data System

1. Introduction

The prevalence of thyroid nodules varies depending on different diagnostic methods [1]: about 5% of individuals may have thyroid nodules detected during routine physical examinations; however, using more sensitive imaging techniques such as computed tomography (CT) or ultrasonography (US) nodules can be detected in up to 15% to 67% of people, respectively [2]. About 95% of thyroid nodules are asymptomatic and are often discovered incidentally during imaging tests performed for other reasons or during routine physical examinations [3]. While most thyroid nodules are benign, for those with suspicious ultrasound characteristics, a fine needle aspiration (FNA) biopsy is indicated to determine whether the nodule is cancerous.

As age increases, thyroid nodules become more prevalent, but their likelihood of being malignant decreases [4]. It has been proposed that several clinical variables, obtained during routine initial thyroid nodule evaluation, should be considered in assessing malignancy potential: younger age, male sex, and nodule size seem to increase malignancy, and "individualization" on thyroid nodule care is recommended [5].

In clinical practice, the risk of malignancy is assessed using ultrasound-based stratification systems, such as the American College of Radiology Thyroid Imaging Reporting and Data System (ACR TI-RADS) [6] and the European Thyroid Imaging Reporting and Data System (EU-TIRADS) [7]. Of note, in both classification systems, nodule stratification is performed regardless of clinical variables and is based solely on ultrasound characteristics. Demographic factors like age or gender are not taken into consideration. For example, in a subgroup of patients, such as older adults (>70), the specificity of TIRADS was low (28%) and the number of unnecessary biopsies increased [8].

Despite these observations, there is a notable gap in the literature regarding how clinical variables interact with ultrasound-based classifications to affect malignancy risk estimates. In particular, it remains unclear whether incorporating factors such as age could improve the diagnostic precision of TI-RADS categories. Therefore, the primary aim of this study was to assess whether clinical variables—particularly age—modify the cytological malignancy risk of thyroid nodules stratified by the ACR TI-RADS system. We also examined the potential influence of gender, Body Mass Index (BMI), the presence of autoimmune thyroid disease, and thyroxine replacement therapy. We hypothesized that age would significantly influence malignancy rates across specific TI-RADS categories, suggesting a need for age-adapted risk stratification in clinical practice.

2. Materials and Methods

2.1. Design and Patients' Characteristics

We performed a retrospective cohort study of patients aged ≥18 years with thyroid nodules evaluated using fine needle aspiration (FNA) at ten endocrine clinics in Greece between January 2023 and January 2024. Cytopathology results from FNA and histopathology results from thyroidectomies were used to classify malignancy. All cases with histologically confirmed malignancy were classified as papillary thyroid carcinoma (PTC); no other histological subtypes were included in the analysis.

Thyroid nodules had been evaluated for composition, margins, echogenicity, shape, presence of echogenic foci, and description of vascularization pattern (color Doppler) in the initial examination by experienced endocrinologists and classified according to the ACR TI-RADS. TIRADS classification was based on the original sonographic report. Cytological findings were reported based on the classification of thyroid nodules according to the criteria of the Bethesda System for Reporting Thyroid Cytopathology into 6 diagnostic categories: (I) nondiagnostic, (II) benign, (III) atypia of undetermined significance (AUS), (IV) follicular neoplasm, (V) suspicious for malignancy (SFM), and (VI) malignant [9].

The exclusion criteria were as follows: Nodules with Bethesda I, III, and IV FNA results, unless cytology was further confirmed by thyroidectomy and operational histopathology reports. This study was approved by the Hellenic Endocrine Network Institutional Review

Board (Protocol Number: 2024/0121314). The Institutional Review Board waived the requirement for written informed consent due to the retrospective nature and the minimal risks associated with this study. The study was conducted under the standards of the Declaration of Helsinki.

Data from patients' records were retrieved, regarding the presence of autoimmune thyroiditis (based on antithyroid antibodies titers) and the potential need for treatment with levothyroxine (LT4) due to hypothyroidism (hypothyroidism was defined as a TSH level greater than 5 mIU/L prior to the initiation of LT4 therapy).

Univariate and multivariate analyses were performed to assess the impact of age, sex, Body Mass Index (BMI), nodule size, presence of autoimmunity, and thyroxine therapy on the malignant cytology rate of thyroid nodules adjusted for the respective ACR TI-RADS category. Secondary analysis included an evaluation of the ACR TI-RADS in the prediction of malignant cytology in different age subgroups of thyroid nodules classified as TR3, TR4, and TR5 (since nodules classified as TR1 and TR2 do not indicate subsequent FNA).

2.2. Statistical Analysis

Data are presented as absolute numbers and percentages for categorical variables, and in median and interquartile range (IQR) for variables with skewed distributions. The Mann–Whitney test was employed to compare medians of the non-normally distributed variables. We utilized Pearson's chi-square test or Yates adjustment for continuity in the study of categorical data.

We used receiver operating characteristic (ROC) analysis to evaluate age as a continuous variable in predicting malignancy, calculating the corresponding sensitivity and specificity. The ideal cutoff age for predicting thyroid nodule malignancy was determined using the Youden index. The Clopper-Pearson technique for binomial distribution was employed to compute confidence bounds for a sample proportion.

For this study, we conducted a univariate analysis to determine the risk variables for malignant cytology, including age, sex, BMI, nodule size, presence of thyroid autoimmune disease, and levothyroxine (LT4) therapy. To determine possible independent risk factors for malignant cytology, a multivariate analytic model was employed. This model utilized logistic regression and considered the ACR TI-RADS categories as a control variable. All thyroid nodules investigated in this study were included in both univariate and multivariate analyses. We further investigated the subgroup of patients where FNA was indicated according to the ACR-TIRADS system.

$p < 0.05$ was used to determine statistical significance and all tests were conducted with a two-tailed approach. The statistical analyses were conducted using MedCalc Statistical Software version 19.2.6 (MedCalc Software Ltd., Ostend, Belgium; https://www.medcalc.org; 2020).

3. Results

A total of 1191 nodules from 1005 patients were initially evaluated. Eight patients were excluded due to age (<18 years) and 55 were excluded due to the absence of ACR-TIRADS classification, resulting in 1128 thyroid nodules from 1001 adult patients who were included in the analysis (Figure 1 for nodules with a clinical indication for FNA). Demographic characteristics of the study population are listed in Table 1. The median age was 48 (IQR, 38–59) years and 865 were females (76.68%). The median nodule diameter was 16.1 mm (IQR, 12–23). The percentage of nodules classified as TR1, TR2, TR3, TR4, and TR5 was 0.1% (n = 1), 1.1% (n = 11), 17.7% (n = 182), 63.8% (n = 656), and 27.1% (n = 278), respectively. The corresponding malignancy rates were 0%, 0%, 8.8%, 22.1%, and 74.1%, respectively (Table 1).

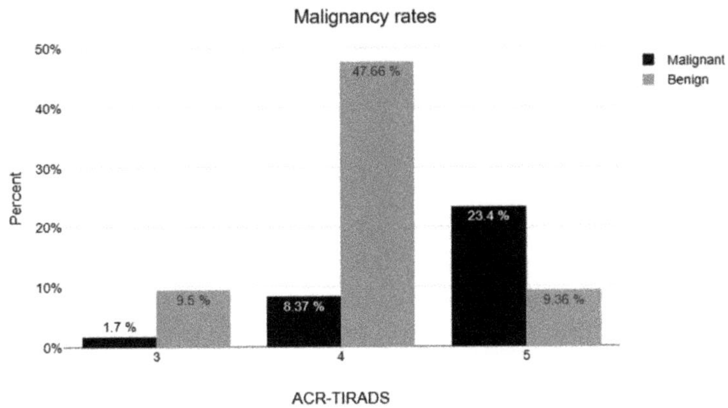

Figure 1. Stratification of the 705 thyroid nodules with an indication for FNA in ACR-TIRADS categories. ACR TI-RADS: American College of Radiology Thyroid Imaging Reporting and Data System. FNA: fine needle aspiration. Percentile refers to the total study population.

Table 1. Characteristics of the study population when categorized based on the ACR TI-RADS risk stratification.

Age, Years	48 (38–59)	
Male sex, n (%)	233 (23.32)	
Nodule size (mm)	16.1 (12–23)	
BMI (kg/m^2)	27.2 (23.9–32)	
Autoimmune thyroiditis, n (%)	269 (23.85)	
Hypothyroidism, n (%)	367 (32.54)	
Indication for FNA, n (%)	705 (62.5)	
ACR TI-RADS categories, n (%)		**Malignant histopathology, n (%)**
1	1 (0.9)	0
2	11 (1.1)	0
3	182 (17.7)	16 (8.8)
4	656 (63.8)	145 (22.1)
5	278 (27.1)	206 (74.1)
Bethesda categories, n (%)		
I	11 (0.9)	1 (9)
II	531 (47.1)	9 (1.7)
III	262 (23.2)	72 (27.5)
IV	33 (2.9)	5 (15.2)
V	145 (12.8)	136 (93.8)
VI	146 (12.9)	144 (98.6)

Stratification revealed a reduction in the malignant cytology rate with advancing age across the subgroups of 18–39, 40–59, and ≥60 years: 37.8%, 21.8%, and 19.1%, respectively (X^2 (2) = 35.49, p < 0.001; Table 2). Details for each Bethesda category are shown in Supplementary Table S1.

Table 2. Age stratification, FNA results, and thyroid malignancy.

Bethesda Category	20–39 y (n = 328)	40–59 y (n = 528)	≥60 y (n = 272)	*p*-Value
Benign (I–II)	110 (33.5%)	272 (51.5%)	160 (58.9%)	<0.001
Indeterminate (III–IV)	94 (28.7%)	141 (26.7%)	60 (22.1%)	0.116
Malignant (V–VI)	124 (37.8%)	115 (21.8%)	52 (19.1%)	<0.001
Confirmed malignancy *	150 (45.7%)	153 (28.9%)	64 (23.5%)	<0.001

Abbreviations: y: age in years, FNA: fine needle aspiration, V, VI: includes both Bethesda V (suspicious for malignancy) and Bethesda VI (malignant) categories, *: malignancy based on the histopathological results.

We also analyzed age as a dichotomous variable and the best cutoff for predicting malignancy was 40.25 years (maximum Youden index: 0.189). The prevalence of malignancy was 45.7% and 26.5% in the <41 (161/352) and ≥41 years (206/776) subgroups, respectively ($p < 0.001$). When adjusted for sex and nodule size, age ≤40.25 years was a risk factor for malignancy compared to age > 40.25 years (odds ratio, OR, 2.26; 95% CI: 1.72–2.97; $p < 0.001$). We conducted a post hoc power analysis to determine whether the sample size was sufficient to detect differences in cytological malignancy rates between age groups in patients where FNA indication exists according to ACR-TIRADS system. With 212 nodules in the younger group (≤40.25 years) and 493 in the older group (>40.25 years), and observed malignancy rates of 48.1% and 27.2% respectively, the calculated statistical power was 100% at a significance level of $\alpha = 0.05$.

Univariate analysis revealed age, sex, and nodule size as risk factors for malignant cytology. For each year of age, there was a 2.33% reduction in the OR for malignant cytology (95% CI: 1.1%–3.1%; $p = < 0.001$). Male sex was associated with increased risk of malignant cytology (OR 1.47, 95% CI: 1.10–1.95; $p = 0.009$), whereas nodule size was a protective factor with OR of 0.94 (0.93–0.96; $p < 0.001$), while BMI, autoimmune thyroiditis, and the use of thyroxine did not show a significant association with malignancy.

The multivariate logistic regression analysis involving 1128 thyroid nodules, adjusted for ACR TI-RADS categories, sex, and nodule size also showed a 2.5% reduction in the OR for malignant cytology for each year of age (Table 3).

Table 3. Risk factors for malignancy, adjusted for the ACR-TIRADS categories.

	Malignancy			**Univariate Analysis**		**Multivariate Analysis**	
	Yes (n = 367)	**No (n = 761)**	**Coefficient B**	**Odds Ratio (95% CI)**	***p***	**Odds Ratio (95% CI)**	***p***
Age, years (median, IQR)	44 (35–55)	50 (40–60)	−0.02	0.98 (0.97–0.99)	<0.001	0.98 (0.97–0.99)	<0.001
Nodule size, mm	13 (10.65–19.2)	18 (13–24)	−0.06	0.94 (0.93–0.96)	<0.001	0.96 (0.95–0.99)	0.01
Male sex, N *	92/324 (28.4)	141/677 (20.8)	0.38	1.47 (1.10–1.95)	0.009	1.42 (0.99–2.01)	0.051
AT, n (%)	92 (25.1)	177 (23.3)			0.504		
Hypothyroidism, n (%)	112 (30.5)	255 (33.5)			0.315		
BMI, kg/m^2	27.00 (23.6–32.42)	27.34 (23.92–31.96)			0.814		

Univariate and multivariate analyses were conducted to assess the influence of age, sex, multinodularity, and nodule size as risk factors for malignant cytology in 1128 thyroid nodules from 1001 patients. These analyses were adjusted for the ACR TI-RADS categories. Data are expressed as median and interquartile range (IQR) and percentiles. Abbreviations: ACR TI-RADS: American College of Radiology Thyroid Imaging Reporting and Data System. AT: autoimmune thyroiditis, BMI: Body Mass Index, n: number of nodules, N *: refers to the number of patients.

We further analyzed data in the subgroup of nodules (705) where FNA was indicated according to their ACR TI-RADS score and diameter (excluding TI-RADS 1 and 2 categories, Figure 1) to estimate potential predictive factors of malignancy in real-world circumstances.

Backward multiple logistic regression analyses were performed to assess the impact of age, sex, nodule size, BMI, autoimmune thyroiditis, and hypothyroidism on the malignant cytology rate of thyroid nodules adjusted for the respective ACR TI-RADS category (Table 4). Intragroup analysis was performed in each group of ACR TI-RADS (TR3, TR4, and TR5) nodules where FNA was indicated (Tables 5–7, respectively).

Table 4. Predictors of malignancy in 705 nodules with indication for FNA according to ACR-TIRADS system.

	Coefficient B	Std. Error	z	OR	95% CI	*p*
Age, years	−0.03	0.01	4.19	0.97	0.96–0.98	<0.001
Hypothyroidism	−0.52	0.24	2.18	0.6	0.37–0.95	0.029
Male sex	0.14	0.24	0.58	1.15	0.72–1.83	0.564
BMI, kg/m^2	0.02	0.02	0.92	1.02	0.98–1.05	0.359
AT	−0.19	0.26	0.72	0.83	0.5–1.38	0.472
Nodule size, mm	0.01	0.01	0.84	1.01	0.98–1.04	0.401

Abbreviations: ACR TI-RADS: American College of Radiology Thyroid Imaging Reporting and Data System. AT: autoimmune thyroiditis, BMI: Body Mass Index, SE: standard error, OR: odds ratio, CI: coefficient interval.

Table 5. Backward logistic regression analysis of predictive factors for malignancy in ACR-TIRADS 3 category nodules.

Variable	Coefficient	Std. Error	Wald	OR	95% CI	*p*
Nodule size, mm	0.16250	0.049951	10.5829	1.176	1.066–1.297	0.001

Significant overall model fit, $p < 0.001$. Variables not included in the model: BMI, Hashimoto, age, hypothyroidism, and gender.

Table 6. Backward logistic regression analysis of predictive factors for malignancy in ACR-TIRADS 4 category nodules.

Variable	Coefficient	Std. Error	Wald	OR	95% CI	*p*
Age	−0.043998	0.011991	13.4629	0.9570	0.934–0.979	0.001
Hypothyroidism	−0.98317	0.39491	6.1981	0.3741	0.172–0.811	0.012

Significant overall model fit. $p < 0.001$. Variables not included in the model: BMI, Hashimoto, nodule size, sex. Prevalence of malignancy is 14.9% (reported by the guidelines: 5–20%).

Table 7. Backward logistic regression analysis of predictive factors for malignancy in ACR-TIRADS 5 category nodules.

Variable	Coefficient	Std. Error	Wald	Odds Ratio	95% CI	*p*
Age	−0.020841	0.010382	4.0295	0.9794	0.9596–0.9995	0.044

Significant overall model fit, $p = 0.043$. Variables not included in the model: BMI, Hashimoto, hypothyroidism, sex, nodule size. Disease prevalence is 71.4% (reported by the guidelines: >20%).

In ACR TI-RADS 3 category nodules, only age was a strong predictor for malignancy (Table 5). ROC analyses revealed a diameter of >34 mm as the cutoff value with the best sensitivity and specificity (Youden index 0.564, sensitivity 83.3%, and specificity 73.1%, Figure 2).

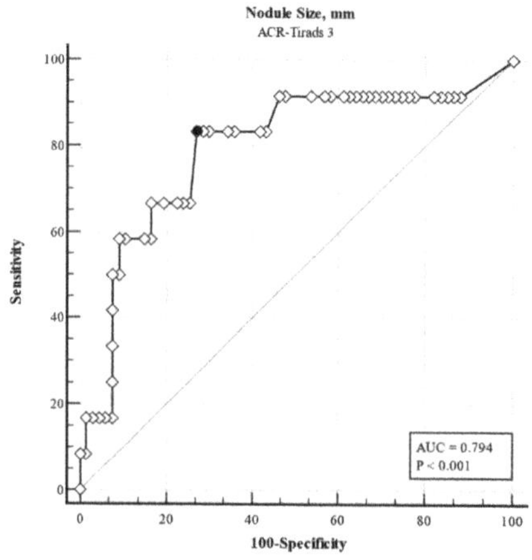

Figure 2. Receiver operating characteristic (ROC) curve illustrating the diagnostic performance of nodule size in predicting cytological malignancy among thyroid nodules classified as ACR TI-RADS category 3 (TR3). The analysis identified an optimal size cutoff of 34 mm, yielding a sensitivity of 83.3% and specificity of 73.1% (area under the curve (AUC) = 0.794). The curve is based on data from 182 nodules with an indication for fine needle aspiration (FNA). Prevalence of malignancy 15.2% (reported by the guidelines: <5%). Youden index 0.564. Abbreviations: ROC, receiver operating characteristic; AUC, area under the curve; TI-RADS, Thyroid Imaging Reporting and Data System; FNA, fine needle aspiration. Black dot = Youden Index.

There was a 4.3% decrease in the odds of malignancy for each year of age increase in patients in the ACR TI-RADS 4 category (Table 6). The odds ratio of 0.374 for hypothyroidism suggested a 62.59% decrease in the odds of the outcome of malignancy in cases without hypothyroidism when the age is the same. For every one-year increase in age, there was a 2.1% decrease in the odds of malignancy for patients in the ACR-TIRADS 5 category (Table 7, Figure 3).

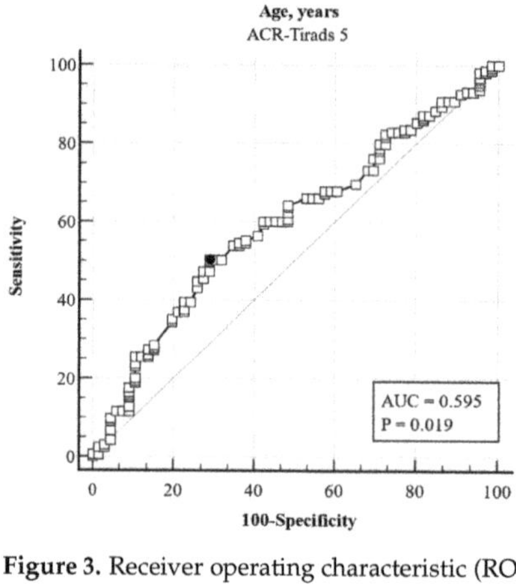

Figure 3. Receiver operating characteristic (ROC) curve assessing the diagnostic value of patient age in predicting cytological malignancy among thyroid nodules classified as ACR TI-RADS category 5 (TR5). The optimal age cutoff, determined by the Youden index (0.215), was ≤43 years. This threshold yielded a sensitivity of 50.3% and specificity of 71.2% for malignancy detection (AUC and 95% CI not shown). Data are derived from a retrospective analysis of 278 nodules evaluated for fine needle aspiration (FNA). Abbreviations: ROC, receiver operating characteristic; TI-RADS, Thyroid Imaging Reporting and Data System; FNA, fine needle aspiration. Black dot = Youden Index.

4. Discussion

Several studies have investigated the impact of clinical variables on the risk of malignancy in fine needle aspiration biopsy (FNAB) cytology of thyroid nodules. Rago et al. found that male sex, single nodularity, and younger age were independent risk factors for malignancy [10]. Angell et al. identified age as a significant predictor with a cutoff of $\leq$52 years associated with increased malignancy risk [5]. Belfiore et al. categorized age into decades and observed higher odds ratios of malignancy in patients $\leq$ 30 years and $\geq$60 years [11]. Similar to our strategy, previous studies that treated age as a continuous variable reported a 2.2% decrease in the relative risk of malignancy per year [4]. There is a growing body of evidence underlying the role of age in sonographic risk estimate of thyroid nodules. Di Fermo et al. demonstrated that while risk stratification systems are applicable in elderly patients, certain systems may underperform in malignancy detection compared to younger cohorts [12]. Similarly, Grani et al. highlighted that sonographic risk stratification systems, including ACR TI-RADS and EU-TIRADS, can serve effectively as rule-out tools in older adults, though their specificity may be influenced by age-related morphological variations [13]. In our study, the age threshold of 40.25 years was statistically derived using the Youden index to optimize discrimination of cytological malignancy risk. Although this cutoff did not directly match previously reported categorical age brackets, it aligns closely with thresholds identified in the literature—such as the $\leq$52-year cutoff reported by Angell et al. [5] and the increased malignancy odds at extreme age groups described by Belfiore et al. [11]. These converging findings suggest that age may affect thyroid cancer risk in a non-linear and possibly complex manner. The biological plausibility of such thresholds may relate to cumulative mutational burden, hormonal shifts, or immune-related mechanisms emerging during the fourth and fifth decades of life. Thus, our data further support the hypothesis that age can meaningfully modify malignancy risk even within standardized ultrasound-based classifications.

Walter et al. reported a significant age-related variation in malignant cytology rates suggesting a lower predictive value of high ACR TI-RADS scores in older populations [14]. Complementing this, Grani et al. validated the ACR TI-RADS performance in transition-age individuals, reinforcing its applicability in younger populations while indirectly pointing to the need for age-adapted thresholds or interpretations in older adults. Collectively, these findings support the integration of age as a modifying factor in the interpretation of ultrasound risk stratification for thyroid nodules [15].

These aforementioned findings, along with our own, highlight the importance of considering age as a key factor in the evaluation and management of thyroid nodules—particularly in cases with suspicious ultrasound features (TR4 and TR5).

Our study also aimed to evaluate the influence of other clinical variables on the malignant cytology rates within the ACR TI-RADS categories, such as BMI, use of thyroxine, and history of autoimmune thyroiditis. Some research suggested that higher BMI may be associated with an increased risk of thyroid cancer, particularly in women [16]. It is hypothesized that this could be due to various factors such as hormonal changes, obesity-related inflammation, and insulin resistance, which are more prevalent in individuals with higher BMI [17]. However, as is the case in our study, higher BMI was found not to be associated with more aggressive tumor features or a greater likelihood of recurrence or persistence over the analyzed period [17].

It is generally believed that higher TSH concentrations are a risk factor for the growth of thyroid nodules and cancer in adults [18], especially in the absence of autoimmunity [19]. Under this aspect, suboptimal thyroxine supplementation may interfere with the prevalence of thyroid malignancy although such a hypothesis has not been demonstrated clinically. Of note, in our cohort, thyroxine use was recommended as a replacement therapy and not as a suppressive therapy for nodular disease. However, TSH levels were not consistently available and were therefore not included in the final analysis. In the subgroup of patients with TR4, the prevalence of malignancy was lower in those with hypothyroidism. Several studies have reported an increased risk of thyroid cancer in patients with primary hypothyroidism [20,21] while others have not [22]. Whether chronic lymphocytic thyroiditis (CLT) is an important risk factor for differentiated thyroid cancer (DTC) remains a topic of debate. Patients with CLT had an increased risk of incidental PTC in studies that investigated surgical specimens [23,24]. Nevertheless, TPO-Ab and Tg-Ab may play a different role in thyroid malignancy. Another study reported that TgAb positivity was significantly associated with an increased risk of papillary thyroid carcinoma (PTC) in females with an OR of 3.532 (95% CI: 1.219–10.233), whereas TPOAb did not show a significant association [25]. In our study, the presence of at least one of the two antithyroid antibodies was considered indicative of autoimmune thyroiditis.

Regarding age-related variation of DTC prevalence, our study has three major strengths compared to the previous report of Walter et al. [14]. First, ACR TI-RADS stratification was performed by each investigator (trained endocrinologist) during the initial comprehensive "real-time" ultrasound examination and was not based on retrospectively examined static images. It is well known that risk stratification systems (RSS) are subject to interobserver variability, which may influence how nodules are categorized [26,27] with agreement ranging from poor to excellent. However, recent reports illustrated an excellent rating agreement between experienced observers [28], such as the well-trained endocrinologists participating in our study. Second, except for ACR TI-RADS categories, we further analyzed the specific predictive factors of malignancy in each ACR TI-RADS group separately. Third, in our cohort, the proportion of undefined cytology was eliminated since we included only patients with Bethesda III and IV in whom a definitive histopathology diagnosis was available after thyroidectomy. However, this criterion inherently favors the selection of surgically managed cases, which are more likely to represent higher-risk nodules. As a result, the malignancy rates observed in these categories may be overestimated and not entirely reflective of the broader population of Bethesda III/IV nodules encountered in routine clinical practice. This selection bias limits the generalizability of our findings and highlights the need for prospective studies that include conservatively managed nodules within these cytological categories.

Although histopathology after thyroid surgery remains the gold standard of the diagnosis of malignancy, FNA is still the first step to evaluate the malignancy potential with significant diagnostic accuracy with sensitivity and specificity ranging between 65 and 98% and 72 and 100%, respectively [29]. As mentioned, it should be noted that our cohort has a limited number of undefined cytology, since in such cases, either FNA was repeated or surgery was performed, diminishing the effect of undetermined samples on the interpretation of our results. Compared to previous studies, the prevalence of suspicious FNA results was higher in our patients [14]. The main difference was observed in the ACR TI-RADS 3 category (15.2% compared to <2.5%). This alteration may be attributed to our focused assessment of the echogenicity of the nodules. Indeed, the assignment of hypoechogenicity ranged from 19 to 69% in a multi-institutional registry [30]. Assignment of hypoechoic or very hypoechoic echogenicity adds a further 2 to 3 points, moving a TR2 nodule that does not warrant FNA to TR3 or even TR4 category. In this subgroup of patients, nodule size heralds further investigation with FNA. We observed a threshold of 34 mm in nodule size, associated with a sensitivity of 83.3% and specificity of 73.1% for thyroid malignancy. This finding suggests that the currently recommended 25 mm cutoff for FNA indication in TR3 nodules may merit further evaluation in future prospective studies.

The ACR TI-RADS White Paper predicts cancer risks of <2%, <5%, 5–20%, and >20% in TR1–2, TR3, TR4, and TR5 thyroid nodules, respectively [6]. Here, we observed higher malignancy rates comparable to those reported in the ACR TI-RADS guidelines: <1.0%, 15%, 31%, and 86% for TR1-2, TR3, TR4, and TR5, respectively. This should be attributed to our selection criteria since over 60% of the enrolled patients in our study fulfilled evidence-based indications for FNA, based on ACR-TIRADS criteria, while other studies might have involved more specimens from unnecessarily performed FNA biopsies.

In the present study, 423 nodules (37.5%) underwent FNA without a clear indication according to the ACR TI-RADS published guidelines; 79 (7%) of them were small nodules (<10 mm) but with suspicious ultrasound characteristics. Clinicians performed FNA for another 129 (30.5%) nodules with diameters >10 mm without following the ACR TI-RADS published guidelines. This discrepancy is in line with other reports [31] showing that using an RSS reduces unneeded biopsies (57 from 100) compared to using published ACR TI-RADS guidelines (80/100). Further, in a prospective analysis of 502 nodules, Grani et al. found that the "right" TI-RADS avoided unnecessary biopsies in more nodules than other systems [32].

Our study has some limitations that should be discussed. The histotype of thyroid cancer can influence the pre-operative neck US results, also when several RSS were considered, including ACR-TIRADS [33]. In the present study, only papillary thyroid carcinoma (PTC) cases were assessed. This should be stated as a limitation, as it may affect the generalizability of the findings. Another limitation of our study is that no comparison was made among cytologists' diagnoses across different centers and no interobserver agreement coefficient was calculated. This may have affected the consistency and reliability of the cytological evaluations. In our study, semantic sonographic features were evaluated based on standard descriptive terms and standardized sonographic lexicon was not applied for the definition of semantic ultrasound features, which could have affected the consistency and reproducibility of the results [34,35]. Additionally, no formal assessment of interobserver variability was performed for the ACR TI-RADS classification of nodules, despite the well-known variability in sonographic interpretation among observers. To mitigate this, all ultrasound evaluations were conducted by board-certified endocrinologists with experience in thyroid imaging, following the official ACR TI-RADS guidelines. Internal training sessions were held at the beginning of the study to align classification practices across centers. Nevertheless, the absence of objective inter-rater agreement analysis remains a limitation and should be addressed in future prospective research. Lastly, as previously reported, in several nodules, fine needle aspiration cytology (FNAC) was performed without strict adherence to the indications of the risk stratification system (RSS) used. Although we did not conduct a separate analysis excluding these cases, future studies should consider doing so to more accurately reflect the real-world applicability and diagnostic performance of the system. For example, the malignancy rate observed for TR3 nodules in our study (~15%) is substantially higher than the <5% rate reported in the ACR TI-RADS guidelines. This likely reflects a referral and diagnostic bias, as our cohort included only nodules that underwent FNA or surgery, potentially skewing the risk estimate toward higher values.

5. Conclusions

Modifications to the current ACR TI-RADS may be warranted as new data become available. Potential modification could involve adjusting point assignments for certain features [36] and nodule location [37]. Given the typically slow-growing nature of thyroid cancer and the success of active surveillance strategies, our findings raise the hypothesis that increasing the size threshold for recommending FNA of TR3 nodules—particularly in certain subgroups—may help reduce unnecessary procedures. Moreover, incorporating clinical variables such as patient age and gender into risk assessment could potentially enhance the performance of the ACR TI-RADS system, as both our data and previous studies [14] have suggested higher malignancy risk in younger individuals and males. However, these observations should be interpreted with caution and viewed as hypothesis-generating. Prospective, multicenter studies are needed to validate whether such modifications can improve risk stratification and clinical decision-making (Figure 4).

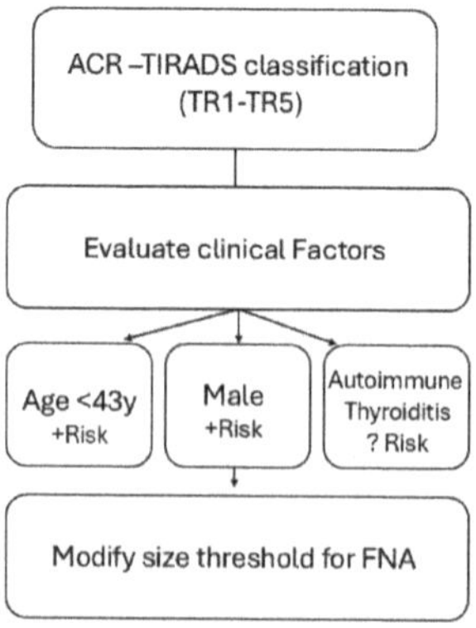

Figure 4. Proposed framework for integrating clinical variables into ACR TI-RADS-based malignancy risk estimation.

Supplementary Materials: The following supporting information can be downloaded at: https://www.mdpi.com/article/10.3390/jcm14155352/s1, Table S1: Age stratification and Malignancy.

Author Contributions: N.A., S.L., R.D.P., and J.C.J. contributed to the conception and design of the study; acquisition, analysis, interpretation of data; and drafting; I.A., D.P.A., N.V., A.B., V.P., D.Z., D.B., and A.R. contributed to acquisition of data. All authors contributed to revision of the article, approved the final version, and had the final responsibility for the decision to submit for publication. All authors have read and agreed to the published version of the manuscript.

Funding: This research received no external funding.

Institutional Review Board Statement: This study was approved by the Hellenic Endocrine Network Institutional Review Board (Protocol Number: 2024/0121314) on 10 March 2024. The Institutional Review Board waived the requirement for written informed consent due to the retrospective nature and the minimal risks associated with this study. The study was conducted under the standards of the Declaration of Helsinki.

Informed Consent Statement: Patient consent was waived due to the nature of the study.

Data Availability Statement: Data are available from the corresponding author upon reasonable request.

Conflicts of Interest: The authors declare no conflicts of interest.

References

1. Russ, G.; Leboulleux, S.; Leenhardt, L.; Hegedüs, L. Thyroid Incidentalomas: Epidemiology, Risk Stratification with Ultrasound and Workup. *Eur. Thyroid J.* **2014**, *3*, 154–163. [CrossRef]
2. Sosa, J.A.; Hanna, J.W.; Robinson, K.A.; Lanman, R.B. Increases in Thyroid Nodule Fine-Needle Aspirations, Operations, and Diagnoses of Thyroid Cancer in the United States. *Surgery* **2013**, *154*, 1420–1426; discussion 1426–1427. [CrossRef] [PubMed]
3. Durante, C.; Grani, G.; Lamartina, L.; Filetti, S.; Mandel, S.J.; Cooper, D.S. The Diagnosis and Management of Thyroid Nodules. *JAMA* **2018**, *319*, 914. [CrossRef] [PubMed]

4. Kwong, N.; Medici, M.; Angell, T.E.; Liu, X.; Marqusee, E.; Cibas, E.S.; Krane, J.F.; Barletta, J.A.; Kim, M.I.; Larsen, P.R.; et al. The Influence of Patient Age on Thyroid Nodule Formation, Multinodularity, and Thyroid Cancer Risk. *J. Clin. Endocrinol. Metab.* **2015**, *100*, 4434–4440. [CrossRef] [PubMed]
5. Angell, T.E.; Maurer, R.; Wang, Z.; Kim, M.I.; Alexander, C.A.; Barletta, J.A.; Benson, C.B.; Cibas, E.S.; Cho, N.L.; Doherty, G.M.; et al. A Cohort Analysis of Clinical and Ultrasound Variables Predicting Cancer Risk in 20,001 Consecutive Thyroid Nodules. *J. Clin. Endocrinol. Metab.* **2019**, *104*, 5665–5672. [CrossRef]
6. Tessler, F.N.; Middleton, W.D.; Grant, E.G.; Hoang, J.K.; Berland, L.L.; Teefey, S.A.; Cronan, J.J.; Beland, M.D.; Desser, T.S.; Frates, M.C.; et al. ACR Thyroid Imaging, Reporting and Data System (TI-RADS): White Paper of the ACR TI-RADS Committee. *J. Am. Coll. Radiol.* **2017**, *14*, 587–595. [CrossRef]
7. Russ, G.; Bonnema, S.J.; Erdogan, M.; Durante, C.; Ngu, R.; Leenhardt, L. European Thyroid Association Guidelines for Ultrasound Malignancy Risk Stratification of Thyroid Nodules in Adults: The EU-TIRADS. *Eur. Thyroid J.* **2017**, *6*, 225–237. [CrossRef]
8. Eidt, L.B.; de Oliveira, C.N.; De Lagos, Y.B.B.; Solera, G.L.M.; Izquierdo, R.; Meyer, E.L.d.S.; Mattevi, V.S.; Golbert, L. A Prospective Comparison of ACR-TIRADS and EU-TIRADS in Thyroid Nodule Assessment for FNA-US. *Clin. Endocrinol.* **2022**, *98*, 415–425. [CrossRef]
9. Cibas, E.S.; Ali, S.Z. The Bethesda System for Reporting Thyroid Cytopathology. *Am. J. Clin. Pathol.* **2009**, *132*, 658–665. [CrossRef]
10. Rago, T.; Fiore, E.; Scutari, M.; Santini, F.; Di Coscio, G.; Romani, R.; Piaggi, P.; Ugolini, C.; Basolo, F.; Miccoli, P.; et al. Male Sex, Single Nodularity, and Young Age Are Associated with the Risk of Finding a Papillary Thyroid Cancer on Fine-Needle Aspiration Cytology in a Large Series of Patients with Nodular Thyroid Disease. *Eur. J. Endocrinol.* **2010**, *162*, 763–770. [CrossRef]
11. Belfiore, A.; La Rosa, G.L.; La Porta, G.A.; Giuffrida, D.; Milazzo, G.; Lupo, L.; Regalbuto, C.; Vigneri, R. Cancer Risk in Patients with Cold Thyroid Nodules: Relevance of Iodine Intake, Sex, Age, and Multinodularity. *Am. J. Med.* **1992**, *93*, 363–369. [CrossRef]
12. Di Fermo, F.; Sforza, N.; Rosmarin, M.; Morosan Allo, Y.; Parisi, C.; Santamaria, J.; Pacenza, N.; Zuk, C.; Faingold, C.; Ferraro, F.; et al. Comparison of Different Systems of Ultrasound (US) Risk Stratification for Malignancy in Elderly Patients with Thyroid Nodules. Real World Experience. *Endocrine* **2020**, *69*, 331–338. [CrossRef] [PubMed]
13. Grani, G.; Brenta, G.; Trimboli, P.; Falcone, R.; Ramundo, V.; Maranghi, M.; Lucia, P.; Filetti, S.; Durante, C. Sonographic Risk Stratification Systems for Thyroid Nodules as Rule-out Tests in Older Adults. *Cancers* **2020**, *12*, 2458. [CrossRef] [PubMed]
14. Walter, L.B.; Fernandes, P.M.; Strieder, D.L.; Scheinpflug, A.L.; Zanella, A.B.; Faccin, C.S.; Farenzena, M.; Xavier, L.F.; Zorzi, B.D.C.; Graudenz, M.S.; et al. Age-Related Variation in Malignant Cytology Rates of Thyroid Nodules: Insights from a Retrospective Observational Study Assessing the ACR TI-RADS. *Eur. J. Endocrinol.* **2023**, *189*, 584–589. [CrossRef] [PubMed]
15. Grani, G.; Stramazzo, I.; Locantore, P.; Virili, C.; Filardi, T.; Lecis, C.; Centello, R.; Cera, G.; Santaguida, M.G.; Gianfrilli, D.; et al. Validation of ACR TI-RADS Performance in Transition Age: Results from a Multicenter Retrospective Study by the TALENT Study Group. *Endocrine* **2024**, *87*, 1131–1140. [CrossRef]
16. Shin, A.; Cho, S.; Jang, D.; Abe, S.K.; Saito, E.; Rahman, S.; Islam, R.; Sawada, N.; Shu, X.-O.; Koh, W.-P.; et al. Body Mass Index and Thyroid Cancer Risk: A Pooled Analysis of Half a Million Men and Women in the Asia Cohort Consortium. *Thyroid* **2022**, *32*, 306–314. [CrossRef]
17. Paes, J.; Hua, K.; Nagy, R.J.; Kloos, R.T.; Jarjoura, D.; Ringel, M.D. The Relationship between Body Mass Index and Thyroid Cancer Pathology Features and Outcomes: A Clinicopathological Cohort Study. *J. Clin. Endocrinol. Metab.* **2010**, *95*, 4244–4250. [CrossRef]
18. Fiore, E.; Vitti, P. Serum TSH and Risk of Papillary Thyroid Cancer in Nodular Thyroid Disease. *J. Clin. Endocrinol. Metab.* **2012**, *97*, 1134–1145. [CrossRef]
19. Paparodis, R.D.; Bantouna, D.; Karvounis, E.; Imam, S.; Jaume, J.C. Higher TSH Is Not Associated with Thyroid Cancer Risk in the Presence of Thyroid Autoimmunity. *J. Clin. Endocrinol. Metab.* **2020**, *105*, e2389–e2397. [CrossRef]
20. Falstie-Jensen, A.M.; Kjærsgaard, A.; Lorenzen, E.L.; Jensen, J.D.; Reinertsen, K.V.; Dekkers, O.M.; Ewertz, M.; Cronin-Fenton, D.P. Hypothyroidism and the Risk of Breast Cancer Recurrence and All-Cause Mortality—A Danish Population-Based Study. *Breast Cancer Res.* **2019**, *21*, 44. [CrossRef]
21. Fiore, E.; Rago, T.; Latrofa, F.; Provenzale, M.A.; Piaggi, P.; Delitala, A.; Scutari, M.; Basolo, F.; Di Coscio, G.; Grasso, L.; et al. Hashimoto's Thyroiditis Is Associated with Papillary Thyroid Carcinoma: Role of TSH and of Treatment with L-Thyroxine. *Endocr.-Relat. Cancer* **2011**, *18*, 429–437. [CrossRef] [PubMed]
22. Kitahara, C.M.; Körmendiné Farkas, D.; Jørgensen, J.O.L.; Cronin-Fenton, D.; Sørensen, H.T. Benign Thyroid Diseases and Risk of Thyroid Cancer: A Nationwide Cohort Study. *J. Clin. Endocrinol. Metab.* **2018**, *103*, 2216–2224. [CrossRef] [PubMed]
23. Krzentowska, A.; Konturek, A.; Gołkowski, F.; Merklinger-Gruchała, A.; Barczyński, M. Risk Stratification for Thyroid Malignancies in Chronic Lymphocytic Thyroiditis. *Cancers* **2025**, *17*, 1964. [CrossRef]
24. Jackson, D.; Handelsman, R.S.; Farrá, J.C.; Lew, J.I. Increased Incidental Thyroid Cancer in Patients with Subclinical Chronic Lymphocytic Thyroiditis. *J. Surg. Res.* **2020**, *245*, 115–118. [CrossRef] [PubMed]
25. Peng, X.; Zhu, X.; Cheng, F.; Zhou, B.; Zhu, X.; Zhu, L. Correlation between Thyroid Autoantibodies and the Risk of Thyroid Papillary Carcinoma. *Gland Surg.* **2020**, *9*, 950–955. [CrossRef]

26. Srinivas, M.N.S.; Amogh, V.N.; Gautam, M.S.; Prathyusha, I.S.; Vikram, N.R.; Retnam, M.K.; Balakrishna, B.V.; Kudva, N. A Prospective Study to Evaluate the Reliability of Thyroid Imaging Reporting and Data System in Differentiation between Benign and Malignant Thyroid Lesions. *J. Clin. Imaging Sci.* **2016**, *6*, 5. [CrossRef]
27. Grani, G.; Lamartina, L.; Ascoli, V.; Bosco, D.; Biffoni, M.; Giacomelli, L.; Maranghi, M.; Falcone, R.; Ramundo, V.; Cantisani, V.; et al. Reducing the Number of Unnecessary Thyroid Biopsies While Improving Diagnostic Accuracy: Toward the "Right" TIRADS. *J. Clin. Endocrinol. Metab.* **2018**, *104*, 95–102. [CrossRef]
28. Seifert, P.; Görges, R.; Zimny, M.; Kreissl, M.C.; Schenke, S. Interobserver Agreement and Efficacy of Consensus Reading in Kwak-, EU-, and ACR-Thyroid Imaging Recording and Data Systems and ATA Guidelines for the Ultrasound Risk Stratification of Thyroid Nodules. *Endocrine* **2019**, *67*, 143–154. [CrossRef]
29. Gharib, H. Fine-Needle Aspiration Biopsy of the Thyroid: An Appraisal. *Ann. Intern. Med.* **1993**, *118*, 282. [CrossRef]
30. Hoang, J.K.; Middleton, W.D.; Langer, J.E.; Schmidt, K.; Gillis, L.B.; Nair, S.S.; Watts, J.A.; Snyder, R.W.; Khot, R.; Rawal, U.; et al. Comparison of Thyroid Risk Categorization Systems and Fine-Needle Aspiration Recommendations in a Multi-Institutional Thyroid Ultrasound Registry. *J. Am. Coll. Radiol.* **2021**, *18*, 1605–1613. [CrossRef]
31. Hoang, J.K.; Middleton, W.D.; Farjat, A.E.; Langer, J.E.; Reading, C.C.; Teefey, S.A.; Abinanti, N.; Boschini, F.J.; Bronner, A.J.; Dahiya, N.; et al. Reduction in Thyroid Nodule Biopsies and Improved Accuracy with American College of Radiology Thyroid Imaging Reporting and Data System. *Radiology* **2018**, *287*, 185–193. [CrossRef]
32. Grani, G.; Lamartina, L.; Cantisani, V.; Maranghi, M.; Lucia, P.; Durante, C. Interobserver Agreement of Various Thyroid Imaging Reporting and Data Systems. *Endocr. Connect.* **2018**, *7*, 1–7. [CrossRef]
33. Matrone, A.; Gambale, C.; Pieroni, E.; De Napoli, L.; Torregrossa, L.; Materazzi, G.; Elisei, R. Ultrasound Features and Risk Stratification System in NIFT-P and Other Follicular-Patterned Thyroid Tumors. *Eur. J. Endocrinol.* **2023**, *189*, 175–182. [CrossRef] [PubMed]
34. Luiz, R.; Assumpção, L.; Paiva, F.; Teixeira, S. Does a Three-Degree Hypoechogenicity Grading Improve Ultrasound Thyroid Nodule Risk Stratification and Affect the TI-RADS 4 Category? A Retrospective Observational Study. *Arch. Endocrinol. Metab.* **2023**, *67*, e000608. [CrossRef]
35. Grant, E.G.; Tessler, F.N.; Hoang, J.K.; Langer, J.E.; Beland, M.D.; Berland, L.L.; Cronan, J.J.; Desser, T.S.; Frates, M.C.; Hamper, U.M.; et al. Thyroid Ultrasound Reporting Lexicon: White Paper of the ACR Thyroid Imaging, Reporting and Data System (TIRADS) Committee. *J. Am. Coll. Radiol.* **2015**, *12*, 1272–1279. [CrossRef] [PubMed]
36. Teefey, S.A.; Middleton, W.D.; Reading, C.C.; Langer, J.E.; Beland, M.D.; Szabunio, M.M.; Desser, T.S. Effect of Decreasing the ACR TI-RADS Point Assignment for Punctate Echogenic Foci When They Occur in Mixed Solid and Cystic Thyroid Nodules. *Am. J. Roentgenol.* **2021**, *216*, 479–485. [CrossRef]
37. Jasim, S.; Baranski, T.J.; Teefey, S.A.; Middleton, W.D. Investigating the Effect of Thyroid Nodule Location on the Risk of Thyroid Cancer. *Thyroid* **2020**, *30*, 401–407. [CrossRef]

Journal of
Clinical Medicine

MDPI

Review

Circulating Biomarkers in Medullary Thyroid Carcinoma: Bridging Laboratory Complexities and Clinical Application Through Algorithm Design

Luca Giovanella [1,2,3,*], Federica D'Aurizio [4] and Petra Petranović Ovčariček [5,6]

1 Department of Nuclear Medicine and Thyroid Diseases, Gruppo Ospedaliero Moncucco, 6900 Lugano, Switzerland
2 Department of Nuclear Medicine and Thyroid Centre, University Hospital of Zurich, 8091 Zurich, Switzerland
3 Department of Clinical Chemistry and Endocrinology, Medysin, 6000 Luzern, Switzerland
4 Department of Laboratory Medicine, Udine University Hospital, 33100 Udine, Italy; federica.daurizio@asufc.sanita.fvg.it
5 Department of Oncology and Nuclear Medicine, University Hospital Center Sestre Milosrdnice, 10000 Zagreb, Croatia; p.petranovic@gmail.com
6 School of Medicine, University of Zagreb, 10000 Zagreb, Croatia
* Correspondence: luca.giovanella@moncucco.ch; Tel.: +41-91-811005; Fax: +41-91-811006

Abstract: Medullary thyroid carcinoma (MTC) is a rare (~2–5% of all thyroid cancers) neuroendocrine thyroid malignancy originating from parafollicular C-cells of the thyroid gland with variable biological behavior and potential for early metastasis. Diagnosis, staging, and surveillance are heavily reliant on circulating biomarkers. We aimed to provide a comprehensive overview of circulating biomarkers in the management of MTC and propose an integrated, evidence-based algorithm to guide clinical decision-making using both established and emerging biomarkers. This is a narrative review on the evolving landscape of biomarker-driven management in MTC with emphasis on analytical advancements, clinical applications, and the prognostic implications of individual and combined biomarkers. Calcitonin remains the cornerstone biomarker for MTC, and new generation immunoassays have addressed several pre-analytical and analytical challenges such as pre-analytical degradation, inter-assay variability, and biological confounders. Procalcitonin (ProCT) has emerged as a stable and less interference-prone alternative or adjunct to calcitonin, which is particularly useful in cases with indeterminate calcitonin levels. Carcinoembryonic antigen (CEA) remains a useful complementary biomarker often correlating with aggressive behavior, advanced disease, and distant metastases. Kinetic evaluation (doubling times) of calcitonin and CEA offers independent prognostic information values and those < 6 months are associated with poor survival, whereas those > 2 years suggest favorable outcomes. Newer biomarkers such as pro-gastrin-releasing peptide (ProGRP) and carbohydrate antigen 19-9 (CA19-9) show potential in monitoring advanced disease and response to therapy. Their role is still under investigation but appears promising, particularly when used in conjunction with calcitonin and CEA. Our work advances a comprehensive and clinically pragmatic framework for the management of MTC by integrating established and emerging biomarkers with evidence-based algorithms, offering greater diagnostic precision, more reliable prognostic stratification, and improved personalization of follow-up and treatment strategies.

Keywords: medullary thyroid carcinoma; calcitonin; procalcitonin; carcinoembryonic antigen; biomarkers; doubling time; immunoassay; pro-gastrin-releasing peptide; diagnostic algorithms

1. Introduction

Medullary thyroid carcinoma is a rare C-cell-derived neuroendocrine tumor accounting for ~0.5–1.5% of thyroid nodules, ~2–5% of thyroid cancers, and ~0.15% of thyroid nodules incidentally discovered during autopsies of subjects who died from thyroid-unrelated conditions [1]. MTC exhibits a strong genetic component, particularly through mutations in the rearranged during transfection (RET) proto-oncogene.

1.1. Hereditary MTC and Related Syndromes

Hereditary MTC forms (~25% of cases) are caused by inherited autosomal dominant germline pathogenic variants in the RET proto-oncogene and are subclassified into Multiple Endocrine Neoplasia (MEN) type 2A and type 2B and Familial MTC (FMTC), respectively. MEN2A includes MTC, pheochromocytoma, and hyperparathyroidism (due to parathyroid hyperplasia or multiple adenomas); MEN2B (more aggressive) combines MTC, pheochromocytoma, mucosal neuromas, and marfanoid habitus; and FMTC presents as isolated MTC without other endocrine tumors [2,3]. Hereditary MTC is typically multifocal and bilateral, with variable penetrance and biological/clinical behavior, respectively [4]. Finally, pediatric MTC is exceedingly rare, and inherited cases of MEN 2 are involved in almost all cases [5]. Notably, identification of different RET pathogenic variants improved understanding of the natural course of disease, allowing predictive diagnosis, prophylactic thyroidectomy in pathogenic variants carriers, and targeted therapy with selective RET inhibitors (i.e., selpercatinib and pralsetinib) in advanced or progressive RET-mutant MTC (Table 1).

Table 1. RET-related syndromes: pathogenic variants/phenotypes correlations.

RET Codon/Exon	Syndrome	Clinical Features	Behavior
634 (Exon 11)	MEN2A	MTC, Pheochromocytoma, Hyperparathyroidism	Aggressive behavior
609, 611, 618, 620 (Exon 10)	MEN2A, FMTC	MTC ± Pheochromocytoma	Moderate aggressiveness
768 (Exon 13), 804 (Exon 14), 891 (Exon 15)	FMTC	MTC (only)	Low–moderate aggressiveness
918 (Exon 16)	MEN2B	Early, aggressive, MTC mucosal neuromas, marfanoid habitus	Early onset, highly aggressive

Legend: RET, rearranged during transfection; MEN, multiple endocrine neoplasia; FMTC, familial medullary thyroid carcinoma; MTC, medullary thyroid carcinoma.

1.2. Sporadic Medullary Thyroid Carcinoma

Sporadic MTC represents ~75% of MTC cases and it is usually unilateral and unifocal and presents later in life, often diagnosed due to thyroid nodules, cervical lymphadenopathy, and/or serum calcitonin screening. Notably, germline RET pathogenic variants (often "de novo") are found in up to 5–7% of sporadic MTC cases that have major implications for familial inherited risk and management decisions. Moreover, about 50–60% of patients with sporadic MTC without germline pathogenic variants may carry somatic pathogenic variants, commonly involving codon M918T, which is associated with more aggressive disease and poorer prognosis. Finally, activating pathogenic variants in RAS genes (HRAS, KRAS, NRAS) have been identified in RET-negative sporadic MTC, often linked with a more indolent course compared to RET-driven tumors. Accordingly, genetic testing for RET pathogenic variants is recommended in all patients with a personal medical history of primary C-cell hyperplasia, MTC, or MEN 2 syndrome, respectively.

1.3. Clinical Presentation and Course of the Disease

MTC typically presents as a thyroid nodule, which is occasionally discovered by patients or physicians during a routine clinical examination. Currently, thyroid nodules are mainly detected during thyroid-unrelated imaging procedures, such as ultrasound (US) and vascular studies, computed tomography (CT), magnetic resonance (MR), and positron emission tomography (PET), coupled with CT (PET/CT) or MR (PET/MR). Diagnostic algorithms for MTC are still debated (see below). MTC can metastasize via both lymphatic and hematogenous routes, which contribute to a clinical course that is generally more aggressive than that of differentiated thyroid carcinomas and typically less severe than anaplastic thyroid carcinoma [6]. Treatment of MTC primarily involves total thyroidectomy with central neck lymph node dissection, as surgery remains the only curative option. More extensive lymphadenectomy may be required in cases of locally advanced or metastatic disease. Unlike differentiated thyroid cancers, MTC does not respond to radioactive iodine or thyroid-stimulating hormone suppression therapy. For patients with progressive or symptomatic metastatic disease, systemic therapies such as tyrosine kinase inhibitors (e.g., vandetanib and cabozantinib) have demonstrated clinical benefit by targeting RET pathogenic variants and other pathways involved in tumor growth. Recently, highly selective RET inhibitors like selpercatinib and pralsetinib have shown promising efficacy in RET-mutated MTC. Supportive care and close biochemical and imaging monitoring are essential for ongoing management and early detection of recurrence. Disease-specific mortality at 10 years has been reported to range between 13% and 40%, with overall 10-year survival potentially declining to as low as 50% in some instances [7]. Several prognostic factors, as older age and advanced tumor stage at presentation, have been associated with increased disease-specific mortality [8]. Conversely, early detection and the absence of extra-thyroidal extension are generally associated with more favorable outcomes, with survival rates reaching up to 90% over a 35-year period, as reported in some series [9,10]. Thyroid parafollicular C-cells produce calcitonin, a highly sensitive circulating biomarker adopted as standard of care for the diagnosis and the follow-up of MTC. Moreover, parafollicular C-cells also produce the calcitonin precursor ProCT and several peptides, such as CEA, ProGRP, chromogranin A, neuron-specific enolase, and CA19-9, respectively. Despite its pivotal role, calcitonin measurement is subject to several analytical limitations and interferences that may lead to false-positive or false-negative results, complicating the interpretation of calcitonin results and potentially impacting clinical decisions [11]. Some alternative biomarkers have been proposed to complement or even substitute calcitonin in evaluating MTC patients. This is a narrative review on the evolving landscape of biomarker-driven management in MTC, with emphasis on analytical advancements, clinical applications, and the prognostic implications of individual and combined biomarkers. We aimed to provide a comprehensive overview of circulating biomarkers in the management of MTC and advance a comprehensive and clinically pragmatic framework for the management of MTC by integrating established and emerging biomarkers with evidence-based algorithms to offer greater diagnostic precision, more reliable prognostic stratification, and improved personalization of follow-up and treatment strategies.

2. Biomarkers of Medullary Thyroid Carcinoma

2.1. Calcitonin

Parafollicular thyroid C-cells uniquely secrete calcitonin, a 32-amino-acid peptide hormone, making serum calcitonin levels pivotal for the management of MTC. Serum calcitonin assays include radioactive (IRMA) and non-radioactive (IMA) immunometric methodologies, each varying in sensitivity, specificity, and susceptibility to interferences. Further complicating quantification, calcitonin circulates as multiple isoforms and fragments that some assays fail to detect, impairing inter-assay comparability. Notably, new-generation calcitonin assays, particularly the latest immunochemiluminometric assays (ICMAs) on automated platforms, have significantly enhanced analytical performance, thereby improving their clinical utility. In particular they minimize interferences with calcitonin precursors, enhancing specificity for mature monomeric calcitonin. Moreover, they enable ultrasensitive detection (i.e., <2 pg/mL), allowing for the reliable identification of subtly elevated basal calcitonin levels [11]. Finally, automated platforms offer high throughput, high sensitivity, and full automation, often integrating with laboratory automation systems. They streamline the testing process, reducing manual intervention and potential errors [12]. Additionally, calcitonin measurement also presents analytical challenges which can reduce assay accuracy and inter-method comparability [13], as detailed here.

- *Pre-analytical factors:* Serum proteases can degrade the calcitonin molecule, necessitating rapid sample processing, refrigerated storage, or use of protease inhibitors [14].
- *Biological confounders:* Hypergastrinemia, chronic renal insufficiency, proton-pump inhibitor therapy, cigarette smoke, pregnancy, and lactation may elevate calcitonin in the absence of MTC [15].

Moreover, mild calcitonin elevations can be observed in non-malignant conditions, including C-cell hyperplasia, various non-thyroid neuroendocrine neoplasms (i.e., pancreatic NETs), leukemias, systemic mastocytosis, small-cell lung carcinoma, breast and pancreatic cancers, renal dysfunction, primary hyperparathyroidism, and autoimmune thyroiditis (even if the latter association is currently debated) [16,17].

- *Inter-assay variability:* Comparability across platforms remains imperfect; consistent laboratory/method use is critical for serial monitoring [18].
- *Immunoassay interferences:* Rare heterophilic antibodies may still skew results, underscoring the importance of selecting the appropriate assay and performing repeat testing. Serum pretreatment in heterophilic antibody blocking tubes may detect the interference by lowering the measured calcitonin [19].
- *Hook effect:* It may paradoxically under-report calcitonin in patients with very high levels; its mitigation requires serial serum dilution protocols in high-range samples [20].

2.1.1. Calcitonin Stimulation Testing

In order to increase the specificity of serum calcitonin values and decrease false-positive results, calcitonin stimulation testing was proposed and widely adopted in the past. Traditionally, stimulation with pentagastrin was used with the intention to exclude MTC in patients with basal calcitonin in the gray zone (i.e., 10–100 pg/mL) and detect a residual response after surgery which indicates the need for additional, more aggressive, reinterventions. Pentagastrin has not been available for many years and high-dose calcium gluconate test (2.5 mg/kg) has been proposed as a reliable alternative. It is an effective stimulus which is even more potent than pentagastrin with fewer side effects. Notably, setting reliable cutoffs for either pentagastrin or calcium-stimulated cutoff values was substantially unsuccessful, with large differences reported in the literature. Recent studies have proven that stimulating calcitonin offers, in general, no additional value compared to basal-CT measurement with new generation immunoassay. On the other hand, it may be useful in selected cases, especially in determining the timing of prophylactic thyroidectomy in carriers of germline pathogenic RET variants [21].

In summary, the new generation calcitonin assays improve early detection, reduce false-positives, and simplify the diagnostic trajectory of MTC. Greater baseline sensitivity and gender-specific thresholds further narrow the "gray zone," making basal-only protocols viable in most cases [1].

2.1.2. Calcitonin Thresholds and Clinical Decision Limits

Notably, men and women exhibit consistent differences in basal calcitonin levels, driven by biological factors that significantly inform both clinical interpretation and diagnostic thresholds. These differences are likely related to the different mass of C-cells in males compared to females (ratio ~2:1). Additionally, testosterone may stimulate C-cell proliferation. In contrast, no analogous effect is observed with female sex hormones [22]. An extensive population study (n ≈ 10,500 subjects) showed a mean calcitonin value of ~2.3 pg/mL in men vs. ~1.9 pg/mL in women ($p < 0.001$), even after excluding confounding conditions, with 95th percentile reference thresholds for healthy non-smoking adults of ~5.7 pg/mL in men and ~3.6 pg/mL in women, respectively. Accordingly, gender-specific **calcitonin** thresholds are required to avoid biochemical misclassifications [23]. Similarly, gender-specific peak thresholds should be generated for pentagastrin/calcium stimulation tests [i.e., ~80 pg/mL (women) vs. ~500 pg/mL (men)] [22]. Finally, smoking slightly elevates **calcitonin** in males (non-smoker ~2.4 pg/mL vs. smoker ~2.8 pg/mL; $p < 0.001$) while women show no smoking-related increase. Thus, in men reference thresholds may be further stratified by smoking status (e.g., smoker cutoff ~7.9 pg/mL vs. 2.8 pg/mL) [23]. All in all, applying higher male thresholds reduces unnecessary follow-ups and surgeries, while maintaining high detection rates for MTC and minimizing overdiagnosis. Accordingly, false-positive rates of ~1.8% in men vs. ~1.3% in women were reported in a large screening cohort [24]. Importantly, with new sensitive assays and sex-adjusted interpretation, many guidelines consider avoiding stimulation tests in truly basal-negative individuals (i.e., basal only protocols). Meta-analyses cite pooled basal calcitonin sensitivity/specificity ~99%, reinforcing the effectiveness of these improved tests [25].

2.1.3. The Diagnostic Performance of Circulating Calcitonin

The sensitivity and specificity of basal calcitonin for detecting MTC range from 83 to 100% and 94 to 100%, respectively [26]. Meta-analyses support its reliability for thyroid nodule evaluation [25] and one Cochrane review reported high accuracy, though it noted heterogeneity and risk of bias [27]. Rarely, MTC may present with normal basal and even stimulated results in about 1–2% of cases [28]. Possible causes include impaired secretion, cryptic calcitonin isoforms undetected by immunoassays, or the analytical hook effect [26]. In such challenging cases, alternative biomarkers and confirmatory assays can unmask occult disease. This **calcitonin**-negative variant may respond well to standard surgical treatment, but rigorous long-term follow-up is essential as poorly differentiated cases may also occur with negative CT and are associated with worse outcomes [29].

2.1.4. The Role of Serum Calcitonin in Screening and Diagnosis of Medullary Thyroid Carcinoma

Elevated basal CT (above gender- and assay-specific thresholds) indicates MTC with a nearly 100% positive predictive value. In the context of thyroid nodules, CT is a marker for early detection of occult MT that might elude US and/or cytology [25]. Notably, thyroid nodules are very common while MTC is a rare tumor and many non-MTC-related conditions may increase CT levels, leading to potential false-positive results. In addition, other conditions such as the hook effect can lower CT levels, leading to false negative results [25,30]. The European Thyroid Association recommends measuring calcitonin levels in patients scheduled for surgery or thermoablation of thyroid nodules, those with indeterminate cytology, or those with suspicious US findings. Cutoff points of 30 pg/mL in females and 34 pg/mL in males are also proposed to distinguish between non-MTC reasons for increased calcitonin and MTC. Such thresholds have been established for one assay platform and several additional variables may affect these results, making these thresholds nonactionable outside the authors' setting [31]. The American Thyroid Association leaves clinicians to decide if and when to measure calcitonin in patients with thyroid nodules [1]. Overall, recommendations on calcitonin screening still differ between available guidelines, and the use of calcitonin screening of MTC varies significantly across different countries, specialties, and clinical centers. A broad consensus exists only on the pivotal role of calcitonin screening in cases with a family history of MTC or multiple endocrine neoplasia type 2, and its use in guiding the timing of prophylactic thyroidectomy in carriers of RET pathogenic variants [32,33].

2.1.5. The Role of Serum Calcitonin in Postoperative Monitoring of Medullary Thyroid Carcinoma

After total thyroidectomy calcitonin levels typically decline within hours, and their normalization within weeks signals biochemical remission. Persistent or rising **calcitonin** postoperatively indicates residual or recurrent disease. Serial measurements allow calculation of doubling time (CDT), a powerful prognostic tool: CDT < 6 months correlates with poor survival, while CDT > 2 years indicates favorable outcomes [34]. Adjunctive biomarkers, especially CEA, may refine follow-up and prognostic stratification. Increased CEA levels and shortened doubling time are early signs of disease progression and the shift toward a more aggressive phenotype [35]. Accordingly, the follow-up of patients without an excellent response is based on the simultaneous measurement of both **calcitonin** and CEA, as well as their doubling time evaluation (Table 2) [1].

Table 2. Follow-up of MTC patients after primary surgery (i.e., thyroidectomy ± neck dissections).

Follow-Up	ER	BIR	BIR	SIR
Early	Negative US Negative calcitonin	Negative US calcitonin ≤ 150 pg/mL	Calcitonin > 150 pg/mL	-Positive imaging -Positive biopsy
Long-term	*FU at 6 months* -Negative: US/CT 1–2/yr -Positive: see BIR or SIR	*Visit at 6 months* US/CT 1/six months calcitonin DT -Negative: check 2/yr -Positive imaging (SIR) -Calcitonin > 150 pg/mL (BIR)	*Imaging* -CT/MR/PET/CT -Positive: (SIR) -Negative: Calcitonin, CEA, and calcitonin DT 2–4/yr	-Surgery -EBRT -Thermal ablations -Systemic therapies

Legend. US, ultrasound; CT, computed tomography; MR, magnetic resonance; PET/CT, positron emission tomography/computed tomography; BIR, biochemical incomplete response; SIR, structural incomplete response; DT, doubling time; CEA, carcinoembryonic antigen; EBRT, external beam radiation therapy.

2.2. *Procalcitonin*

Procalcitonin (ProCT) is a 116-amino acid prohormone, normally cleaved to calcitonin in thyroid parafollicular C-cells. Under normal physiological conditions, ProCT expression is limited to thyroid C-cells and circulates at low concentrations. Unlike calcitonin, ProCT exhibits a stable and concentration-independent half-life of ~20–24 h in vivo [36] and it shows excellent in vitro stability when collected as serum or plasma samples, reducing pre-analytical variability [37]. Kratzsch and colleagues tested two fully automated and one non-automated calcitonin assays, comparing these results with those from ProCT (Brahms Kryptor) [38]. They evaluated pre-analytical factors and ProCT cross-reactivity in serum samples from 437 patients presenting with clinical conditions linked to elevated calcitonin levels. Their study also included 60 post-thyroidectomy patients and established calcitonin cutoff values for pentagastrin stimulation tests in 13 patients with chronic kidney disease and 10 patients with MTC.

Their findings revealed several key points. Serum calcitonin concentrations showed significant degradation when stored at room temperature for over 2 h or at 4 °C for more than 6 h. The cutoff values for both baseline and stimulated calcitonin varied depending on the specific disease state and assay methodology employed. Proton pump inhibitor treatment was the most common cause of elevated calcitonin levels. Notably, ProCT concentrations were elevated in MTC patients compared to those with chronic kidney disease who did not have concurrent infections.

The study concluded that elevated calcitonin concentrations occur frequently in patients without MTC and advocated for incorporating ProCT assessment when evaluating unexplained calcitonin elevations in ambiguous clinical scenarios. ProCT testing proves valuable when calcitonin measurements are compromised by pre-analytical or analytical limitations, or when calcitonin values fall within indeterminate ranges [39]. Moreover, in contrast with the weak agreement between different calcitonin assays [12,40] a high degree of agreement was demonstrated between ProCT assays, making it possible to establish general ProCT thresholds in a clinical setting. Lippi and colleagues showed that 10 fully automated commercial ProCT assays deliver acceptable correlations in 176 routine lithium heparin plasma samples, suggesting that other ProCT assays may also be appropriate for the purpose [41]. All in all, ProCT circumvents many of the analytical and pre-analytical problems associated with calcitonin measurement and has recently emerged as a potential complementary or alternative MTC biomarker.

Procalcitonin in Diagnosis and Monitoring of Medullary Thyroid Carcinoma

Multiple studies have robustly demonstrated that ProCT identifies MTC cases with high diagnostic accuracy. Results of a pivotal paper in the field [41] and the largest published series in either diagnostic [42,43] or postoperative settings [44,45] are summarized in Table 3, as well as those of the largest meta-analysis on the role of ProCT in MTC patients [46].

Table 3. Evaluation of the diagnostic performance of ProCT in MTC patients [different clinical settings].

Reference	Study (No of Patients)	Patients Cohort	ProCT Cutoff	Sensitivity	Specificity
Algeciras 2009 [42]	Retrospective (835)	Mixed benign vs. active and inactive MTC	0.10 pg/mL	91%	96%
Giovanella 2013 [43]	Retrospective (1236)	Thyroid nodules	0.10 pg/mL	100%	100%
Giovanella 2018 [44]	Prospective (2705)	Thyroid nodules	0.155 pg/mL	100%	99.7%
Trimboli 2018 [45]	Retrospective (55)	Postoperative/follow-up	0.32 pg/mL	92%	98%
Censi 2023 [46]	Retrospective (90)	Postoperative/follow-up	0.12 pg/mL	100%	84%
Giovanella 2021 [47]	Meta-analysis (5817)	Diagnosis/follow-up	0.10 pg/mL	90%	100%

Legend: ProCT; procalcitonin; MTC; medullary thyroid cancer.

Algeciras-Schimnich and colleagues firstly demonstrated the potential role of ProCT as an alternative biomarker of MTC in a study including 835 patients with active MTC, cured MTC, neuroendocrine tumors, active and cured follicular cell-derived thyroid carcinoma, benign thyroid diseases, mastocytosis, and normal volunteers, respectively [42]. The Receiver Operating Characteristic (ROC) curve analysis revealed no significant difference in diagnostic performance between calcitonin and ProCT. A comparison of calcitonin and ProCT in stability studies showed that calcitonin was very unstable in vitro (i.e., a decrease of 35–50% from the original value 24 h after sampling). In contrast, ProCT concentrations did not significantly change during this time.

Giovanella and colleagues evaluated the role of routine measurement of ProCT in a sample of 1236 patients and reported serum calcitonin levels > 10 pg/mL in 14 (1.1%) patients [43]. Among them, two were found to have MTC, one a C-cell hyperplasia, while MTC was excluded in the remaining patients by subsequent clinical and histological follow-up. Basal levels of calcitonin were >100 pg/mL in two MTC patients, and pentagastrin-stimulated calcitonin was >100 pg/mL in two MTC patients and two non-MTC patients, respectively. Moreover, basal and stimulated ProCT values were elevated in only two MTC patients, resulting in 100% accuracy. As the main result, ProCT was detectable in MTC patients and undetectable in the remaining ones (100% sensitivity and 100% negative predictive values).

In a large prospective study Giovanella and colleagues evaluated 2705 patients with thyroid nodules, measuring only ProCT as a screening test. A ProCT cutoff of 0.155 pg/mL yielded 100% sensitivity and 99.7% specificity in diagnosing MTC [44]. Finally, Clausi and colleagues recently reported results obtained in 478 patients undergoing thyroidectomy [48]. Serum levels of ProCT and calcitonin were measured before surgery. Overall, 23/478 (4.8%) patients tested positive for MTC. Calcitonin values > 10 pg/mL demonstrated a sensitivity of 0.91, specificity of 0.98, PPV of 0.70, and NPV of 0.99. ProCT showed sensitivity, specificity, PPV, and NPV of 0.87, 0.96, 0.56, and 0.99 using a cutoff of 0.04 ng/mL, and 0.78, 0.98, 0.72, and 0.99 using a cutoff of 0.07 ng/mL, respectively. Interestingly, 80.9% of patients with a calcitonin value between 10 and 100 pg/mL would have been correctly identified as MTC or non-MTC by positive or negative ProCT using the cutoff 0.04 ng/mL. The authors concluded that calcitonin demonstrates superior sensitivity compared to ProCT as a diagnostic marker for MTC; however, implementing a two-step approach with ProCT as an adjunctive marker can enhance diagnostic precision and prevent overtreatment, especially when calcitonin serum concentrations fall between 10 and 100 pg/m. Such results are in line with those obtained by Giovanella and colleagues measuring calcitonin and ProCT in 16 patients with active (i.e., primary tumor before surgery or post-surgical recurrent disease) and 23 with inactive (i.e., complete remission) MTC, 125 patients with non-MTC benign thyroid disease, and 62 patients with non-MTC thyroid cancers [49]. Both calcitonin and ProCT median values were significantly higher in active (94 pmol/L and 1.17 ng/mL) than inactive (0.28 pmol/L ng/mL and 0.06 ng/mL), benign (0.37 pmol/L and 0.06 ng/mL), and malignant non-MTC diseases (0.28 pmol/L and 0.06 ng/mL), respectively. Notably, undetectable ProCT was found in five non-MTC patients with false-positive calcitonin results. The authors concluded that, at the very least, ProCT is useful in patients with positive calcitonin results, as negative ProCT values securely exclude active MTC (i.e., a rule-out test). As both markers are available on the same automated platforms, a reflex or reflective strategy can be easily adopted to refine the laboratory diagnosis.

Postoperative monitoring also benefits from ProCT measurements: among 55 patients under surveillance a 0.32 ng/mL threshold achieved 92% sensitivity and 98% specificity for residual or recurrent disease [45].

More recently, Censi and colleagues retrospectively evaluated 90 MTC patients during postoperative follow-up and found a strong relationship between calcitonin and ProCT, corroborating the relevant role of ProCT as an adjunctive biomarker to calcitonin, especially to exclude MTC structural recurrences in patients with a slight to moderate increase in calcitonin concentrations [46]. Importantly, the ProCT-to-calcitonin ratio has also demonstrated predictive value for progression-free survival, further validating its clinical utility as a prognostic indicator [50]. Collectively, available evidence indicates that ProCT measurement offers excellent diagnostic sensitivity, specificity, accuracy, and prognostic information, while providing significant pre-analytical and analytical advantages. Notably, a recent meta-analysis including 5817 individuals (335 with MTC) reported a pooled sensitivity of

90% and specificity of 100% for ProCT in MTC, providing robust evidence in favor of the use of ProCT in diagnosis and follow-up of MTC [47].

Indeed, ProCT levels can become markedly elevated during severe bacterial infections and sepsis due to ectopic production by non-thyroidal tissues. The Food and Drug Administration has approved ProCT assays for risk stratification in critically ill patients at risk for severe sepsis and septic shock [51]. Nonetheless, elevations due to bacterial infections necessitate careful interpretation, as in inflammatory states ProCT can markedly increase [52]. Table 4 summarizes the role of ProCT in different clinical settings and practical advantages.

Table 4. Procalcitonin: clinical role and practical advantages in medullary thyroid cancer.

Screening/diagnosis	Most studies consistently showed similar sensitivity/specificity of calcitonin and ProCT, with better NPV of the latter. Other studies showed superior sensitivity of calcitonin with ProCT serving as a rule-out test in patients with calcitonin concentrations within the gray area (i.e., 10–100 pg/mL)
Postoperative follow-up	Strong ability to detect residual/relapsing disease
Prognosis/Prediction	The ProCT/calcitonin ratio correlates with outcomes (overall and disease-free survival)
Technical advantages	Greater assay stability and less susceptible to pre-analytical issues

Legend: ProCT, procalcitonin.

Regarding the sensitivity of ProCT, which has been found inferior to that of calcitonin by some authors, it is worth noting that serum calcitonin measurement is integral (and often the only diagnostic biomarker) in establishing the diagnosis and referring patients to surgery. Obviously, the diagnostic sensitivity of calcitonin is biased toward 100% (i.e., a slight increase in calcitonin levels prompts diagnostic work-up while normal calcitonin, in the presence of detectable ProCT not measured at that time, would not have required further controls). Accordingly, the best performance an alternative marker can achieve is equal to that of calcitonin, and for statistical reasons, it cannot surpass the current calcitonin standard. Indeed, a potential reservation against replacing calcitonin monitoring as the gold standard for MTC may be related to the opposition/resistance of the medical community. Indeed, ProCT is FDA-approved as a marker for lower respiratory tract infection. Because MTC is rare and obtaining regulatory approval for new indications is costly and complex, manufacturers currently favor its off-label use in this setting. Therefore, ProCT may reasonably be considered as a complementary marker in patients with thyroid nodules and positive calcitonin results (as a rule-out test) and in MTC patients with unclear postoperative calcitonin trends.

2.3. Carcinoembryonic Antigen

Medullary thyroid carcinoma arises from parafollicular C-cells, which express and release CEA in approximately half of cases. CEA is a ~200 kDa onco-fetal glycoprotein involved in cell adhesion and part of the CEACAM immunoglobulin family. CEA is normally expressed during fetal gastrointestinal development, with minimal expression in healthy adults (<2–4 ng/mL) [53]. It is typically quantified via standardized immunometric assays, which are analytically robust, reproducible, and less affected by interferences and the hook effect than calcitonin. Notably, CEA measurement is affected by benign conditions (i.e., inflammation, smoking, liver dysfunction conditions) and other malignancies (colorectal or lung cancer), requiring cautious interpretation. In particular, postoperative CEA is widely adopted as a reliable tumor marker and prognostic factor for colon cancer [54]. Even if CEA is not a specific MTC biomarker, its measurement remains useful in assessing the extension and progression of the disease before and after thyroidectomy. Baseline CEA levels are low in early, thyroid-limited MTC, precluding its use in screening and early diagnosis of MTC. However, CEA remains a valuable adjunct marker to monitor patients after surgery and stratify the risk of recurrence and death in patients with advanced disease. Preoperative CEA values > 30 ng/mL indicate a larger size of the primary tumor and extra-thyroid tumor extension. Moreover, CEA values greater than 100 ng/mL are associated with lymph node involvement, distant metastases, and a poorer prognosis [55]. Accordingly, serum CEA should be systematically measured before surgery in patients with confirmed or suspected MTC to inform the extent of resection and, particularly, lymph node dissection(s) [56]. Following surgery, MTC patients require evaluation for residual disease presence, localization of metastases, and progressive disease identification. Postoperative restaging is essential to distinguish low-risk MTC patients from those at high risk of disease recurrence. Postoperative calcitonin and CEA levels should be systematically documented. Postoperative undetectable calcitonin levels correlate with favorable outcomes. In patients with basal serum calcitonin levels below 150 pg/mL after thyroidectomy, persistent or recurrent disease is typically limited to cervical lymph nodes. Conversely, postoperative serum calcitonin elevation above 150 pg/mL necessitates comprehensive imaging studies, including neck and chest CT, contrast-enhanced MRI, hepatic US, bone scintigraphy, bone MRI, and PET/CT. The integration of CEA measurement is useful in this context as post-thyroidectomy failure of CEA levels to normalize—or an increase in levels—suggests residual disease, offering an early warning for recurrence even when calcitonin remains low [1]. Notably, CEA demonstrates relatively stable kinetics compared to CT, displaying less diurnal fluctuation and thus serving as a robust indicator of tumor mass. Additionally, a rising CEA, even in the absence of a CT increase, suggests a more aggressive disease phenotype (i.e., dedifferentiated disease) and may prompt more comprehensive metastatic workups using advanced imaging modalities such as [^{18}F]FDG PET/CT [57,58]. Among patients with advanced disease, structural disease growth rate can be estimated and monitored through sequential imaging studies using RECIST criteria to document tumor size increases over time, and by measuring serum calcitonin or CEA levels at multiple time points to determine tumor marker doubling time (DT) [1].

2.4. *Pro-Gastrin-Releasing Peptide*

As reported in previous sections of the present paper, calcitonin is the standard of care in the diagnosis and monitoring of MTC, while serum ProCT is a potential alternative or at least complementary test to calcitonin in unclear cases being free from analytical limitations and interferences that may lead to false-positive or negative calcitonin results. The pro-gastrin-releasing peptide (ProGRP) is a stable precursor of gastrin-releasing peptide (GRP), a neuropeptide involved in tumor growth and differentiation. ProGRP is principally employed as a tumor marker of small-cell lung cancer [59]. ProGRP is generally measured using fully automated, non-competitive IMAs, which provide high reproducibility and offer pre-analytical advantages. Furthermore, it is stable in serum, is not subject to the hook effect, and is measurably preserved even with delayed processing. To date no reference method or international standard has been identified in the literature regarding the analytical performance of IMAs, and comparisons between them are sparse [60]. More recently, ProGRP has emerged as a promising adjunct biomarker in MTC, with initial studies demonstrating diagnostic performance similar to that of established markers (Table 5).

Table 5. Available studies on ProGRP in MTC patients (8 studies, 3886 patients).

Study	Patients	Sensitivity	Specificity	TP	FN	FP	TN
Han XD 2021 [61]	360	96.2	99.3	101	4	2	253
Giovanella 2021 [62]	254	75.9	97.9	51	16	4	183
Liang 2020 [63]	2446	53.8	96.7	114	98	73	2161
Parra-Robert 2017 [64]	38	88.9	76.9	20	2	4	12
Torsetnes 2014 [65]	190	80.0	90.0	48	12	13	117
Miao 2023 [66]	236	71.4	92.7	71	29	10	126
Martins Fernandes 2025 [67]	64	88.9	97.9	17	2	1	44
Schonebaum 2023 [68]	278	70.4	99.6	59	24	1	194

Legenda: TP, true-positive; FP, false-positive; FN, false-negative; TN, true-negative; ProGRP, pro-gastrin-releasing peptide. Sensitivity and specificity are expressed as %.

Overall, ProGRP has only moderate sensitivity (~80%) and cannot be used in MTC screening and diagnosis, considering the sensitivity of ~100% robustly demonstrated by either calcitonin or ProCT. Considering the high specificity, it should be considered to rule out false-positive calcitonin results, but again, ProCT already demonstrated a quite absolute negative predictive value in patients with indeterminate calcitonin results. Interestingly, ProGRP correlates with metastatic burden, and ProGRP levels are significantly higher in patients with nodal or distant metastatic MTC than in those with limited disease. Additionally, ProGRP levels drop post-surgery, aligning with effective resection, and serial ProGRP measurements mirror imaging responses more closely than calcitonin or CEA in patients under tyrosine kinase inhibitor therapy (i.e., vandetanib), making it a potential early indicator of therapy response or resistance [62]. Evidence remains fragmented and insufficient to support or refute its implementation in clinical protocols as available studies were retrospective with small sample sizes. Generally speaking, serum ProGRP is likely of limited value in the diagnosis of MTC with some promising preliminary data suggesting its application in advanced disease, especially in therapy response assessment. All in all, ProGRP can currently be considered as a candidate MTC biomarker, and its inclusion in advanced MTC management protocols needs to be studied in a large prospective cohort of patients with progressive disease and active systemic treatment.

2.5. Carbohydrate Antigen 19.9

Carbohydrate antigen 19.9 (CA 19.9) is a sialyl Lewis-A glycan, classically used in monitoring pancreatic and gastrointestinal malignancies. Its aberrant expression was reported in subgroups of MTC characterized by aggressive or metastatic behavior [69]. CA 19.9 is measured by immunoassays employing monoclonal antibodies against the sialyl Lewis-A epitope. Inter-method variability persists even after standardization due to epitope heterogeneity, differences in proprietary antibodies, and technical variations. Additionally, approximately 5–10% of individuals lack the Lewis antigen and cannot produce CA 19-9, yielding potentially false-negative results [70]. CA 19.9 elevations may also be noted in benign hepatobiliary and pancreatic diseases and benign respiratory diseases, which may complicate interpretation in MTC patients [69]. Notably, CA 19.9 is not sensitive to early or localized MTC, as only 5–6% of intra-thyroid tumors overexpress it and fewer present with elevated CA 19.9 serum levels. Vice versa, serum CA 19.9 increases in advanced MTC and its serum concentration correlates with structural disease progression and total tumor volume. Immunohistochemical analyses confirmed CA 19.9 expression in metastatic MTC tissue, affirming the tumor origin of the circulating marker [71]. In a series of 122 MTC patients, mean CA 19.9 levels were significantly higher in those with progressive disease (median ~21.4 U/mL vs. ~7.3 U/mL; $p = 0.01$) and in those who died from MTC ($p < 0.001$) [69]. Additionally, prospective data identify CA 19.9 positivity and fast CA 19.9 DT (i.e., <6 months) in advanced MTC as independent predictors of mortality, regardless of imaging findings. In these patients, systemic treatment (e.g., with cabozantinib or vandetanib) may be considered sooner than imaging alone would indicate [72]. In conclusion, due to limited sensitivity and specificity CA 19.9 cannot replace established MTC biomarkers (i.e., calcitonin and CEA) but may serve as a useful adjunct in select CA 19.9-positive cases. Its elevation and rapid doubling convey increased mortality risk and may prompt earlier therapeutic intervention independent of imaging findings. Additional multicentric, prospective studies are needed to define optimal thresholds, assay standardization, and integration into MTC care algorithms.

3. Doubling Time of Calcitonin and Carcinoembryonic Antigen

Calcitonin and CEA DTs are used to assess tumor burden, the aggressiveness of MTC, and predict the likelihood of recurrence or progression. They help monitor the effectiveness of treatment and guide decisions about further treatment strategies. Patients with shorter DTs may be considered higher risk and may benefit from intensified surveillance and/or additional imaging and/or treatments. Calcitonin and CEA levels are assumed to increase exponentially in MTC, doubling over a specific timeframe. Reliable DT calculation requires a well-standardized procedure. First, serial tumor marker measurements (i.e., every 6 months) with a minimum of four values (ideally over 2 years) are recommended. Second, methodological consistency is essential: all measurements should utilize the same laboratory and assay platforms to ensure accuracy. Third, DT should be calculated using the following formula: $DT = \ln(2)/b$, where "b" represents the exponential growth rate constant derived from regression analysis of measured Calcitonin and CEA levels. Fourth, values below the limit of quantitation (LoQ) of the assay are reported as "equal to the LoQ" (i.e., if the LoQ of a calcitonin assay is 2 pg/mL and the patients' value is rendered as <2 pg/mL then the value inputted for calculation will be 2 pg/mL). Finally, undetectable values and detectable values that do not double are designated as "never doubled". Multiple reliable platforms are freely available to calculate DTs. The Kuma Hospital DT Calculator (Kuma Hospital, Kobe, Japan) is widely employed and was also adopted by the authors of the present review [73]. A note of caution is necessary when using DTs in clinical practice as they can vary significantly between patients and other factors (i.e., tumor grade, stage, and site of metastasis). Accordingly, DT results should always be considered in the general clinical context, taking into account the results of other diagnostic tools. Interpretation criteria of calcitonin and CEA doubling times are summarized in Table 6.

Table 6. Interpretation of calcitonin and CEA doubling times.

Doubling Time (Years)	Risk of Structural Recurrence	Prognosis
<1/2	Present	Very poor, short survival times
<1	High/Present	Poor
1–2	Intermediate	Intermediate
>2	Low	Favorable
Never doubling	Very low	Good

Finally, absolute levels of calcitonin and CEA, as well as the ratio of DTs, are very useful in guiding advanced molecular imaging in patients with relapsing or advanced MTC. In general, [^{18}F]DOPA PET/CT appears to be superior to [^{18}F]FDG PET/CT in detecting and locating lesions in patients with recurrent MTC, especially when calcitonin exceeds 150 pg/mL, CEA is ≥5 ng/mL, or calcitonin DT is between 1 and 2 years. [^{18}F]FDG PET/CT showed a better accuracy in patients with very high calcitonin levels (>500 pg/mL), those with a disproportionate CEA increase compared to calcitonin, and/or calcitonin/CEA DTs are <1 year. Patients with rapidly shortening calcitonin/CEA doubling times may also benefit from [^{68}Ga]DOTA-peptides PET/CT for the detection of occult recurrence. Overall, calcitonin and CEA kinetics can serve as a trigger for advanced molecular imaging, improving the localization of small-volume or occult disease and better identifying high-risk patients who require more careful surveillance [74–76].

4. Measurement of MTC Biomarkers in Fine-Needle Aspiration Washouts

The measurement of **calcitonin** in fine-needle aspiration washout fluids (FNA-calcitonin) from thyroid nodules and/or lymph nodes suspected of MTC or lymph nodes has been proposed to circumvent limitations of cytology in detecting MTC with a sensitivity of only 55% to 65%. Despite numerous criticisms (i.e., interferences, lack of standards, analytical variability of different assays) affecting the accuracy of the results and making it hard to compare studies, all available studies show significantly high sensitivity and specificity of FNA-calcitonin which are clearly better than that of cytopathology (Table 7) [77].

Table 7. Diagnostic accuracy of FNA-**calcitonin** reported in the main studies.

	Lesions (n)	Assay	Cutoff, ng/L	Sensitivity, %	Specificity, %
Boi, 2007 [78]	36	CLIA	36	100	100
Kudo, 2007 [79]	14	NR	67	100	NR
Diazzi, 2013 [80]	60	CLIA	17	100	88.8
Trimboli, 2014 [81]	90	CLIA	39.6	100	100
De Crea, 2014 [82]	62	CLIA	10.4	89	100

Legend: CLIA, chemiluminescence immunoassay; NR, not reported.

Obviously, the appropriate sampling is key, and samples should be representative of the approached lesion in the thyroid nodules, thyroid bed, or lymph node, respectively [83]. Unlike FNA cytology, diagnosis remains possible using FNA-calcitonin even when no thyroid cells are aspirated since calcitonin exhibits high concentrations both within and surrounding the lesion area [77].

Finally, detectable levels of FNA-calcitonin (i.e., higher than the functional sensitivity of the employed assay) were found in most non-medullary thyroid nodules, likely due to normal C-cells entrapped in the FNA sample, especially from the middle/upper thyroid lobes, highlighting the relevance of an appropriate cutoff selection [83].

Relevant practical points for FNA-calcitonin measurement and interpretation are summarized in Table 8.

Table 8. Key points for standardization of FNA marker measurement in washout fluids.

Sampling	Representative of the lesion [lymph node or thyroid nodule]
Washing solution	0.9% saline solution [1 mL]
Collection	Rinse the needle $\geq$ 2 times, collect the amount of washout fluid and keep on ice
Pre-treatment	Mix and centrifuge the sample
Measurement	Consider interferences and perform dilution or batching to detect "hook effect" in case of undetectable FNA-**calcitonin**
Interpretation	Use an assay-specific cutoff adapted to the local population

Legend: FNA; fine-needle aspiration.

Recently, ProGRP measurement was tested in 212 patients with 235 thyroid nodules, classified into chronic thyroiditis, nodular goiter, papillary thyroid carcinoma, thyroid follicular neoplasm, follicular thyroid carcinoma, and MTC. Serum ProGRP and FNA-ProGRP were measured. The median serum ProGRP concentration was 124.40 pg/mL in MTC, significantly higher than in other tested groups. The serum ProGRP cutoff value was 68.30 pg/mL, yielding 53.85% sensitivity, 96.98% specificity, and a kappa value of 0.51 in MTC. The median concentration of FNA-ProGRP in MTC nodules was 2096.00 pg/mL, significantly higher than in other groups. ROC analysis of MTC nodules versus non-MTC nodules revealed a cutoff value of 22.77 pg/mL, achieving 94.12% sensitivity, 98.27% specificity, and a kappa value of 0.85. The authors suggested FNA-ProGRP measurement as an ancillary method for differential diagnosis between MTC and non-MTC thyroid nodules [63]. Further studies are required to confirm or refute this preliminary observation and accurately evaluate the diagnostic advantage over FNA-calcitonin. As a consequence, FNA-ProGRP measurement should only be considered in the context of clinical trials.

5. Integrated Use of Circulating Markers of Medullary Thyroid Carcinoma

This paper presents the biochemical and analytical characteristics of currently available MTC biomarkers, analyzing their diagnostic performance and clinical applications. Algorithms for the rational and integrated use of various biomarkers, as outlined in current guidelines, are presented below.

5.1. Screening and Diagnosis of MTC

Calcitonin proved to be a useful screening test for the presence of MTC in patients with thyroid nodules, exhibiting a high diagnostic sensitivity. This practice remains debated due to the low prevalence of MTC and the non-negligible rate of false-positive calcitonin results [1]. Recently, ProCT has been shown to be highly accurate in excluding MTC in patients with indeterminate calcitonin values (i.e., 10–100 pg/mL), making a two-step procedure actionable. In turn, human, social, and economic costs associated with false-positive calcitonin results (i.e., imaging, FNA, additional laboratory tests) will be reduced by applying a reflex test procedure to safely rule out MTC in patients with undetectable ProCT (Figure 1) [47].

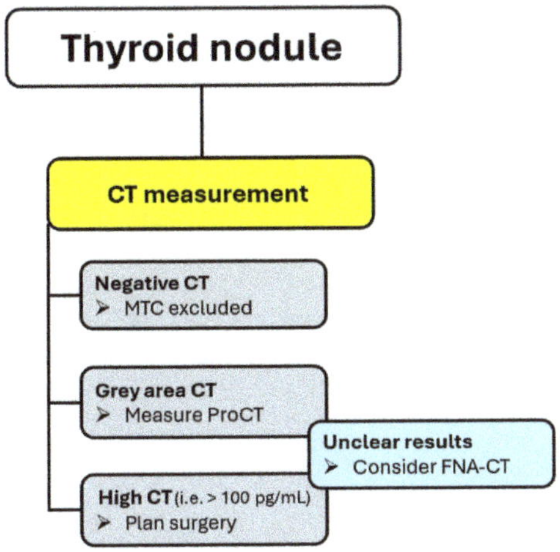

Figure 1. Screening and diagnosis of MTC in patients with thyroid nodules. **Legend**: MTC, medullary thyroid cancer; ProCT, procalcitonin; FNA-CT, fine-needle aspiration-calcitonin.

5.2. Preoperative Assessment

Patients with diagnosed MTC should be assessed before surgery to map neck lymph nodes and detect/exclude distant metastasis. Distant metastases are unlikely in patients with negative US and calcitonin levels below 500 pg/mL. In such cases, no additional imaging is recommended, and total thyroidectomy should be planned with additional lymph node dissections informed by US, absolute calcitonin levels, and intraoperative findings. The risk of advanced disease and distant metastasis significantly increases in patients with calcitonin levels greater than 500 pg/mL, and level II imaging (i.e., ceCT, MR, PET/CT) is required to refine disease staging and detect or exclude distant metastases (Figure 2) [1].

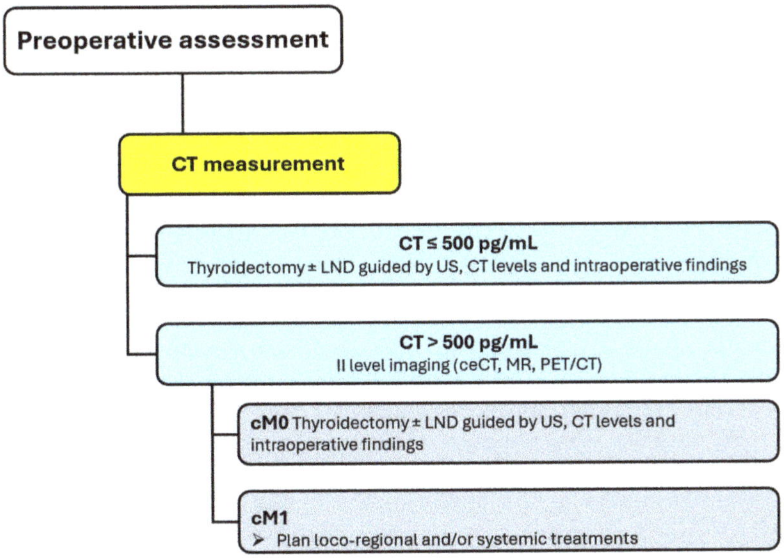

Figure 2. Preoperative assessment of MTC in patients. **Legend**: CT, calcitonin; LND, lymph node dissection; US, ultrasound; ceCT, contrast-enhanced computed tomography; MR, magnetic resonance; PET/CT, positron emission tomography/computed tomography.

5.3. Postoperative Monitoring

Following surgery, serum calcitonin and CEA levels should be measured 3 months postoperatively, and if undetectable or within normal range, should be measured every 6 months for 1 year, and then annually. In patients with detectable serum levels of calcitonin and CEA following thyroidectomy, the levels of the markers should be measured at least every 6 months to determine their doubling time. Patients with elevated postoperative serum calcitonin levels of less than 150 pg/mL should undergo a physical examination and US of the neck. If these studies are negative, the patients should be followed up through physical examinations, measurement of serum levels of calcitonin and CEA, and US every 6 months. If the postoperative serum calcitonin level exceeds 150 pg/mL, patients should be examined by imaging procedures, including neck US, ceCT, MR, three-phase ceCT of the liver, and PET/CT (Figure 3) [1].

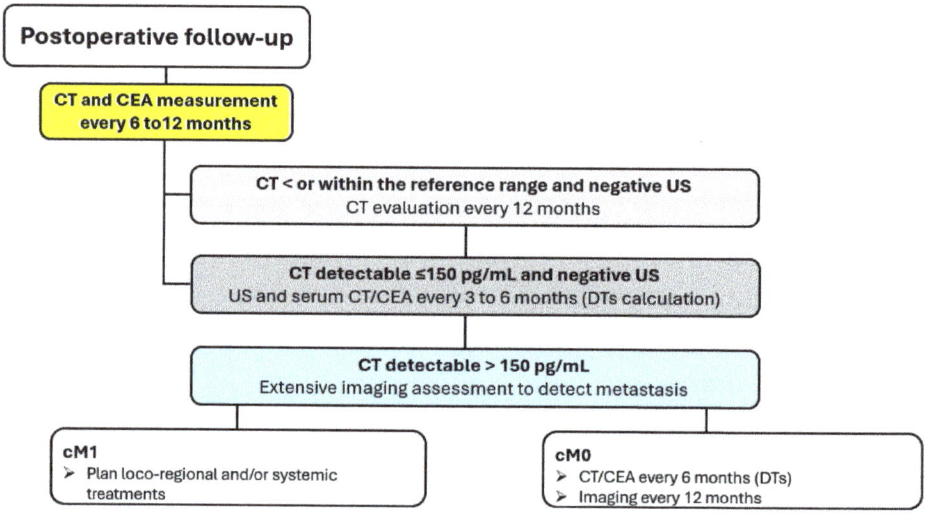

Figure 3. Postoperative assessment and follow-up of MTC patients. **Legend**: CT, calcitonin; CEA, carcinoembryonic antigen; US, ultrasound; DTs, doubling times.

5.4. Analytical and Technical Challenges

Currently, fully automated immunoassays are widely used to evaluate MTC biomarkers across various analytical platforms, which are commercially available from different manufacturers. These highly automated systems offer an optimal balance of high throughput, rapid turnaround time, minimal sample volume, and cost-effectiveness [84]. Although significant advances have been made over the years in the analytical performance of various immunoassays, substantial inter-method variability still persists [85]. This variability necessitates the use of method-specific reference intervals, making it challenging to compare results obtained from different assays. Consequently, the use of the same immunoassay method is essential for reliable patient follow-up [84]. Although extensive research has been conducted over the years, challenges remain in terms of standardization and harmonization. Variability between methods can often be attributed to the use of primary antibodies with different epitope specificities. Indeed, significant discrepancies have also been observed between assays that utilize the same monoclonal antibodies, as seen in CA 19-9 assays employing the Centocor monoclonal antibody, indicating that other methodological factors also play a critical role [86]. In such cases, elements related to the assay's architectural format must be considered when assessing inter-method variability. These include differences in incubation times, reaction kinetics, washing procedures, and the nature of the tracer system used. Together, these parameters influence the final numerical result, potentially leading to a lack of interchangeability between methods. To improve comparability and progress towards the harmonization and standardization of immunoassays for markers of MTC, efforts should focus on the development and implementation of reference materials and reference measurement procedures for each analyte. In addition to the development of methodological references, a key factor for harmonization between methods is the commutability of control materials, particularly those used in External Quality Assessment (EQA) schemes [85,87]. In order to improve this aspect, it is necessary to develop control materials prepared from authentic human samples or with advanced reconstitution technologies; check the commutability of EQA materials before distribution to laboratories (i.e., according to guidelines); use materials that are traceable to primary reference standards where available; and, overall, promote collaborations between reagent manufacturers, laboratories, and international laboratory medicine societies to create reference networks. Investment in this aspect would bring not only technical but also clinical benefits, improving the reliability of diagnostic results.

Table 9 summarizes the main aspects of the pre-analytical, analytical, and post-analytical phases concerning the tests used for determining circulating blood biomarkers of medullary thyroid carcinoma.

Table 9. Main laboratory characteristics of biomarkers used in medullary thyroid carcinoma.

Biomarker	Pre-Analytical Aspects		Analytical Aspects		Post-Analytical Aspects
	Healthy Subject	**Sample**	**Methods**	**WHO IS**	**Reference Interval Clinical Decision Cutoff**
CA 19-9	No peculiar preparation	No peculiar recommendations [88]	Immunoassay	Not available	Method-dependent [89,90]
CEA	No peculiar preparation Blood levels influenced by smoking	No peculiar recommendations [88]	Immunoassay	WHO 1st IS 73/601	Method-dependent [87,91]
Calcitonin	No peculiar preparation Blood levels influenced by age, sex, BMI, and smoking	Instability at RT, ice-bath storage after blood collection Centrifuge and analyze preferably within 30 min of sampling	Immunoassay	WHO 2nd IS 89/620	Method-dependent [92,93]
ProCT	No peculiar preparation	Greater stability at RT than CT	Immunoassay	Not available	0.1 ng/mL [44]
proGRP	No peculiar preparation Blood levels influenced by age, BMI, and smoking	No peculiar recommendations [88]	Immunoassay	Not available	Method- and matrix-dependent [94]

Legend: BMI, body mass index; Ca 19-9, carbohydrate antigen 19-9; CEA, carcinoembryonic antigen; IS, international standard; ProCT, procalcitonin; proGRP, pro-gastrin-releasing peptide; RT, room temperature; WHO, World Health Organization.

6. Discussion

Medullary thyroid carcinoma (MTC) is a neuroendocrine malignancy originating in the parafollicular C-cells of the thyroid and is characterized by the secretion of specific peptide markers. The biochemical profile of MTC serves as a cornerstone for diagnosis, risk stratification, and longitudinal monitoring. In addition to tumor markers such as calcitonin, ProCT, CEA and CA19.9, neuroendocrine MTC cells may also secrete different bioactive peptides and hormones that, in turn, can give rise to paraneoplastic syndromes (PNSs) [1]. Overall, PNSs are rare and mostly involve patients with extensive metastases and/or aggressive tumor biology. High levels of circulating calcitonin (>1000 pg/mL) are the most common biochemical cause of secretory diarrhea in MTC (prevalence ~5%), a debilitating condition with electrolyte imbalances (e.g., hypokalemia) and weight loss. Facial or generalized flushing (prevalence 2–5%) is associated with secretion of serotonin, prostaglandins, and CGRP, and mimics carcinoid syndrome. Elevated urinary 5-HIAA can support diagnosis. Ectopic ACTH syndrome (EAS) is a rare (<1% of MTC cases) but serious paraneoplastic phenomenon. It presents with rapid-onset hypertension, hypokalemia, proximal muscle weakness, and hyperglycemia. Diagnosis involves demonstration of inappropriately elevated plasma ACTH in front of increased cortisol levels, with lack of suppression on high-dose dexamethasone testing. Finally, MTC may also secrete histamine, contributing to flushing, and chromogranin A (CgA), a general marker of neuroendocrine activity. Elevated CgA has limited specificity and is not recommended for routine monitoring in MTC but may reflect tumor burden in select cases. Notably, paraneoplastic manifestations predict a worse outcomes, requiring intensive surveillance and early systemic intervention [1].

Regarding tumor markers "strictu senso", which have been the central focus of our review, we can state that calcitonin remains the most specific and sensitive biomarker for MTC. Its serum concentration correlates well with tumor burden, lymph node involvement, and the presence of distant metastases. Moreover, postoperative calcitonin levels and doubling time are predictive of recurrence and survival, forming the basis for risk-adapted follow-up strategies. However, the utility of calcitonin is challenged in certain clinical scenarios and false-positive results may occur in various non-thyroid malignancies and non-malignant conditions or be induced by some pharmacologic agents. Furthermore, the lack of global assay standardization complicates inter-laboratory comparisons and undermines its longitudinal utility across different healthcare settings. In such a context ProCT has emerged as a promising biomarker with expanding utility beyond its traditional role in infectious diseases, and correlates significantly with MTC tumor burden, stage, and metastatic dissemination. Importantly, in cases where calcitonin levels are discordant with imaging findings or clinical progression, ProCT may provide additional insight. Its longer half-life and greater biochemical stability compared to calcitonin enhance its reproducibility and analytical robustness. Overall, the combination of calcitonin and ProCT measurements appears to improve diagnostic accuracy, particularly in patients with atypical biochemical profiles or aggressive disease variants. Despite its promise, ProCT's utility is hindered by its potential for confounding elevations in the context of acute infection, systemic inflammation, or post-surgical stress. Nevertheless, these limitations can often be mitigated through clinical correlation and judicious interpretation. Carcinoembryonic antigen is frequently co-secreted with calcitonin and serves as a valuable adjunct in MTC, particularly for prognostic evaluation. Unlike calcitonin, CEA levels tend to rise in dedifferentiated or metastatic disease and may remain elevated in tumors that secrete little to no calcitonin. Short CEA doubling time (<2 years) has been associated with poor prognosis, making it a useful surveillance tool. However, its limited specificity due to non-MTC malignant and non-malignant causes of elevation precludes its use as a primary diagnostic marker. In contrast, markers such as pro-gastrin-releasing peptide (ProGRP) and carbohydrate antigen 19-9 (CA19-9) remain of limited clinical relevance in MTC but may have contextual significance in aggressive or dedifferentiated disease. ProGRP, a biomarker widely used in the diagnosis of small-cell lung carcinoma, has been sporadically investigated in MTC due to its neuroendocrine origins. Although some studies have suggested elevated ProGRP levels in advanced or poorly differentiated MTC, the evidence remains limited, and no standardized diagnostic thresholds or prognostic algorithms have been established. Similarly, CA19-9, a sialylated Lewis antigen primarily used in gastrointestinal and pancreatic malignancies, has shown rare and inconsistent elevation in MTC. Overall, these markers may be of interest in research settings or in patients with atypical tumor behavior but are not currently recommended for routine clinical use.

7. Integrated Approaches and Future Directions

The complex biology of MTC necessitates a multimodal monitoring strategy. The integration of calcitonin, ProCT, and CEA, particularly with attention to their respective doubling times, enables more nuanced disease tracking and risk stratification. Future efforts should focus on defining MTC-specific cutoffs and establishing standardized algorithms that incorporate biochemical, imaging, and molecular parameters. The integration of biochemical and molecular markers, inflammatory/immunologic signatures, and molecular imaging represents a promising step toward personalized risk stratification and tailored treatments in MTC. Ongoing clinical trials evaluating RET inhibitors and immunotherapy in MTC provide an opportunity to validate multi-marker panels that complement and extend beyond traditional biochemical biomarkers. Next-generation sequencing (NGS) has become an important tool in the molecular characterization of MTC. While RET proto-oncogene pathogenic variants are the defining genetic hallmark of hereditary MTC, NGS allows comprehensive analysis of both germline and somatic alterations, offering insights beyond conventional RET testing. It may also inform eligibility for selective RET inhibitors which show high response rates in RET-mutant MTC. Ongoing studies are also exploring the predictive value of co-mutational landscapes (e.g., TP53, TERT promoter pathogenic variants) for resistance to targeted therapies. Finally NGS of circulating tumor DNA (ctDNA) is emerging as a non-invasive tool to monitor minimal residual disease and assess clonal evolution under therapy (i.e., liquid biopsy). Integration of NGS data with immunogenomic profiling may further refine risk models and identify patients who could benefit from immunotherapy in combination with RET inhibition (i.e., VEGF, soluble immune-checkpoint molecules, markers of angiogenesis). Moreover biochemical and molecular marker panels are increasingly used in conjunction with functional and imaging methods to improve detection sensitivity and informs therapeutic timing. Until such technologies become widely accessible, optimizing the use of currently available markers remains essential to improving outcomes in this challenging thyroid malignancy.

8. Conclusions

We provided a robust analysis and a structured guide for serum biomarker deployment in MTC management, balancing established markers (i.e., calcitonin and CEA) and emerging tools to enhance clinical decision-making (i.e., ProCT, CA 19.9, ProGRP). The currently available panel of different markers is well-suited to manage MTC patients and guide treatments. Standardization of methods should be further ameliorated and large prospective multicentric validation is desirable to refine clinical thresholds of different markers, evaluate candidate biomarkers, and address rare clinical scenarios, such as calcitonin-negative MTC.

Author Contributions: Conceptualization, L.G.; methodology, L.G.; data curation, L.G., F.D., and P.P.O.; writing—original draft preparation, L.G.; writing—review and editing, L.G., F.D., and P.P.O.; supervision, L.G. All authors have read and agreed to the published version of the manuscript.

Funding: This research received no external funding.

Institutional Review Board Statement: Not applicable.

Informed Consent Statement: Not applicable.

Data Availability Statement: Not applicable.

Conflicts of Interest: The authors declare no conflicts of interest.

References

1. Wells, S.A.; Asa, S.L.; Dralle, H.; Elisei, R.; Evans, D.B.; Gagel, R.F.; Lee, N.; MacHens, A.; Moley, J.F.; Pacini, F.; et al. Revised American Thyroid Association Guidelines for the Management of Medullary Thyroid Carcinoma. *Thyroid* **2015**, *25*, 567–610. [CrossRef]
2. Matrone, A.; Gambale, C.; Prete, A.; Elisei, R. Sporadic Medullary Thyroid Carcinoma: Towards a Precision Medicine. *Front. Endocrinol.* **2022**, *13*, 864253. [CrossRef] [PubMed]
3. Donis-keller, H.; Dou, S.; Chi, D.; Carlson, K.M.; Toshima, K.; Lairmore, T.C.; Howe, J.R.; Moley, J.F.; Goodfellow, P.; Wells, S.A. Mutations in the RET Proto-Oncogene Are Associated with MEN 2a and FMTC. *Hum. Mol. Genet.* **1993**, *2*, 851–856. [CrossRef] [PubMed]
4. Mulligan, L.M.; Marsh, D.J.; Robinson, B.G.; Schuffenecker, I.; Zedenius, J.; Lips, C.J.M.; Gagel, R.F.; Takai, S.I.; Noll, W.W.; Fink, M.; et al. Genotype-Phenotype Correlation in Multiple Endocrine Neoplasia Type 2: Report of the International RET Mutation Consortium. *J. Intern. Med.* **1995**, *238*, 343–346. [CrossRef]
5. Sanso, G.E.; Domene, H.M.; Garcia Rudaz, M.C.; Pusiol, E.; De Mondino, A.K.; Roque, M.; Ring, A.; Perinetti, H.; Elsner, B.; Iorcansky, S.; et al. Very Early Detection of RET Proto-Oncogene Mutation Is Crucial for Preventive Thyroidectomy in Multiple Endocrine Neoplasia Type 2 Children: Presence of C-Cell Malignant Disease in Asymptomatic Carriers. *Cancer* **2002**, *94*, 323–330. [CrossRef]
6. Molinaro, E.; Romei, C.; Biagini, A.; Sabini, E.; Agate, L.; Mazzeo, S.; Materazzi, G.; Sellari-Franceschini, S.; Ribechini, A.; Torregrossa, L.; et al. Anaplastic Thyroid Carcinoma: From Clinicopathology to Genetics and Advanced Therapies. *Nat. Rev. Endocrinol.* **2017**, *13*, 644–660. [CrossRef]
7. Christensen, S.B.; Ljungberg, O. Mortality from Thyroid Carcinoma in Malmö, Sweden 1960–1977. A Clinical and Pathologic Study of 38 Fatal Cases. *Cancer* **1984**, *54*, 1629–1634. [CrossRef] [PubMed]
8. Matrone, A.; Gambale, C.; Prete, A.; Piaggi, P.; Cappagli, V.; Bottici, V.; Romei, C.; Ciampi, R.; Torregrossa, L.; De Napoli, L.; et al. Impact of Advanced Age on the Clinical Presentation and Outcome of Sporadic Medullary Thyroid Carcinoma. *Cancers* **2021**, *13*, 94. [CrossRef]
9. Gharib, H.; Mcconahey, W.M.; Tiegs, R.D.; Bergstralh, E.J.; Goellner, J.R.; Grant, C.S.; van Heerden, J.A.; Sizemore, G.W.; Hay, I.D. Medullary Thyroid Carcinoma: Clinicopathologic Features and Long-Term Follow-Up of 65 Patients Treated During 1946 Through 1970. *Mayo Clin. Proc.* **1992**, *67*, 934–940. [CrossRef] [PubMed]
10. Kebebew, E.; Ituarte, P.H.G.; Siperstein, A.E.; Duh, Q.Y.; Clark, O.H. Medullary Thyroid Carcinoma: Clinical Characteristics, Treatment, Prognostic Factors, and a Comparison of Staging Systems. *Cancer* **2000**, *88*, 1139–1148. [CrossRef]
11. Bae, Y.J.; Schaab, M.; Kratzsch, J. Calcitonin as Biomarker for the Medullary Thyroid Carcinoma. *Recent Results Cancer Res.* **2015**, *204*, 117–137. [CrossRef]
12. Bieglmayer, C.; Vierhapper, H.; Dudczak, R.; Niederle, B. Measurement of Calcitonin by Immunoassay Analyzers. *Clin. Chem. Lab. Med.* **2007**, *45*, 662–666. [CrossRef]
13. Schiettecatte, J.; Strasser, O.; Anckaert, E.; Smitz, J. Performance Evaluation of an Automated Electrochemiluminescent Calcitonin (CT) Immunoassay in Diagnosis of Medullary Thyroid Carcinoma. *Clin. Biochem.* **2016**, *49*, 929–931. [CrossRef] [PubMed]
14. Ou, G.; Chen, Q.; Liu, W.; Li, X.; Chen, S.; Wu, X.; Chen, H. Study on the Degradation Rule of Calcitonin in Vitro in Patients with Medullary Thyroid Carcinoma. *Biochem. Biophys. Res. Commun.* **2018**, *507*, 106–109. [CrossRef]
15. d'Herbomez, M.; Caron, P.; Bauters, C.; Do Cao, C.; Schlienger, J.L.; Sapin, R.; Baldet, L.; Carnaille, B.; Wémeau, J.L. Reference Range of Serum Calcitonin Levels in Humans: Influence of Calcitonin Assays, Sex, Age, and Cigarette Smoking. *Eur. J. Endocrinol.* **2007**, *157*, 749–755. [CrossRef] [PubMed]
16. Hypercalcitoninemia in Conditions Other than Medullary Cancers of the Thyroid. Available online: https://pubmed.ncbi.nlm.nih.gov/8734284/ (accessed on 27 June 2025).
17. Cvek, M.; Punda, A.; Brekalo, M.; Plosnić, M.; Barić, A.; Kaličanin, D.; Brčić, L.; Vuletić, M.; Gunjača, I.; Torlak Lovrić, V.; et al. Presence or Severity of Hashimoto's Thyroiditis Does Not Influence Basal Calcitonin Levels: Observations from CROHT Biobank. *J. Endocrinol. Investig.* **2022**, *45*, 597–605. [CrossRef] [PubMed]
18. Ramachandran, R.; Benfield, P.; Dhillo, W.S.; White, S.; Chapman, R.; Meeran, K.; Donaldson, M.; Martin, N.M. Need for Revision of Diagnostic Limits for Medullary Thyroid Carcinoma with a New Immunochemiluminometric Calcitonin Assay. *Clin. Chem.* **2009**, *55*, 2225–2226. [CrossRef]
19. Papapetrou, P.D.; Polymeris, A.; Karga, H.; Vaiopoulos, G. Heterophilic Antibodies Causing Falsely High Serum Calcitonin Values. *J. Endocrinol. Investig.* **2006**, *29*, 919–923. [CrossRef]
20. Leboeuf, R.; Langlois, M.F.; Martin, M.; Ahnadi, C.E.; Fink, G.D. "Hook Effect" in Calcitonin Immunoradiometric Assay in Patients with Metastatic Medullary Thyroid Carcinoma: Case Report and Review of the Literature. *J. Clin. Endocrinol. Metab.* **2006**, *91*, 361–364. [CrossRef] [PubMed]
21. Băetu, M.; Olariu, C.A.; Stancu, C.; Caragheorgheopol, A.; Ioachim, D.; Moldoveanu, G.; Corneci, C.; Badiu, C. Thresholds of Basal- And Calcium-Stimulated Calcitonin for Diagnosis of Thyroid Malignancy. *Horm. Metab. Res.* **2021**, *53*, 779–786. [CrossRef]

22. Machens, A.; Hoffmann, F.; Sekulla, C.; Dralle, H. Importance of Gender-Specific Calcitonin Thresholds in Screening for Occult Sporadic Medullary Thyroid Cancer. *Endocr. Relat. Cancer* **2009**, *16*, 1291–1298. [CrossRef]
23. Song, E.; Jeon, M.J.; Yoo, H.J.; Bae, S.J.; Kim, T.Y.; Kim, W.B.; Shong, Y.K.; Kim, H.K.; Kim, W.G. Gender-Dependent Reference Range of Serum Calcitonin Levels in Healthy Korean Adults. *Endocrinol. Metab.* **2021**, *36*, 365. [CrossRef] [PubMed]
24. Broecker-Preuss, M.; Simon, D.; Fries, M.; Kornely, E.; Weber, M.; Vardarli, I.; Gilman, E.; Herrmann, K.; Görges, R. Update on Calcitonin Screening for Medullary Thyroid Carcinoma and the Results of a Retrospective Analysis of 12,984 Patients with Thyroid Nodules. *Cancers* **2023**, *15*, 2333. [CrossRef]
25. Vardarli, I.; Weber, M.; Weidemann, F.; Führer, D.; Herrmann, K.; Görges, R. Diagnostic Accuracy of Routine Calcitonin Measurement for the Detection of Medullary Thyroid Carcinoma in the Management of Patients with Nodular Thyroid Disease: A Meta-Analysis. *Endocr. Connect.* **2021**, *10*, 358–370. [CrossRef]
26. Abaalkhail, M.; Alorainy, J.; Alotaibi, O.; Albuhayjan, N.; Alnuwaybit, A.; Alqaryan, S.; Alessa, M. Diagnostic Challenges in Calcitonin Negative Medullary Thyroid Carcinoma: A Systematic Review of 101 Cases. *Gland. Surg.* **2024**, *13*, 1785–1804. [CrossRef]
27. Verbeek, H.H.; de Groot, J.W.B.; Sluiter, W.J.; Kobold, A.C.M.; van den Heuvel, E.R.; Plukker, J.T.; Links, T.P. Calcitonin Testing for Detection of Medullary Thyroid Cancer in People with Thyroid Nodules. *Cochrane Database Syst. Rev.* **2020**, *3*, CD010159. [CrossRef]
28. Schmid, K.W.; Ensinger, C. "Atypical" Medullary Thyroid Carcinoma with Little or No Calcitonin Expression. *Virchows Arch.* **1998**, *433*, 209–215. [CrossRef] [PubMed]
29. Trimboli, P.; Giovanella, L. Serum Calcitonin Negative Medullary Thyroid Carcinoma: A Systematic Review of the Literature. *Clin. Chem. Lab. Med.* **2015**, *53*, 1507–1514. [CrossRef]
30. Costante, G.; Meringolo, D.; Durante, C.; Bianchi, D.; Nocera, M.; Tumino, S.; Crocetti, U.; Attard, M.; Maranghi, M.; Torlontano, M.; et al. Predictive Value of Serum Calcitonin Levels for Preoperative Diagnosis of Medullary Thyroid Carcinoma in a Cohort of 5817 Consecutive Patients with Thyroid Nodules. *J. Clin. Endocrinol. Metab.* **2007**, *92*, 450–455. [CrossRef] [PubMed]
31. Fugazzola, L. Medullary Thyroid Cancer—An Update. *Best Pract. Res. Clin. Endocrinol. Metab.* **2023**, *37*, 101655. [CrossRef]
32. Costante, G.; Durante, C.; Francis, Z.; Schlumberger, M.; Filetti, S. Determination of Calcitonin Levels in C-Cell Disease: Clinical Interest and Potential Pitfalls. *Nat. Clin. Pract. Endocrinol. Metab.* **2009**, *5*, 35–44. [CrossRef]
33. Medullary Thyroid Carcinoma: Practice Essentials, Pathophysiology, Etiology. Available online: https://emedicine.medscape.com/article/282084-overview (accessed on 28 June 2025).
34. Miyauchi, A.; Onishi, T.; Morimoto, S.; Takai, S.; Matsuzuka, F.; Kuma, K.; Maeda, M.; Kumahara, Y. Relation of Doubling Time of Plasma Calcitonin Levels to Prognosis and Recurrence of Medullary Thyroid Carcinoma. *Ann. Surg.* **1984**, *199*, 461–466. [CrossRef]
35. Barbet, J.; Campion, L.; Kraeber-Bodéré, F.; Chatal, J.F. Prognostic Impact of Serum Calcitonin and Carcinoembryonic Antigen Doubling-Times in Patients with Medullary Thyroid Carcinoma. *J. Clin. Endocrinol. Metab.* **2005**, *90*, 6077–6084. [CrossRef]
36. Meisner, M.; Schmidt, J.; Hüttner, H.; Tschaikowsky, K. The Natural Elimination Rate of Procalcitonin in Patients with Normal and Impaired Renal Function. *Intensive Care Med.* **2000**, *26*, S212–S216. [CrossRef] [PubMed]
37. Meisner, M.; Tschaikowsky, K.; Schnabel, S.; Schmidt, J.; Schüttler, J.; Katalinic, A. Procalcitonin—Influence of Temperature, Storage, Anticoagulation and Arterialor Venous Asservation of Blood Samples on Procalcitonin Concentrations. *Clin. Chem. Lab. Med.* **1997**, *35*, 597–602. [CrossRef] [PubMed]
38. Kratzsch, J.; Willenberg, A.; Frank-Raue, K.; Kempin, U.; Rocktäschel, J.; Raue, F. Procalcitonin Measured by Three Different Assays Is an Excellent Tumor Marker for the Follow-up of Patients with Medullary Thyroid Carcinoma. *Clin. Chem. Lab. Med.* **2021**, *59*, 1861–1868. [CrossRef] [PubMed]
39. Giovanella, L.; Giordani, I.; Imperiali, M.; Orlandi, F.; Trimboli, P. Measuring Procalcitonin to Overcome Heterophilic-Antibody-Induced Spurious Hypercalcitoninemia. *Clin. Chem. Lab. Med.* **2018**, *56*, e191–e193. [CrossRef]
40. Giovanella, L.; Imperiali, M.; Ferrari, A.; Palumbo, A.; Lippa, L.; Peretti, A.; Graziani, M.S.; Castello, R.; Verburg, F.A. Thyroid Volume Influences Serum Calcitonin Levels in a Thyroid-Healthy Population: Results of a 3-Assay, 519 Subjects Study. *Clin. Chem. Lab. Med.* **2012**, *50*, 895–900. [CrossRef] [PubMed]
41. Lippi, G.; Salvagno, G.L.; Gelati, M.; Pucci, M.; Lo Cascio, C.; Demonte, D.; Faggian, D.; Plebani, M. Two-Center Comparison of 10 Fully-Automated Commercial Procalcitonin (PCT) Immunoassays. *Clin. Chem. Lab. Med.* **2020**, *58*, 77–84. [CrossRef] [PubMed]
42. Algeciras-Schimnich, A.; Preissner, C.M.; Theobald, J.P.; Finseth, M.S.; Grebe, S.K. Procalcitonin: A Marker for the Diagnosis and Follow-up of Patients with Medullary Thyroid Carcinoma. *J. Clin. Endocrinol. Metab.* **2009**, *94*, 861–868. [CrossRef]
43. Giovanella, L.; Verburg, F.A.; Imperiali, M.; Valabrega, S.; Trimboli, P.; Ceriani, L. Comparison of Serum Calcitonin and Procalcitonin in Detecting Medullary Thyroid Carcinoma among Patients with Thyroid Nodules. *Clin. Chem. Lab. Med.* **2013**, *51*, 1477–1481. [CrossRef]

44. Giovanella, L.; Imperiali, M.; Piccardo, A.; Taborelli, M.; Verburg, F.A.; Daurizio, F.; Trimboli, P. Procalcitonin Measurement to Screen Medullary Thyroid Carcinoma: A Prospective Evaluation in a Series of 2705 Patients with Thyroid Nodules. *Eur. J. Clin. Investig.* **2018**, *48*, e12934. [CrossRef] [PubMed]
45. Trimboli, P.; Lauretta, R.; Barnabei, A.; Valabrega, S.; Romanelli, F.; Giovanella, L.; Appetecchia, M. Procalcitonin as a Postoperative Marker in the Follow-up of Patients Affected by Medullary Thyroid Carcinoma. *Int. J. Biol. Markers* **2018**, *33*, 156–160. [CrossRef] [PubMed]
46. Censi, S.; Manso, J.; Benvenuti, T.; Piva, I.; Iacobone, M.; Mondin, A.; Torresan, F.; Basso, D.; Crivellari, G.; Zovato, S.; et al. The Role of Procalcitonin in the Follow-up of Medullary Thyroid Cancer. *Eur. Thyroid. J.* **2023**, *12*, e220161. [CrossRef] [PubMed]
47. Giovanella, L.; Garo, M.L.; Ceriani, L.; Paone, G.; Campenni', A.; D'Aurizio, F. Procalcitonin as an Alternative Tumor Marker of Medullary Thyroid Carcinoma. *J. Clin. Endocrinol. Metab.* **2021**, *106*, 3634–3643. [CrossRef]
48. Clausi, C.; Censi, S.; Zanin, E.; Messina, G.; Piva, I.; Basso, D.; Merante Boschin, I.; Bertazza, L.; Torresan, F.; Iacobone, M.; et al. Combining Procalcitonin and Calcitonin for the Diagnosis of Medullary Thyroid Cancer: A Two-Step Approach. *Clin. Endocrinol.* 2025; *early view*. [CrossRef]
49. Giovanella, L.; Fontana, M.; Keller, F.; Verburg, F.A.; Ceriani, L. Clinical Performance of Calcitonin and Procalcitonin Elecsys ® Immunoassays in Patients with Medullary Thyroid Carcinoma. *Clin. Chem. Lab. Med.* **2020**, *59*, 743–747. [CrossRef] [PubMed]
50. Walter, M.A.; Meier, C.; Radimerski, T.; Iten, F.; Kränzlin, M.; Müller-Brand, J.; De Groot, J.W.B.; Kema, I.P.; Links, T.P.; Müller, B. Procalcitonin Levels Predict Clinical Course and Progression-Free Survival in Patients with Medullary Thyroid Cancer. *Cancer* **2010**, *116*, 31–40. [CrossRef] [PubMed]
51. Chambliss, A.B.; Patel, K.; Colón-Franco, J.M.; Hayden, J.; Katz, S.E.; Minejima, E.; Woodworth, A. AACC Guidance Document on the Clinical Use of Procalcitonin. *J. Appl. Lab. Med.* **2023**, *8*, 598–634. [CrossRef]
52. Schuetz, P. How to Best Use Procalcitonin to Diagnose Infections and Manage Antibiotic Treatment. *Clin. Chem. Lab. Med.* **2023**, *61*, 822–828. [CrossRef]
53. Kankanala, V.L.; Zubair, M.; Mukkamalla, S.K.R. *Carcinoembryonic Antigen*; StatPearls, 2024. Available online: https://www.ncbi.nlm.nih.gov/books/NBK578172/ (accessed on 7 July 2025).
54. Morimoto, Y.; Takahashi, H.; Arita, A.; Itakura, H.; Fujii, M.; Sekido, Y.; Hata, T.; Fujino, S.; Ogino, T.; Miyoshi, N.; et al. High Postoperative Carcinoembryonic Antigen as an Indicator of High-Risk Stage II Colon Cancer. *Oncol. Lett.* **2021**, *23*, 167. [CrossRef]
55. Machens, A.; Ukkat, J.; Hauptmann, S.; Dralle, H. Abnormal Carcinoembryonic Antigen Levels and Medullary Thyroid Cancer Progression: A Multivariate Analysis. *Arch. Surg.* **2007**, *142*, 289–293. [CrossRef] [PubMed]
56. Passos, I.; Stefanidou, E.; Meditskou-Eythymiadou, S.; Mironidou-Tzouveleki, M.; Manaki, V.; Magra, V.; Laskou, S.; Mantalovas, S.; Pantea, S.; Kesisoglou, I.; et al. A Review of the Significance in Measuring Preoperative and Postoperative Carcinoembryonic Antigen (CEA) Values in Patients with Medullary Thyroid Carcinoma (MTC). *Medicina* **2021**, *57*, 609. [CrossRef]
57. Raue, F.; Frank-Raue, K. Long-Term Follow-Up in Medullary Thyroid Carcinoma Patients. *Recent Results Cancer Res.* **2025**, *223*, 267–291. [CrossRef] [PubMed]
58. Terroir, M.; Caramella, C.; Borget, I.; Bidault, S.; Dromain, C.; El Farsaoui, K.; Deandreis, D.; Grimaldi, S.; Lumbroso, J.; Berdelou, A.; et al. F-18-Dopa Positron Emission Tomography/Computed Tomography Is More Sensitive Than Whole-Body Magnetic Resonance Imaging for the Localization of Persistent/Recurrent Disease of Medullary Thyroid Cancer Patients. *Thyroid* **2019**, *29*, 1457–1464. [CrossRef] [PubMed]
59. La Salvia, A.; Fanciulli, G. Progastrin-Releasing Peptide As a Diagnostic Biomarker of Pulmonary and Non-Pulmonary Neuroendocrine Neoplasms. *Endocr. Res.* **2024**, *49*, 243–250. [CrossRef]
60. Sainz de Medrano, J.I.; Laguna, J.; Julian, J.; Filella, X.; Fabregat, A.; Luquin, M.; Hurtado, H.H.; García Humanes, A.; Morales-Ruiz, M.; Fernández-Galán, E. Comparison of Two Automated Immunoassays for Quantifying ProGRP, SCC and HE4 in Serum: Impact on Diagnostic Accuracy. *Scand. J. Clin. Lab. Investig.* **2025**, *85*, 116–124. [CrossRef]
61. Han, X.; Lu, R.; Hu, H.; Guo, L. Application of Serum Markers in Medullary Thyroid Carcinoma. *Chin. J. Prev. Med.* **2021**, *55*, 1468–1474. [CrossRef]
62. Giovanella, L.; Fontana, M.; Keller, F.; Campenni', A.; Ceriani, L.; Paone, G. Circulating Pro-Gastrin Releasing Peptide (ProGRP) in Patients with Medullary Thyroid Carcinoma. *Clin. Chem. Lab. Med.* **2021**, *59*, 1569–1573. [CrossRef]
63. Liang, X.; Zhu, J.; Cai, M.; Dai, Z.; Fang, L.; Chen, H.; Yu, L.; Lin, Y.; Lin, E.; Wu, G. ProGRP as a Novel Biomarker for the Differential Diagnosis of Medullary Thyroid Carcinoma in Patients with Thyroid Nodules. *Endocr. Pract.* **2020**, *26*, 514–522. [CrossRef] [PubMed]
64. Parra-Robert, M.; Orois, A.; Augé, J.M.; Halperin, I.; Filella, X.; Molina, R. Utility of ProGRP as a Tumor Marker in the Medullary Thyroid Carcinoma. *Clin. Chem. Lab. Med.* **2017**, *55*, 441–446. [CrossRef]
65. Torsetnes, S.B.; Broughton, M.N.; Paus, E.; Halvorsen, T.G.; Reubsaet, L. Determining ProGRP and Isoforms in Lung and Thyroid Cancer Patient Samples: Comparing an MS Method with a Routine Clinical Immunoassay. *Anal. Bioanal. Chem.* **2014**, *406*, 2733–2738. [CrossRef]

66. Miao, Q.; Lv, X.; Luo, L.; Zhang, J.; Cai, B. Exploring the Application Value of Pro-Gastrin-Releasing Peptide in the Clinical Diagnosis and Surgical Treatment of Medullary Thyroid Carcinoma. *Cancer Med.* **2023**, *12*, 19576–19582. [CrossRef]
67. Martins, F.A.; Batista, M.; Augusto, S.L.; Rita, E.A.; Couto, J.; Martins, R.G.; Santos, J.; Martins, T.; Cunha, N.; Rodrigues, F. The Role of Procalcitonin and ProGRP in the Follow-up of Medullary Thyroid Carcinoma. *Endocr. Abstr.* **2025**, *110*, e220161. [CrossRef]
68. Schonebaum, L.; van Balkum, M.; Edward, V.W.; van den Berg, S.; Peeters, R. PRO-Gastrin-Releasing Peptide as an Additional Screening Marker in the Diagnostic Work up for Medullary Thyroid Carcinoma. *Endocr. Abstr.* **2023**, *92*. [CrossRef]
69. Alencar, R.; Kendler, D.B.; Andrade, F.; Nava, C.; Bulzico, D.; Cordeiro De Noronha Pessoa, C.; Corbo, R.; Vaisman, F. CA19-9 as a Predictor of Worse Clinical Outcome in Medullary Thyroid Carcinoma. *Eur. Thyroid. J.* **2019**, *8*, 186–191. [CrossRef] [PubMed]
70. Codrich, M.; Biasotto, A.; D'Aurizio, F. Circulating Biomarkers of Thyroid Cancer: An Appraisal. *J. Clin. Med.* **2025**, *14*, 1582. [CrossRef] [PubMed]
71. Elisei, R.; Lorusso, L.; Romei, C.; Bottici, V.; Mazzeo, S.; Giani, C.; Fiore, E.; Torregrossa, L.; Insilla, A.C.; Basolo, F.; et al. Medullary Thyroid Cancer Secreting Carbohydrate Antigen 19-9 (Ca 19-9): A Fatal Case Report. *J. Clin. Endocrinol. Metab.* **2013**, *98*, 3550–3554. [CrossRef] [PubMed]
72. Lorusso, L.; Romei, C.; Piaggi, P.; Fustini, C.; Molinaro, E.; Agate, L.; Bottici, V.; Viola, D.; Pellegrini, G.; Elisei, R. Ca19.9 Positivity and Doubling Time Are Prognostic Factors of Mortality in Patients with Advanced Medullary Thyroid Cancer with No Evidence of Structural Disease Progression According to Response Evaluation Criteria in Solid Tumors. *Thyroid* **2021**, *31*, 1050–1055. [CrossRef]
73. Kuma Hospital—Tools. Available online: https://en.kuma-h.or.jp/tools (accessed on 28 June 2025).
74. Yang, J.H.; Camacho, C.P.; Lindsey, S.C.; Valente, F.O.F.; Andreoni, D.M.; Yamaga, L.Y.; Wagner, J.; Biscolla, R.P.M.; Maciel, R.M.B. The Combined Use of Calcitonin Doubling Time and 18f-Fdg Pet/Ct Improves Prognostic Values in Medullary Thyroid Carcinoma: The Clinical Utility of 18f-Fdg Pet/Ct. *Endocr. Pract.* **2017**, *23*, 942–948. [CrossRef]
75. Romero-Lluch, A.R.; Cuenca-Cuenca, J.I.; Guerrero-Vázquez, R.; Martínez-Ortega, A.J.; Tirado-Hospital, J.L.; Borrego-Dorado, I.; Navarro-González, E. Diagnostic Utility of PET/CT with 18F-DOPA and 18F-FDG in Persistent or Recurrent Medullary Thyroid Carcinoma: The Importance of Calcitonin and Carcinoembryonic Antigen Cutoff. *Eur. J. Nucl. Med. Mol. Imaging* **2017**, *44*, 2004–2013. [CrossRef]
76. Wang, B.; Huang, J.; Chen, L. Management of Medullary Thyroid Cancer Based on Variation of Carcinoembryonic Antigen and Calcitonin. *Front. Endocrinol.* **2024**, *15*, 1418657. [CrossRef]
77. Trimboli, P.; D'Aurizio, F.; Tozzoli, R.; Giovanella, L. Measurement of Thyroglobulin, Calcitonin, and PTH in FNA Washout Fluids. *Clin. Chem. Lab. Med.* **2017**, *55*, 914–925. [CrossRef]
78. Boi, F.; Maurelli, I.; Pinna, G.; Atzeni, F.; Piga, M.; Lai, M.L.; Mariotti, S. Calcitonin Measurement in Wash-out Fluid from Fine Needle Aspiration of Neck Masses in Patients with Primary and Metastatic Medullary Thyroid Carcinoma. *J. Clin. Endocrinol. Metab.* **2007**, *92*, 2115–2118. [CrossRef] [PubMed]
79. Kudo, T.; Miyauchi, A.; Ito, Y.; Takamura, Y.; Amino, N.; Hirokawa, M. Diagnosis of Medullary Thyroid Carcinoma by Calcitonin Measurement in Fine-Needle Aspiration Biopsy Specimens. *Thyroid* **2007**, *17*, 635–638. [CrossRef] [PubMed]
80. Diazzi, C.; Madeo, B.; Taliani, E.; Zirilli, L.; Romano, S.; Granata, A.R.M.; De Santis, M.C.; Simoni, M.; Cioni, K.; Carani, C.; et al. The Diagnostic Value of Calcitonin Measurement in Wash-out Fluid from Fine-Needle Aspiration of Thyroid Nodules in the Diagnosis of Medullary Thyroid Cancer. *Endocr. Pract.* **2013**, *19*, 769–779. [CrossRef] [PubMed]
81. Trimboli, P.; Cremonini, N.; Ceriani, L.; Saggiorato, E.; Guidobaldi, L.; Romanelli, F.; Ventura, C.; Laurenti, O.; Messuti, I.; Solaroli, E.; et al. Calcitonin Measurement in Aspiration Needle Washout Fluids Has Higher Sensitivity than Cytology in Detecting Medullary Thyroid Cancer: A Retrospective Multicentre Study. *Clin. Endocrinol.* **2014**, *80*, 135–140. [CrossRef]
82. De Crea, C.; Raffaelli, M.; Maccora, D.; Carrozza, C.; Canu, G.; Fadda, G.; Bellantone, R.; Lombardi, C.P. Calcitonin Measurement in Fine-Needle Aspirate Washouts vs. Cytologic Examination for Diagnosis of Primary or Metastatic Medullary Thyroid Carcinoma. *Acta Otorhinolaryngol. Ital.* **2014**, *34*, 399. [PubMed]
83. Giovanella, L.; Ceriani, L.; Bongiovanni, M. Calcitonin Measurement on Fine Needle Washouts: Preanalytical Issues and Normal Reference Values. *Diagn. Cytopathol.* **2013**, *41*, 226–229. [CrossRef]
84. Cho, H.W.; Kim, S.H.; Cho, Y.; Jeong, S.H.; Lee, S.G. Concordance of Three Automated Procalcitonin Immunoassays at Medical Decision Points. *Ann. Lab. Med.* **2021**, *41*, 419–423. [CrossRef]
85. Huynh, H.H.; Bœuf, A.; Pfannkuche, J.; Schuetz, P.; Thelen, M.; Nordin, G.; Van Der Hagen, E.; Kaiser, P.; Kesseler, D.; Badrick, T.; et al. Harmonization Status of Procalcitonin Measurements: What Do Comparison Studies and EQA Schemes Tell Us? *Clin. Chem. Lab. Med.* **2021**, *59*, 1610–1622. [CrossRef] [PubMed]
86. Partyka, K.; Maupin, K.A.; Brand, R.E.; Haab, B.B. Diverse Monoclonal Antibodies against the CA 19-9 Antigen Show Variation in Binding Specificity with Consequences for Clinical Interpretation. *Proteomics* **2012**, *12*, 2212–2220. [CrossRef] [PubMed]

87. Kremser, M.; Weiss, N.; Kaufmann-Stoeck, A.; Vierbaum, L.; Schmitz, A.; Schellenberg, I.; Holdenrieder, S. Longitudinal Evaluation of External Quality Assessment Results for CA 15-3, CA 19-9, and CA 125. *Front. Mol. Biosci.* **2024**, *11*, 1401619. [CrossRef]
88. Handling, C. *Transport, Processing and Storage of Blood Specimens for Routine Laboratory Examinations*; Clinical and Laboratory Standards Institute: Wayne, PA, USA, 2023; 84p.
89. Fu, W.; Yue, Y.; Song, Y.; Zhang, S.; Shi, J.; Zhao, R.; Wang, Q.; Zhang, R. Comparable Analysis of Six Immunoassays for Carcinoembryonic Antigen Detection. *Heliyon* **2024**, *10*, e25158. [CrossRef] [PubMed]
90. Wojtalewicz, N.; Vierbaum, L.; Kaufmann, A.; Schellenberg, I.; Holdenrieder, S. Longitudinal Evaluation of AFP and CEA External Proficiency Testing Reveals Need for Method Harmonization. *Diagnostics* **2023**, *13*, 2019. [CrossRef]
91. La'ulu, S.L.; Roberts, W.L. Performance Characteristics of Five Automated CA 19-9 Assays. *Am. J. Clin. Pathol.* **2007**, *127*, 436–440. [CrossRef] [PubMed]
92. Kahaly, G.J.; Algeciras-Schimnich, A.; Davis, T.E.; Diana, T.; Feldkamp, J.; Karger, S.; König, J.; Lupo, M.A.; Raue, F.; Ringel, M.D.; et al. United States and European Multicenter Prospective Study for the Analytical Performance and Clinical Validation of a Novel Sensitive Fully Automated Immunoassay for Calcitonin. *Clin. Chem.* **2017**, *63*, 1489–1496. [CrossRef] [PubMed]
93. Kiriakopoulos, A.; Giannakis, P.; Menenakos, E. Calcitonin: Current Concepts and Differential Diagnosis. *Ther. Adv. Endocrinol. Metab.* **2022**, *13*, 20420188221099344. [CrossRef]
94. Korse, C.M.; Holdenrieder, S.; Zhi, X.Y.; Zhang, X.; Qiu, L.; Geistanger, A.; Lisy, M.R.; Wehnl, B.; van den Broek, D.; Escudero, J.M.; et al. Multicenter Evaluation of a New Progastrin-Releasing Peptide (ProGRP) Immunoassay across Europe and China. *Clin. Chim. Acta* **2015**, *438*, 388–395. [CrossRef]

MDPI AG
Grosspeteranlage 5
4052 Basel
Switzerland
Tel.: +41 61 683 77 34

Journal of Clinical Medicine Editorial Office
E-mail: jcm@mdpi.com
www.mdpi.com/journal/jcm

www.ingramcontent.com/pod-product-compliance
Lightning Source LLC
Chambersburg PA
CBHW061559210926
51850CB00009B/2157
* 9 7 8 3 7 2 5 8 5 8 6 5 1 *